Dedication

To dear Joy, whom I love so dearly – who, through
thick and thin, has patiently allowed my obsession
to freely flow and who has never once complained
about the hours, days and months of absence in
my search for the final goal.

Foreword

When it first appeared, *The Lumbar Spine* was a slim edition that announced a new concept. It postulated what might be happening in patients with low back pain, and it provided a system of assessment and treatment.

Since its inception, the McKenzie system has grown into a movement. The system captured the imagination of therapists and others, who adopted it. Their numbers grew to form an international organisation that offers training programmes and postgraduate degrees in several countries around the world. The system also attracted the attention of opponents, critics and non-aligned investigators.

Over the years, tensions have developed as the McKenzie system has tried to keep pace with advances in spine science, but also as spine science has tried to keep pace with advances in McKenzie. In basic sciences, our understanding of the structure, function and pathology of the lumbar intervertebral disc has increased enormously. In clinical sciences, the advent of evidence-based medicine has demanded that interventions have evidence of reliability, validity and efficacy. These developments have challenged the McKenzie system, but have not threatened it. Indeed, in many respects, the McKenzie movement has led the way in undertaking research into its precepts, and has implicitly called upon other concepts in physical therapy to catch up. No other system in physical therapy has attracted as much research both from among its proponents and from its detractors.

This new edition of *The Lumbar Spine* has become a tome. It still describes the original concept, albeit updated and revised, but the edition provides students and other readers with a compendium of all the literature pertaining to the lumbar intervertebral disc and the massive literature that now pertains to the McKenzie system.

Readers receive an up-to-date review of information on the structure and function of the disc, its pathology, and new data on its patho-biomechanics. Related entities, such a zygapophysial joint pain and sacro-iliac joint, are comprehensively reviewed.

As befitting a text on this subject, *The Lumbar Spine* contains a complete collection of all studies that have examined the McKenzie system. These studies have sought the evidence for its reliability, validity and efficacy.

Its reliability is now beyond doubt. Whereas research has shown that other methods of assessment lack reliability, McKenzie assessment has moved from strength to strength. Its reliability, however, is contingent upon training. While anyone can assess according to the system, it cannot be mastered by hearsay or assumption.

Some steps have been taken towards establishing validity. The early studies have been encouragingly positive, but perhaps self-fulfilling. The critical studies have yet to be performed and depend on establishing the efficacy of the treatment.

The Lumbar Spine provides an exhaustive but honest and responsible appraisal of studies of the efficacy of McKenzie treatment. Much of the world finds the evidence insufficiently compelling, but the treatment has not been refuted. Proponents retain the prospect of still vindicating the treatment if and once putatively confounding factors can be eliminated or controlled.

To some observers McKenzie therapy may seem to be a glorified system of special manoeuvres and exercises, but such a view mistakes and understates its virtues. Throughout its history, McKenzie treatment has emphasised educating patients and empowering them to take charge of their own management. Not only did this approach pre-empt contemporary concepts of best practice, it has been vindicated by the evidence. Empowering the patient is seminal to the success of any programme of management.

Although I am not a McKenzie disciple or enthusiast, we have in our own research borrowed from the McKenzie system. In studying the efficacy of evidence-based practice for acute low back pain in primary care,[1] we talked to our patients and we addressed their fears; but to complement that we needed something more for the patients to take with them. For this purpose we drew on some of the simpler exercises described in *The Lumbar Spine*. Not that we believed that these were therapeutic in their own right, but they empowered the patients with sensible things that they could do to cope with their pain and maintain, if not improve, their mobility and function. This approach, a not-too-distant cousin of what McKenzie promotes, was not only successful in a clinical sense, but received great approval from the consumers.

The patho-anatomic concepts and the mechanical aspects of McKenzie therapy may or may not be absolutely material. They may or may not be vindicated in time. But what is already clearly evidence-based is the central theme of McKenzie therapy: to enable patients confidently to care for themselves.

Nikolai Bogduk MD, PhD, DSc
Professor of Pain Medicine
University of Newcastle
Royal Newcastle Hospital
Newcastle, Australia

[1]McGuirk B, King W, Govind J, Lowry J, Bogduk N. The safety, efficacy, and cost-effectiveness of evidence-based guidelines for the management of acute low back pain in primary care. Spine 2001; 26.2615-2622.

Acknowledgments

I would like to give special thanks to my co-author and colleague, Stephen May, MA, MCSP, Dip MDT, MSc, who has provided the necessary expertise to make this second edition an evidence-based text of importance to all health professionals involved in non-operative care of the lower back.

I am also greatly indebted to the many faculty of the McKenzie Institute International, who have either directly or indirectly influenced the refinements that have been made to the descriptions of the procedures of assessment and examination. The value of these contributions is immeasurable.

I would also like to express my gratitude to Kathy Hoyt, a founder of the Institute in the United States, and Helen Clare of Australia, the Institute's Director of Education, who gave so much of their time to read the manuscripts and provide invaluable commentary and criticism.

To Vert Mooney, who opened so many doors, to Ron Donelson for his continued support of the system and the Institute, and to those members of the International Society for the Study of the Lumbar Spine who have encouraged and supported my work, I give my thanks.

Finally, to Jan, my daughter, who reorganised me and coordinated the various specialists required to successfully complete this major task, I give my heartfelt love and thanks.

Robin McKenzie
March 2003

About the Authors

Robin McKenzie was born in Auckland, New Zealand, in 1931 and graduated from the New Zealand School of Physiotherapy in 1952. He commenced private practice in Wellington, New Zealand in 1953, specialising in the diagnosis and treatment of spinal disorders.

During the 1960s, Robin McKenzie developed new concepts of diagnosis and treatment derived from a systematic analysis of patients with both acute and chronic back problems. This system is now practised globally by specialists in physiotherapy, medicine and chiropractic.

The success of the McKenzie concepts of diagnosis and treatment for spinal problems has attracted interest from researchers worldwide. The importance of the diagnostic system is now recognised and the extent of the therapeutic efficacy of the McKenzie Method is subject to ongoing investigation.

Robin McKenzie is an Honorary Life Member of the American Physical Therapy Association "in recognition of distinguished and meritorious service to the art and science of physical therapy and to the welfare of mankind". He is a member of the International Society for the Study of the Lumbar Spine, a Fellow of the American Back Society, an Honorary Fellow of the New Zealand Society of Physiotherapists, an Honorary Life Member of the New Zealand Manipulative Therapists Association, and an Honorary Fellow of the Chartered Society of Physiotherapists in the United Kingdom. In the 1990 Queen's Birthday Honours, he was made an Officer of the Most Excellent Order of the British Empire. In 1993, he received an Honorary Doctorate from the Russian Academy of Medical Sciences. In the 2000 New Year's Honours List, Her Majesty the Queen appointed Robin McKenzie as a Companion of the New Zealand Order of Merit.

In 2003, the University of Otago, in a joint venture with the McKenzie Institute International, instituted a Post Graduate Diploma /Masters programme endorsed in Mechanical Diagnosis and Therapy. Robin McKenzie has been made a Fellow in Physiotherapy at Otago and will be lecturing during the programme.

Robin McKenzie has authored four books: *Treat Your Own Back; Treat Your Own Neck; The Lumbar Spine: Mechanical Diagnosis and Therapy;* and *The Cervical and Thoracic Spine: Mechanical Diagnosis and Therapy.* With the publication of *Mechanical Diagnosis & Therapy of the Human Extremities,* Robin McKenzie, in collaboration with Stephen May, describes the application of his methods for the management of musculoskeletal disorders in general. As with his publications dealing with spine-related problems, the emphasis in this text is directed at providing self-treatment strategies for pain and disability among the general population.

Stephen May was born in Kent, England, in 1958. His first degree was in English Literature from Oxford University. He trained to be a physiotherapist at Leeds and graduated in 1990. Since qualifying, he has worked for the National Health Service in England, principally in Primary Care. In 2002 he became a Senior Lecturer at Sheffield Hallam University.

He developed a special interest in musculoskeletal medicine early in his career and has always maintained a diligent interest in the literature. One of the results of this was a regular supply of articles and reviews to the McKenzie newsletter (UK). In 1995 Stephen completed the McKenzie diploma programme. In 1998 he completed an MSc in Health Services Research and Technology Assessment at Sheffield University.

Stephen is author or co-author of several articles published in international journals. He has previously collaborated with Robin McKenzie on *The Human Extremities: Mechanical Diagnosis & Therapy*.

Contents

List of Figures

List of Tables

Introduction

Many years have passed since the publication of the first edition of my monograph, *The Lumbar Spine: Mechanical Diagnosis and Therapy*. Since 1981, when the book was first released, the conceptual models for the identification of subgroups in the non-specific spectrum of back pain and the methods of treatment I recommended have internationally received wide acceptance.

The extent of the acceptance for what I chose to call Mechanical Diagnosis and Therapy (MDT) was never anticipated. I did not, as a result of dissatisfaction with existing methods, deliberately construct a new system of diagnosis and treatment to manage common mechanical back problems. Rather, from everyday observation and contact with large numbers of patients, I learned from them, unconsciously at first I suspect, that different patients with apparently similar symptoms reacted quite differently when subjected to the same mechanical loadings. On grouping together all those whose symptomatic and mechanical responses to loading were identical, three consistent patterns emerged and became in turn the syndromes whose identification and management are described within these pages.

Because of the stable population in the city of Wellington in New Zealand, many patients with recurrent and chronic problems returned for help over time. Thus I had the opportunity to observe in many individuals the passing spectrum of mechanical and symptomatic changes that progressed during two or even three decades of life. From this experience I learned how to make the changes in management that were dictated by the gradual structural changes resulting from the natural ageing process. The eventual refinement of my observations and techniques of loading were thus merely a function of evolution.

I have recounted the story of "Mr Smith", described later in this volume, on many courses and at many conferences around the world. I do so because it describes an actual event that has had an enormous impact on my life and has, and continues to have, an impact on the way health professionals worldwide think about and manage the spine and musculoskeletal problems in general.

Occasionally I am asked, "Was there really a Mr Smith, or did you invent him to provide an amusing story to go with the effects of extension?" I can only reply that, yes, it is a true story, and no, I did not make it up, but his real name is long forgotten.

Prior to the encounter with Mr Smith, I, along with a few other physiotherapists at that time, was exploring and mastering the multitude of manipulative techniques and the philosophies that lay behind them. Cyriax, Mennell, Stoddard and the chiropractors were the flavour of that period. Maitland and Kaltenborn were yet to appear. In my mind, the only rational explanation to account for the centralisation of Mr Smith's symptoms was to be found in the first volume (1954), written by one James Cyriax, MD.

Cyriax attributed sudden and slow onset back pain respectively to tearing of the annulus and bulging or displacement of the nucleus. If the bulge was large enough, compression of the root would follow. Thus it suggested to me that Mr Smith's centralisation occurred because the pressure on his sciatic nerve was removed. Extension, I thought, was therefore a good thing to apply in these cases. It might even be more effective than the manipulations we practised, which sometimes did – and many times did not – produce a benefit for the patient.

Following the encounter with Mr Smith, the hypothesis to explain the varying responses to loading crystallised and formed the basis of the conceptual models upon which the treatments were developed. Without the conceptual model of displacement and its sequelae, I doubt that I could have developed the explanations and eventually provided the solutions for many of the mechanical disorders presenting in daily practice.

Belief in the conceptual model provided an explanation and better understanding of centralisation and peripheralisation. It explained the changes in pain location and intensity that follow prolonged or repetitive sagittal loading and led to the discovery that offset loading (hips off centre) was required when symptoms were unilateral or asymmetrical. The model suggested that it could be possible, by applying lateral forces, to entice low back and cervical pains to change sides. That phenomenon is now clinically repeatable in certain selected patients.

Identification of the most effective direction for applying therapeutic exercise – the use of prolonged positioning and repeated rather than single movements in assessment; the progressions of force; differentiation between the pain of displacement, from the pain of contracture, and pain arising from normal tissue; the three syndromes; differentiation of limb pain caused by root adherence, entrapment or disc protrusion – all arose directly or indirectly from the conceptual model.

The disc model, the theories and clinical outcomes relative to mechanical diagnosis and therapy are under investigation worldwide. The models are as yet unproven scientifically; even so they provide a sound basis for the management of non-specific disorders of the lower back. Much to my intense satisfaction, the experiments, the conclusions and the results I recorded have successfully been replicated by others.

To this day, belief in the conceptual model, acting on its suggestions and obeying its warnings, guide me in the management of the patient. Many things indirectly arose from the model. Mr Smith was the catalyst. We no longer have to manipulate all patients in order to deliver the procedure to the very few requiring it. We no longer have to apply manipulation to our patients to determine retrospectively if it was indicated. I would never be without the model and Mr Smith is never far from my thoughts.

Mechanical Diagnosis and Therapy is now one of the most commonly used treatment approaches utilised by physiotherapists in the United Kingdom, New Zealand and the United States. It is an approach also utilised and recommended by chiropractors, physicians and surgeons. The increasing interest is reflected in the substantial body of research that has been conducted into aspects of "The McKenzie Method", as it has come to be known. The very nature of MDT lends itself to measurement.

There have been numerous studies into centralisation, symptom response and reliability, as well as studies into the efficacy of MDT. More studies are needed, but much research already strongly endorses aspects of this system of assessment and management. Further recent endorsement of MDT has been given by its inclusion in national back pain guidelines from Denmark and systematic musculoskeletal guidelines from the United States.

Centralisation has been shown to have clear prognostic as well as diagnostic significance. It is one of the few clinical factors that have been found to have more prognostic implications than psychosocial factors. Study after study has asserted the poor reliability of assessment that is based on palpation or observation, while symptom response consistently shows good reliability.

Education in MDT has now been structured to enable the formalised teaching of clinicians and provide a base upon which rigorous scientific inquiry may proceed. Educational programmes are provided under the auspices of the McKenzie Institute International and its branches and are conducted in all continents and attended annually by thousands of clinicians. Some appreciation of the extent of the adoption of MDT can be seen from the request by the Director of the Chinese Ministry of Health, Department of Rehabilitation, to provide the Institute's education programme for Chinese physicians and surgeons involved in the management of back disorders throughout the world's most populous country.

It is now common knowledge that management of musculoskeletal problems must involve patient understanding, including a knowledge of the problem and proffered solution. Patients must be actively involved in treatment. This was a message first stated over twenty years ago in the first edition of this title. Sadly, it seems, with the continued usage of ultrasound and other passive treatment modalities by clinicians, despite clear evidence for lack of efficacy; this is a message that health professionals have still not clearly heard. "How many randomised controlled trials does it take to convince clinicians about the lack of efficacy for ultrasound and other passive treatments?" (Nachemson, 2001).

The clinical utility and worth of the system is attested to by the thousands of 'studies of one' conducted by clinicians on their patients throughout the world every year. It is used and continues to be used because it is effective.

Ultimately, do we wish to make the patient feel 'better', albeit briefly, or do we wish to offer the patient a means of self-treatment and understanding so that there is a strong possibility they will benefit from our services in the long-term? Are we creating patient dependence on therapy, or providing a chance of independence through self-management? A key role for clinicians must be as educators, rather than 'healers'.

The second edition of this title is presented to the reader with the knowledge and hindsight of experience gained since the production of the first. In the first edition of 1981, there were few, if any, references to quote in support of the methods and theories I propounded. Prior descriptions of the use of repetitive end-range motion and its effects on pain location and intensity; the phenomenon of clinically induced centralisation and peripheralisation; the prognostic value of centralisation and non-centralisation; the theoretical models; identification of subgroup syndromes; the progressions of therapeutic forces; and most importantly self-treatment and management strategies did not exist in the literature of the day. Fortunately that is not the case today.

I believe that with the involvement of Stephen May in the writing of this edition, the imperfections that abound in my first excursion into the literary world have been eliminated. Stephen's understanding of "McKenzie", combined with his literary talents and global familiarity with the scientific literature, have brought to this edition a quality that far exceeds my own capabilities. This will become apparent to the reader on advancing through the chapters within.

We have provided for you in this second edition, a monograph that describes in explicit detail what the "McKenzie Method" is, how to apply it and the evidence that substantiates and justifies its use for the management of non-specific low back pain.

I believe these chapters will allow better understanding and more appropriate investigation of MDT. Above all, I trust it will serve its prime purpose in helping our patients.

Robin McKenzie
Raumati Beach
New Zealand

1: The Problem of Back Pain

Introduction

It is important to understand the extent to which any health problem impacts upon the population. This provides an understanding of that problem, as well as suggestions as to how it should be addressed by health care providers. Clearly it is inappropriate for health professionals to deal with a benign, self-limiting and endemic problem such as the common cold in the same way that they address possibly life-threatening disorders such as heart attacks. The study and description of the spread of a disease in a population is known as *epidemiology*.

Modern clinical epidemiology is concerned with the distribution, natural history and clinical course of a disease, risk factors associated with it, the health needs it produces and the determination of the most effective methods of treatment and management (Streiner and Norman 1996). Epidemiology thus offers various insights that are critical to an understanding of any health problem (Andersson 1991; Nachemson *et al.* 2000). It provides information about the extent of a problem and the resultant demand on services. An understanding of the natural history informs patient counselling about prognosis and helps determine the effects of treatment. Associations between symptoms and individual and external factors allow the identification and modification of risk factors. Outcomes from studies about interventions should provide the evidence for the most effective management strategies.

The sections in this chapter are as follows:

- prevalence
- natural history
- disability
- cost
- health care
- treatment
- effectiveness.

Risk and prognostic factors are discussed in the next chapter. This information provides a background understanding that should influence the management that health professionals provide.

Prevalence

Trying to measure the frequency of back pain, its clinical course or the rate of care-seeking related to back pain is not straightforward. There is considerable variability in the way data has been gathered – in different countries, at different times, employing different definitions, asking slightly different questions and using different methods to gather this information. There is often a lack of objective measurement, the problem is frequently intermittent and recall can be plagued by bias. Thus there is a problem with the validity and reliability of the data, and the figures offered should be seen as estimations rather than exact facts (Andersson 1991; Nachemson *et al.* 2000). Nonetheless, certain figures appear consistently enough to give a reasonably reliable overall picture of the extent of the problem and its natural history.

Despite all methodological difficulties, it can be stated that back pain is about the most prevalent pain complaint, possibly along with headaches (Raspe 1993). In adults, between one-half and three-quarters of the population will experience back pain at some point in their life. About 40% will experience an episode of back pain in any one year, and about 15 – 20% are experiencing back pain at any given time. Similar figures are given in reviews and primary research from different countries around the world (Croft *et al.* 1997; Klaber Moffett *et al.* 1995; Evans and Richards 1996; Waddell 1994; Shekelle 1997; Papageorgiou and Rigby 1991; Papageorgiou *et al.* 1995; Linton *et al.* 1998; Brown *et al.* 1998; Leboeuf-Yde *et al.* 1996; McKinnon *et al.* 1997; Szpalski *et al.* 1995; Heliovaara *et al.* 1989; Toroptsova *et al.* 1995; Cassidy *et al.* 1998). Apparently only 10 – 20% of the adult population seems to have never had back problems (Raspe 1993).

Table 1.1 contains a sample of international studies that have been conducted in great numbers of the general population. Large representative surveys are the best evidence for a problem in the greater population (Nachemson *et al.* 2000). Commonly these surveys describe the proportion of people who report back pain at the time or that month (point prevalence), in that year (year prevalence) or back pain ever (lifetime prevalence).

Table 1.1   Prevalence of back pain in selected large
             population-based studies

Reference	Country	Point prevalence	Year prevalence	Lifetime prevalence
Hillman *et al.* 1996	UK	19%	39%	59%
Papageorgiou *et al.* 1995	UK	39%		
Brown *et al.* 1984	Canada (police force)		42%	
Heliovaara *et al.* 1989	Finland	20%		75%
Toroptsova *et al.* 1995	Russia	11%	31%	48%
Leboeuf-Yde *et al.* 1996	Nordic countries (review)		50%	66%
Linton *et al.* 1998	Sweden		66%	
McKinnon *et al.* 1997	UK	16%	48%	62%
Skovron *et al.* 1994	Belgium	33%		59%
Walsh *et al.* 1992	UK		36%	58%
Dodd 1997	UK	15%	40%	
Waxman *et al.* 2000	UK		41%	59%
Average rates of selected studies		**22%**	**44%**	**61%**

These gross figures disguise differences in the characteristics of different episodes of back pain relative to duration, severity and effect on a person's lifestyle.

Clearly back pain is an endemic problem, widespread throughout the community. It is a problem that will affect the majority of adults at some point in their lives. Back pain is normal.

Natural history

The traditional concept of back pain was the acute/chronic dichotomy, in which it was thought that most patients have brief finite episodes and only a few progress to a chronic problem. It is frequently stated that for most people the prognosis is good (Klaber Moffett *et al.* 1995; Evans and Richards 1996; Waddell 1994): *"80 – 90% of attacks of low back pain recover in about 6 weeks"* regardless of the treatment applied, or lack of it (Waddell 1987). However, a picture of the natural history of back pain that suggests the majority will have a brief self-limiting episode denies recent epidemiological evidence and paints an over-optimistic summary of many individuals' experience of this problem.

It is certainly true that a great number of acute episodes of back pain resolve quickly and spontaneously (Coste *et al.* 1994; Carey *et al.* 1995a). Coste *et al.* (1994) followed 103 acute patients in primary care for three months and found that 90% had recovered in two weeks and that only two developed chronic back pain. However, this study sample contained patients with a very brief history of back pain (less than 72 hours), no referral of pain below the gluteal fold and excluded those who had experienced a previous episode in the last three months – all characteristics with a good prognosis.

Dillane *et al.* (1966) reported that the duration of the episode in over 90% of those who visited their GP with acute back pain was less than four weeks. However, the duration was defined as the time between the first and last consultation with the doctor. An episode of back pain cannot be defined in this way. Although patients may stop attending their medical practitioner, this does not necessarily mean that their back pain has resolved. More recently it was found that while most patients only visited their GP once or twice because of the problem, one year later 75% of them were still not symptom-free (Croft *et al.* 1998).

Other studies that have looked at the natural history of new episodes of back pain in primary care settings also paint a more pessimistic picture, although outcome depends partly on what is being measured (Carey *et al.* 1995a; Cherkin *et al.* 1996a). Studies have found that only 30 – 40% of their sample are completely resolved at about two to three months, with little further improvement at six or twelve months (Cherkin *et al.* 1996a; Philips and Grant 1991; Klenerman *et al.* 1995). Thomas *et al.* (1999) interviewed patients who had presented to primary care with new episodes of back pain – 48% still reported disabling symptoms at three months, 42% at one year and 34% were classified as having persistent disabling back pain at both reporting times.

Recurrences in the following year after onset are extremely common, reported in about three-quarters of samples (Klenerman *et al.* 1995; van den Hoogen *et al.* 1998). In a large group of patients in primary care studied (von Korff *et al.* 1993) one year after seeking medical treatment for back pain, the majority with both recent and non-recent onset of back problems reported pain in the previous month (69% and 82% respectively). In those whose problem had started recently, only 21% were pain-free in the previous month; in those whose problem was of a longer duration, only 12% were pain-free in the previous month.

Table 1.2 gives a selection of studies that have described relapse rates and persistent symptoms. Relapse rates refer to those in the back pain population who report more than one episode in a year, and persistence refers to back pain that has lasted for several months or more. Exact definitions vary between different studies, but a history of recurrences and non-resolving symptoms is clearly a very common experience.

Table 1.2   Relapse rate and persistent symptoms in selected studies

Reference	Relapse rate	Persistent symptoms
Linton *et al.* 1998	57%	43%
Brown *et al.* 1998	55%	
Szpalski *et al.* 1995		36%
Heliovaara *et al.* 1989	45%	
Toroptsova *et al.* 1995	65%	23%
Hillman *et al.* 1996		47%
Philips and Grant 1991		40%
Klenerman *et al.* 1995	71%	
Thomas *et al.* 1999		48%
Van den Hoogen *et al.* 1998	76%	35%
Miedema *et al.* 1998		28%
Croft *et al.* 1998		79%
Carey *et al.* 1999	39%	
Waxman *et al.* 2000		42%
Average rates from selected studies	**58%**	**42%**

"The message from the figures is that, in any one year, recurrences, exacerbations and persistence dominate the experience of low back pain in the community" (Croft *et al.* 1997, p. 14).

It is clear that for many individuals, recovery from an acute episode of backache is not the end of their back pain experience. The strongest known risk factor for developing back pain is a history of a previous episode (Croft *et al.* 1997; Shekelle 1997; Smedley *et al.* 1997). The chance of having a recurrence of back pain after a first episode is greater than 50%. Many recurrences are common and more than one-third of the back pain population have a long-term problem (Croft *et al.* 1997; Evans and Richards 1996; Waddell 1994;

Papageorgiou and Rigby 1991; Linton *et al.* 1998; Brown *et al.* 1998; Szpalski *et al.* 1995; Heliovaara *et al.* 1989; Toroptsova *et al.* 1995). There is also the suggestion from one population study that those with persistent or episodic pain may gradually deteriorate, being significantly more likely to report chronic low back pain and associated disability at a later date (Waxman *et al.* 2000). However, the risk of recurrence or persistence of back pain appears to lessen with the passage of time since the last episode (Biering-Sorensen 1983a).

The inference from these figures is clear – an individual's experience of back pain may well encompass their life history. The high rate of recurrences, episodes and persistence of symptoms seriously challenges the myth of an acute/chronic dichotomy. Back pain is *"a recurrent condition for which definitions of acute and chronic pain based on a single episode are inadequate, characterised by variation and change, rather than an acute, self-limiting episode. Chronic back pain, defined as back pain present on at least half the days during an extended period is far from rare..."* (Von Korff and Saunders 1996).

It would appear from the evidence that the much-quoted speedy recovery of back pain does not conform to many people's experience and that the division of the back pain population into chronic and acute categories presents a false dichotomy (Figure 1.1). This is not to deny that many people have brief acute episodes that resolve in days, nor that there is a small group of seriously disabled chronic sufferers, but that for large numbers, *"low back pain should be viewed as a chronic problem with an untidy pattern of grumbling symptoms and periods of relative freedom from pain and disability interspersed with acute episodes, exacerbations, and recurrences"* (Croft *et al.* 1998). Back pain should be viewed from the perspective of the sufferer's lifetime – and given such a perspective, the logic of self-management is overwhelming.

Figure 1.1   The assumed and real natural history of back pain

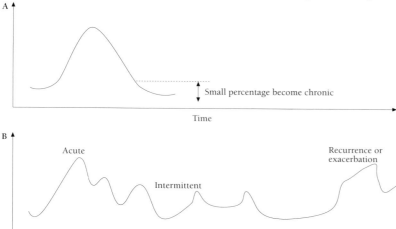

A: Assumed course of acute low back pain
B: Real course of back pain

Reproduced with permission from Croft P, Papageorgiou A and McNally R (1997) *Low Back Pain*. In: A Stevens and J Raftery (eds) Health Care Needs Assessment. Second Series: Radcliffe Medical Press, Oxford.

In summary, many episodes of back pain are brief and self-limiting; however, a significant proportion of individuals will experience persistent symptoms, while a minority develop chronic pain. The natural improvement rate stabilises after the first few months, and after this time resolution is much less likely. Up to one-third of new episodes result in prolonged periods of symptoms. Half of those having an initial episode of back pain will experience relapses. Lack of clinical follow-up creates the mistaken impression that there is common resolution of problems, which is not confirmed by more stringent research methods.

Disability

Not all back pain is the same. There is variability between individuals in the persistence of symptoms, in severity and in functional disability (von Korff *et al.* 1990). One review of the literature found that between 7% and 18% of population samples that have been studied are affected frequently, daily or constantly by back pain (Raspe 1993). Persistent symptoms have been reported by about 40% and longstanding, disabling backache by about 10% of all those who suffer from the problem (Croft *et al.* 1997; Evans and Richards 1996; Fordyce 1995;

Waddell 1994; Linton *et al.* 1998; Szpalski *et al.* 1995; Heliovaara *et al.* 1989; Toroptsova *et al.* 1995; Carey *et al.* 2000). Levels of disability, even among those with persistent symptoms, vary widely.

Musculoskeletal disorders are the most common cause of chronic incapacity, with back pain accounting for a significant proportion of this total (Bennett *et al.* 1995; Badley *et al.* 1994). Back pain is thus one of the most common causes of disability, especially during the productive middle years of life. It has been estimated (Waddell 1994) that 10% of the adult population, or 30% of those with back pain, report some limitation of their normal activity in the past month because of it. Work loss due to backache occurs for 2% of the adult population each month, just less than 10% each year and in 25 – 30% of the working population across their lifetimes (Waddell 1994).

Heliovaara *et al.* (1989) reported from a population survey that 40% of those with back pain had been forced to reduce leisure activities permanently, 20% had marked limitation of daily activities and 5% had severe limitations. In a one-year period, 22% of those with back pain who were employed went on sick leave because of it, representing a prevalence rate in the adult population of 6% (Hillman *et al.* 1996). According to one study, serious disability and work loss affects 5 – 10% of the population in any year, and in a lifetime over one-quarter of the population take time off work due to back pain (Walsh *et al.* 1992).

Table 1.3   Disability and work loss due to back pain in general population

	Men One year	*Men Lifetime*	*Women One year*	*Women Lifetime*
Disability	5%	16%	4.5%	13%
Work loss	11%	34%	7%	23%

Source: Walsh *et al.* 1992

Disability due to back pain has varied over time. In the UK during the 1980s, the payment of sickness and invalidity benefit rose by 208%, compared to an average rise of 54% for all incapacities (Waddell 1994). There is no evidence of an increased prevalence of back pain over recent decades (Nachemson *et al.* 2000; Leboeuf-Yde *et al.* 1996); the increased incapacity is thought to relate to changed attitudes and expectations, changed medical ideas and management, and changed social provision (Waddell 1994). It might also be seen to reflect a time of high unemployment and social change within the UK. Indeed, more recent evidence from the US reports that rather than being on the increase, the estimate of annual occupational back pain for which workers claimed compensation actually declined by 34% between 1987 and 1995 (Murphy and Volinn 1999).

It is important to be aware that patients with chronic back pain represent a diverse group, not all of whom are fated to a poor prognosis. When ninety-four individuals with chronic back pain were questioned about work and social disability, less than 8% indicated an interruption of normal activities over a six-month period (McGorry *et al.* 2000). Attempts have been made to classify chronic pain states relative to severity and associated disability, which indicated that over half of those with chronic pain report a low level of restriction on their lifestyle and low levels of depression.

Several large population-based studies of chronic pain and back pain (von Korff *et al.* 1990, 1992; Cassidy *et al.* 1998) and a study of chronic back pain patients (Klapow *et al.* 1993) reveal reasonably consistent levels of limitation of activity due to persistent pain problems. About half of those with chronic pain report a low level of disability and a good level of coping. About a quarter report moderate levels of disability, and another quarter report severe incapacity due to the problem (see Table 1.4). In those attending primary care for back pain, about 60% had low disability and about 40% had high disability at presentation (von Korff *et al.* 1993). After one year, less than 20% were pain-free, 65% had minimal disability and between 14% and 20% had high disability, so even in those with persistent symptoms the severity and disability is variable, with the majority reporting minimal reduction of function.

Table 1.4   Grading of chronic back pain

Grade	*von Korff et al. 1992 (N = 1213)*	*Klapow et al. 1993 (N = 96)*	*Cassidy et al. 1998 (N = 1110)*
Low disability and low intensity	35%	49%	48%
Low disability and high intensity	28%	25%	12%
High disability	37% (Moderate 20%; Severe 17%)	26%	11%

"There was considerable heterogeneity in manifestations of pain dysfunction among persons with seemingly comparable pain experience. A considerable proportion of persons with severe and persistent pain did not evidence significant pain-related disability. Some persons with severe and persistent pain did not evidence psychological impairment, although many did" (Von Korff *et al.* 1990).

The pain status of individuals is not static, but dynamic (Table 1.5). Symptoms and associated disability fluctuate over time, and many patients leave the pool of persistent pain sufferers if followed over a few years. The overall pool of those with chronic pain appears to stay about the same, but a proportion leave that group and either become pain-free or are less severely affected, while a similar number join it over a period of a year or more (Cedraschi *et al.* 1999; Croft *et al.* 1997; Troup *et al.* 1987; von Korff *et al.* 1990; McGorry *et al.* 2000).

Table 1.5   The dynamic state of chronic back pain

	CLBP or chronic pain who become pain-free	CLBP who improve	CLBP who remain ISQ
Croft *et al.* 1997		33%	67%
Cedraschi *et al.* 1999		53%	47%
Troup *et al.* 1987	8%	9%	83%
Crook *et al.* 1989	13% (pain clinic) 36% (primary care)		

CLBP = chronic low back pain

ISQ = in status quo

Back pain is a symptom that describes a heterogeneous and dynamic state. Individuals vary in their experience of backache relative to time, severity and disability. Many individuals have persistent problems. Most chronic back pain is of low intensity and low disability; high levels of severity and disability affect only the minority. Some of those with chronic backache do become pain-free; however, because of high prevalence rates, back pain produces extensive disability and work loss and thus impacts considerably on individuals and on society.

Cost

Even though not everyone with back pain seeks health care, the prevalence of the problem is so great that high numbers of patients are entering the health services. A major concern is the cost associated with back pain, although this is difficult to calculate. It is made up of the direct cost of health care borne by society or by the patient and the indirect costs associated with absence from work. In the UK costs to the NHS alone in 1992/3 have been estimated at between £265 and £383 million, which constitutes 0.65 – 0.93% of total NHS spending (Klaber Moffett *et al.* 1995). A more recent estimate of the direct health care costs of back pain in the UK for 1998 put the cost at £1,632 million (Maniadakis and Gray 2000). In the US, medical care costs have been estimated at between $8 and $18 billion (Shekelle *et al.* 1995).

The medical costs of back pain, however, are only a part of the whole cost of the problem that society pays. Indirect costs, such as disability or compensation payments, production losses at workplaces and informal care, dwarf the amount that is spent directly on patient care. The total societal cost of back pain in the US has been estimated at $75 – $100 billion in 1990 (Frymoyer and Cats-Baril 1991). Cost data from insurance companies from two separate studies shows that medical care represents about 34% of the total costs, while indemnity costs make up about 66% (Webster and Snook 1990; Williams *et al.* 1998a). Total employment-related costs in the UK have been estimated at between £5 and £10 billion (Maniadakis and Gray 2000), which means that direct costs only account for between 13% and 24% of the total costs (Figure 1.2). In the Netherlands, the direct health care costs have been estimated as only 7% of the total cost, with the total cost representing 1.7% of the gross national product (van Tulder *et al.* 1995).

Figure 1.2   The direct and indirect costs of back pain

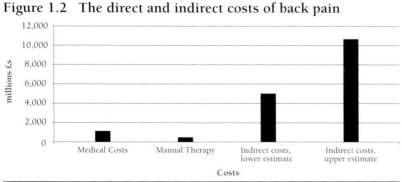

Source: Maniadakis and Gray 2000

Medical costs include medicines and x-rays; manual therapy includes physiotherapy, osteopathy and chiropractic; indirect costs include production losses and informal care. Some of these costs can only be estimated. The direct and indirect costs of back pain are so great that the economic burden is larger than for any other disease for which economic analysis was available in the UK in 1998 (Maniadakis and Gray 2000). It is more costly than coronary heart disease and the combined costs of rheumatoid arthritis, respiratory infections, Alzheimer's disease, stroke, diabetes, arthritis, multiple sclerosis, thrombosis and embolism, depression, diabetes, ischaemia and epilepsy.

A minority of patients consume the majority of health care and indirect costs for low back pain. Combining data from multiple studies suggests that about 15% of the back pain population account for about 70% of costs (Spitzer *et al.* 1987; Webster and Snook 1990; Williams *et al.* 1998a; Linton *et al.* 1998).

Thus, not only is the cost of back pain huge, but the majority of this money is not spent directly on patient care, but on indirect societal 'costs'. Furthermore, it is the chronic few who consume the largest proportion of this expense.

Health care

Not everybody with back pain seeks professional help. Most surveys reveal that about a quarter to a half of all people with back pain will consult their medical practitioner (Croft *et al.* 1997; Papageorgiou and Rigby 1991; McKinnon *et al.* 1997; Carey *et al.* 1996). A survey in Belgium found that 63% of those with back pain had seen a health professional for the most recent episode (Szpalski *et al.* 1995). Where chiropractic care is available, 13% of back pain sufferers seek their help (Linton *et al.* 1998; Carey *et al.* 1996). Seeking care appears to vary widely; one survey in the UK found those seeking consultation with local physicians to range from 24 – 59% of those with back pain in different areas (Walsh *et al.* 1992). Care-seeking among those with chronic back pain may be slightly higher (Carey *et al.* 1995b, 2000). Many people with low back pain cope independently in the community and do not seek help, whether medical or alternative.

Table 1.6   **Proportion of back pain population who seek health care**

Reference	Country	% who consult GP	% who consult osteopath	% who consult chiropractor	% who consult physio-therapist
Dodd 1997	UK	38%	6%	3%	9%
Walsh *et al.* 1992	UK	40%			
Hillman *et al.* 1996	UK	37%	4.5%	1%	10%
Linton *et al.* 1998	Sweden	8%		13%	5%
Carey *et al.* 1996	US	24%		13%	
McKinnon *et al.* 1997	UK	24%			
Santos-Eggimann *et al.* 2000	Switzerland	25%			

In the UK, Waddell (1994) estimated a population prevalence of 16.5 million people with back pain in 1993. Of these he estimated that 18 – 42% consult their GP, 10% attend a hospital outpatient department, 6% are seen by NHS physiotherapists, 4% by osteopaths, less than 2% each by private physiotherapists and chiropractors, 0.2% become inpatients and 0.14% go to surgery.

Even though many people with back pain do not attend a health professional, because of the large prevalence rate in the community the numbers actually seeking health care are considerable and constitute a significant burden in primary care. For instance, in the US it is estimated that it is the reason for 15 million visits to physicians annually, the fifth-largest reason for attendance, representing nearly 3% of all visits (Hart *et al.* 1995). In a rural primary care setting in Finland and practices in the UK, low back pain patients make up about 5% of all GP consultations (Rekola *et al.* 1993; Hackett *et al.* 1993; Waddell 1994). In the UK it has been estimated that one-third of those attending primary care with back pain will present with a new episode, one-third will present with a recurrence and one-third will present with a persistent disabling problem (Croft *et al.* 1997).

There are no clear clinical features that distinguish those patients who seek health care from those who do not. Hillman *et al.* (1996) found that those who consult tended to report higher levels of pain, greater disability and longer episodes, but also that some individuals with the same characteristics did not seek health care. Carey *et al.* (1999) found that recurrences of back pain, the presence of sciatica and greater disability were associated with care-seeking. Longer duration of an episode of back pain is more likely to cause people to consult (Santos-Eggimann *et al.* 2000), and failure to improve is associated with seeking care from multiple providers of health care (Sundararajan *et al.* 1998).

Those who attend tertiary care tend to be at the more severe end of the spectrum of symptoms. However, one-fifth of non-consulters had constant pain and needed bed-rest, one-third had had pain for over three months in the previous year and nearly half had leg pain and restricted activity (Croft *et al.* 1997).

In the US, Carey *et al.* (1996) found that those who sought care were more likely to have pain for longer than two weeks that radiated into the leg and had come on at work. However, considerable numbers of those not seeking care also had these characteristics. Szpalski *et al.* (1995) found that back pain frequency, health beliefs and sociocultural factors influenced health care-seeking. Other studies have also found that psychosocial factors have some impact on care-seeking for back pain (Wright *et al.* 1995; Vingard *et al.* 2000). The type of health provider that patients first see may have an effect on subsequent consultation rates, with those who see a chiropractor being twice as likely to seek further help compared to those who saw a medical doctor (Carey *et al.* 1999).

The message in the epidemiological literature – that many people with back pain cope independently from professional help – is reinforced by evidence from qualitative research using interviews of people with back pain. Skelton *et al.* (1996) in the UK found a large number of his sample to be actively working on their problem by adopting various preventive strategies. These included use of certain body postures when bending, sitting and lifting; taking light exercise; resting; doing back and abdominal exercises; and, for some, constant awareness of a back problem in day-to-day activities. In contrast, a smaller group of patients reported taking a minimalist approach to self-management, despite having some knowledge about preventive measures. In between these two extremes were a few who reported that they were in the process of recognising a need to do something about their problem and were beginning to perceive the need to adopt self-management strategies.

Borkan *et al.* (1995) also found patients adopting a range of intellectual and behavioural strategies that were designed to minimise pain or maximise function. Information about back care is a common expectation of those who do seek professional help (Fitzpatrick *et al.* 1987).

Less than half of those in the community with back pain actually seek health care. It is thus clear that self-management of back problems is both attainable and practised by many. Some of those who do not seek health care have constant, persistent and referred pain with reduced function. The majority of people with back pain manage independently of health professionals. Of those who do seek help, many are looking for things that they can do to help themselves to manage their problem better. There are others who are neglectful of adopting the necessary strategies, but who may be convinced of the necessity of doing so if they are sufficiently informed. Nonetheless, because of the high prevalence rate, back pain constitutes a considerable burden to primary care.

Treatment

The range of treatments offered to patients with back pain varies considerably. There is no consensus on the best type of treatment for back pain, and so the treatment given is chosen on the inclination of the practitioner. It depends more on whom the patient sees than their clinical presentation (Deyo 1993).

A back pain patient in the United States is five times more likely to be a surgical candidate than if they were a patient in England or Scotland (Figure 1.3 from Cherkin *et al.* 1994a). Back surgery rates increased almost linearly with the local supply of orthopaedic and neurosurgeons.

Figure 1.3   Ratios of back surgery rates to back surgery rate in the US (1988 – 1989)

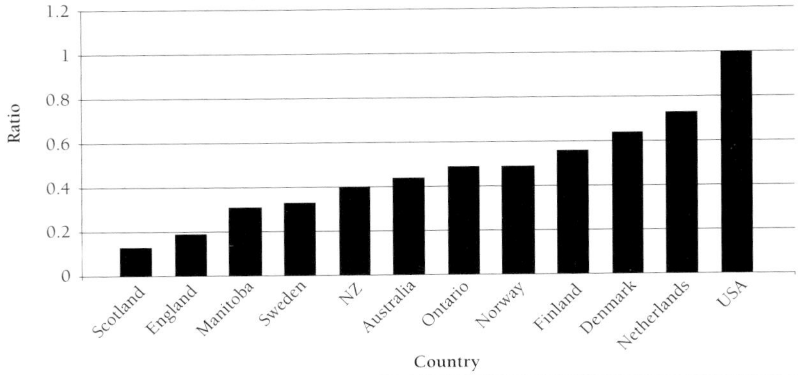

Source: Cherkin *et al.* 1994.

In the US, non-surgical hospitalisation and surgery rates vary considerably, both over time and place. For instance, patients are twice as likely to be hospitalised in the south than in the west, and between 1979 and 1990 there was a 100% increase in the rate of fusion operations (Taylor *et al.* 1994).

In the Netherlands, a descriptive study of general practitioners' approaches to chronic back pain patients has shown that there is little consistency between clinicians (van Tulder *et al.* 1997a). Cherkin *et al.* (1994b) found there was little consensus among physicians about which diagnostic tests should be used for back pain patients with certain clinical presentations and concluded that, for the patient, 'who you see is what you get'.

Equally, in physical therapy there is no standardised management of back pain. Surveys of reported management styles have been conducted in the US (Battie *et al.* 1994; Jette *et al.* 1994; Jette and Delitto 1997; Mielenz *et al.* 1997), in the Netherlands (van Baar *et al.* 1998) and in the UK (Foster *et al.* 1999). These surveys show that a wide range of thermal and electrotherapy modalities, massage, mobilisation and manipulation, exercises and mixed treatment regimes are used. Exercises are commonly used, but these are frequently combined with the use of passive treatment modalities, such as ultrasound, heat or electrical stimulation and, less frequently, with the use of manual therapy. Passive treatment modalities tend to be used by some clinicians, whatever the duration of symptoms.

In a survey in the US, The McKenzie Method was deemed the most useful approach for managing back pain, although in practice clinicians were likely to use a variety of treatment approaches (Battie *et al.* 1994). In the UK and Ireland, the Maitland and McKenzie approaches were reportedly used most often to manage back problems, although electrotherapy modalities (interferential, ultrasound, TENS and short-wave diathermy) and passive stretching and abdominal exercises are also commonly used (Foster *et al.* 1999). Internationally, physiotherapy practice is eclectic and apparently little influenced by the movement towards evidence-based practice.

Back care regimes are clearly eclectic and non-standardised. When so much variety of treatment is on offer, what patients get is more likely to reflect the clinicians' biases rather than to be based on their clinical presentation or the best evidence. Under these circumstances there must be occasions when the management offered is sub-optimal and is not in the best long-term interest of the patient.

Effectiveness

Unfortunately, seeking health care does not, for many, solve their back problem (Von Korff *et al.* 1993; Linton *et al.* 1998; van den Hoogen *et al.* 1997; Croft *et al.* 1998). Despite the vast numbers who are treated for this condition by different health professionals, the underlying epidemiology of back pain, with its high prevalence and recurrence rates, remains unchanged (Waddell 1994). Indeed, there is even the accusation that traditional methods of care, involving rest and passive treatment modalities rather than activity, have been partly implicated in the alarming rise of those disabled by back pain (Waddell 1987).

Some studies have challenged the notion that outcomes are necessarily better in those who are treated with physiotherapy or chiropractic (Indahl *et al.* 1995; van den Hoogen *et al.* 1997). For instance, Indahl *et al.*'s study (1995,) followed nearly 1,000 patients who were randomised either to normal care or to a group who were given a thorough explanation of the importance of activity and the negative effects of being 'too careful'. At 200 days, 60% of the normal care group were still on sick leave, compared to 30% of those instructed to keep active. Of those in the normal care group, 62% received physical therapy and 42% chiropractic, of which 79% and 70%

respectively reported that treatment made the situation worse or had little or no effect.

Various reviews and systematic reviews have been undertaken into interventions used in the treatment of back pain. These universally only include prospective randomised controlled trials, which, with their supposed adherence to strict methodological criteria, are seen as the 'gold standard' by which to judge interventions. This adherence to specific study designs is rarely achieved, but the focus on study design tends to distract from the intervention itself. Restricted recruitment and follow-up may limit generalisability; interventions may not reflect clinical practice, because mostly they are given in a standardised way with no attempt at assessment of individual suitability for that treatment regime; the outcome measures may not be appropriate for the condition.

Nonetheless, the underlying message is impossible to evade – no intervention to date offers a straightforward, curative resolution of back problems (Spitzer *et al.* 1987; AHCPR 1994; Evans and Richards 1996; Croft *et al.* 1997; van Tulder *et al.* 1997b). These are all major reviews conducted in the last decade or so that question the efficacy of a wide range of commonly used interventions.

"Research to date has been insufficiently rigorous to give clear indications of the value of treatment for non-specific LBP patients. No treatment has been shown beyond doubt to be effective. .... There is ... no clear indication of the value of treatments compared to no treatment, or of the relative benefit of different treatments" (Evans and Richards 1996, pp. 2–3).

Specific systematic reviews have been conducted on individual interventions. The use of ultrasound in the treatment of musculoskeletal problems in general has been seriously challenged by all comprehensive systematic reviews to date, which report that active ultrasound is no more effective than placebo (van der Windt *et al.* 1999; Gam and Johannsen 1995; Robertson and Baker 2001). There is no clear evidence for the effectiveness of laser therapy (de Bie *et al.* 1998).

A systematic review found the evidence concerning traction to be inconclusive (van der Heijden *et al.* 1995a), so a randomised sham-controlled trial was constructed avoiding earlier study flaws. Despite favourable results in a pilot study (van der Heijden *et al.* 1995b), larger numbers and short and long-term follow-up revealed lack of efficacy for lumbar traction (Beurskens *et al.* 1995, 1997).

Results of another systematic review show there was no evidence that acupuncture is more effective than no treatment and some evidence to show it is no more effective than placebo or sham acupuncture for chronic back pain (van Tulder *et al.* 1999).

A recent systematic review of the use of TENS for chronic back pain found no difference in outcomes between active and sham treatments (Milne *et al.* 2001). There would appear to be little role in the management of back pain for such passive therapies.

"No controlled studies have proved the efficacy of physical agents in the treatment of patients who have acute, subacute, or chronic low back pain. The effect of using a passive modality is equal to or worse than a placebo effect" (Nordin and Campello 1999, p. 80).

The lack of efficacy of passive therapies is reinforced by systematic reviews of bed-rest compared to keeping active. There is a consistent finding that bed-rest has no value, but may actually delay recovery in acute back pain. Advice to stay active and resume normal activities as soon as possible results in faster return to work, less chronic disability and fewer recurrent problems. If patients are forced to rest in the acute stage, this should be limited to two or three days (Koes and van den Hoogen 1994; Waddell *et al.* 1997; Hagen *et al.* 2000). Even for sciatica the same rules apply (Vroomen *et al.* 1999).

There is some evidence that non-steroidal anti-inflammatory drugs (NSAIDs) might provide short-term symptomatic relief in cases of acute back pain, but these are not clearly better than ordinary analgesics, and no NSAID is better than another. There is no evidence to suggest that NSAIDs are helpful in chronic back pain or in sciatica (Koes *et al.* 1997; van Tulder *et al.* 2000b).

Several systematic reviews found little evidence for the efficacy of group education or 'back schools' (Di Fabio 1995; Cohen *et al.* 1994; Linton and Kamwendo 1987), but there was some evidence for benefit to chronic back pain patients, especially in an occupational setting (van Tulder *et al.* 1999b).

Several more recent randomised controlled trials would suggest that there is a role for education in the management of back pain (Indahl *et al.* 1998; Burton *et al.* 1999; von Korff *et al.* 1998; Moore *et al.* 2000; Roland and Dixon 1989). These studies used a variety of methods to provide appropriate information about normal activity, self-management and removal of fear of movement, and affected the attitudes and beliefs of several patients, as well as function and behaviour.

In line with the emergence of the concept of patients' attitudes and beliefs influencing illness behaviour, there have been attempts to reduce chronic disability through the modification of environmental contingencies and patients' cognitive processes using behavioural therapy. Systematic reviews suggest that behavioural therapy can be effective when compared to no treatment, but is less clearly so when compared to other active interventions (Morley *et al.* 1999; van Tulder *et al.* 2000c). Compared to a 'treatment as usual' group, one cognitive-behavioural intervention produced a range of improved outcomes of clinical importance, including reducing the risk of long-term sick leave by threefold (Linton and Ryberg 2001).

There have been multiple reviews of manipulation for back pain; there are more reviews than trials (Assendelft *et al.* 1995). Some reviews suggest that manipulation is effective (Anderson *et al.* 1992; Shekelle *et al.* 1992; Bronfort 1999), but others suggest that its efficacy is unproven because of contradictory results (Koes *et al.* 1991, 1996). Even when the conclusion favours manipulation, there are limitations to its value. Most reviews note that the benefit of manipulation is short-term only, and also largely confined to a sub-acute group with back pain only. The value of manipulation in other sub-groups of the back pain population is unclear. If the individual trials are examined in detail, it is also apparent that the treatment effect, when present, is mostly rather trivial, with clinically unimportant differences between the treatment groups. Furthermore, many of the trials reviewed as being about manipulation in fact include non-thrust mobilisation as part of the treatment – often it is unclear exactly which of these interventions is being judged.

Some systematic reviews suggest that the evidence for specific exercises does not indicate they are effective (Koes *et al.* 1991; van Tulder *et al.* 2000a). These reviews include a heterogeneous collection of different types of exercises from which they seek a generalised interpretation of all exercise. Most trials fail to prescribe exercise in a rational manner to suitable patients, but rather exercises are given in a standardised way. The reviewers show great concern for methodological correctness, but display less understanding of the interventions they are seeking to judge – trials that use extension exercises are considered to be using the McKenzie approach. Hilde and Bo (1998) failed to reach a conclusion regarding the role of exercise in chronic back pain.

Other reviews have been more positive, especially concerning exercises used during the sub-acute and chronic phases (Faas 1996; Haigh and Clarke 1999; Maher *et al.* 1999; Nordin and Campello 1999). Maher *et al.* (1999) concluded that acute back patients should be advised to avoid bed-rest and return to normal activity in a progressive way and that this basic approach could be supplemented with manipulative or McKenzie therapy. For chronic back patients there is strong evidence to encourage intensive exercises.

This brief overview of the literature makes for sobering reading concerning normal physiotherapy practice. For a wide range of passive therapies still being dispensed by clinicians on a regular basis, there is scant supporting evidence. Even for the interventions that receive some support from the literature, namely manipulation, exercise, behavioural therapy and information provision, there is sometimes contradictory or limited evidence.

Informed both by this evidence and by the role that psychosocial factors have in affecting chronic disability, the outlines of an optimal management approach begin to emerge:

- avoidance of bed-rest and encouragement to return to normal activity

- information aimed at making patients less fearful

- seeking to influence some of their attitudes and beliefs about pain

- advising patients how they can manage what may be an ongoing or recurrent problem

- informing patients that their active participation is vital in restoring full function

- encouraging self-management, exercise and activity

- providing patients with the means to affect symptoms and thus gain some control over their problem.

These would appear to be the main themes that should be informing clinical management of back pain.

Conclusions

Our understanding of the problem of low back pain must be guided by certain irrefutable truths:

- Back pain is so common it may be said to be normal. In the way of other endemic problems, such the common cold or dental hygiene problems, resistance to the medicalisation of a normal experience should be allied to a self-management approach in which personal responsibility is engendered.

- The course of back pain is frequently full of episodes, persistence, flare-ups, reoccurrences and chronicity. It is important to remember this in the clinical encounter. Management must aim at long-term benefits, not short-term symptomatic relief.

- Many people with back pain manage independently and do not seek health care. They do this using exercises and postural or ergonomic strategies. Some patients find the adoption of this personal responsibility difficult and may need encouragement. Successful self-management involves the adoption of certain intellectual and behavioural strategies that minimise pain and maximise function.

- The cost of back pain to the health industry and society as a whole is vast. Indirect 'societal' costs absorb the majority of this spending. The direct medical costs are dominated by spending on the chronic back pain population. Therefore, management should be directed to trying to reduce the disability and need for care-seeking in this group by encouraging a self-reliant and coping attitude.

- Back pain is not always a curable disorder and for many is a lifelong problem. No intervention has been shown to alter the underlying prevalence, incidence or recurrence rates. Consequently, management must – and should always – be offering models of self-management and personal responsibility to the patient.

- Passive modalities appear to have no role in the management of back pain. There is some evidence that favours exercise, manipulation, information provision and behavioural therapy.

Given these aspects of back pain, perhaps it should be viewed in light of other chronic diseases in which management rather than curative therapy is on offer. A therapeutic encounter needs to equip the sufferer with long-term self-management strategies as well as short-term measures of symptomatic improvement. It may also be suggested that to do otherwise and treat patients with short-term passive modalities or manipulation, but not equip them with information and strategies for self-management, is ill-conceived and is not in the patients' best interests. If a condition is very common, persistent, often episodic and resistant to easy remedy, it is time patients were fully empowered to deal with these problems in an optimal and realistic fashion. As clinicians, we should be offering this empowerment to our patients.

2: Risk and Prognostic Factors in Low Back Pain

Introduction

Aetiological factors are variables relating to lifestyle, occupation, genetics, individual characteristics and so on that are associated with a higher risk of developing a specific health problem. These factors are identified for study and their occurrence is noted in those who have the outcome of interest (in this case back pain) compared to those who do not. A *risk factor* is a characteristic that is associated with a higher rate of back pain onset. After the onset of symptoms, certain factors may affect the future course of the problem. Again comparisons are made, this time between those who recover quickly and those who have a protracted problem. A *prognostic factor* may be used to predict outcome once an episode has started (Bombardier *et al.* 1994). A poor prognostic factor is suggestive of someone who will have a protracted period of back pain.

Sections in this chapter are as follows:

- risk factors
- individual risk factors
- biomechanical risk factors
- psychosocial risk factors
- all risk factors
- onset
- individual and clinical prognostic factors
- biomechanical prognostic factors
- psychosocial prognostic factors
- all prognostic factors.

Risk factors

Epidemiological studies have generally considered risk factors for the onset of back pain to relate to three dimensions: individual and lifestyle factors, physical or biomechanical factors and psychosocial factors. Examples of each are given in Table 2.1 (Bombardier *et al.* 1994; Frank *et al.* 1996; Ferguson and Marras 1997).

Table 2.1   Three major classes of risk factors for back pain

Class of risk factor	Examples
Individual and lifestyle factors	History of back pain, age, sex, weight, muscle strength, flexibility, smoking status, marital status
Physical or biomechanical factors	Lifting, heavy work, posture, vibration, driving, bending, sitting, twisting
Psychosocial factors	Depression, anxiety, beliefs and attitudes, stress, job satisfaction, relationships at work, control at work

Individual factors have in the past received most scientific attention, but in general their predictive value was low. Ergonomic epidemiology emphasised physical factors, but research has provided only limited evidence of their importance; the focus more recently is upon psychosocial dimensions (Winkel and Mathiassen 1994). This chapter considers the variables that may be risk factors in the onset of back pain, as well as variables that may be prognostic factors in the outcome of an episode of back pain once it has started.

Individual risk factors

The strongest risk factor for future back pain is history of past back pain. This factor is found consistently across numerous studies, indicating its vital predictive role in future episodes (Frank *et al.* 1996; Ferguson and Marras 1997). Frank *et al.* (1996) estimated that an individual with a previous history is three to four times more likely to develop back pain than someone without that history. The epidemiology reviewed in Chapter 1 suggests that more than half of those who have an episode of back pain will have a recurrence.

The association of increasing age and female gender to back pain are less well established. For the majority of other individual factors, such as obesity, smoking or fitness, the evidence is contradictory or scant (Frank *et al.* 1996; Ferguson and Marras 1997; Burdorf and Sorock 1997). In a review of individual risk factors for back pain, the following variables were considered: age, gender, height, weight, strength, flexibility, exercise fitness, leg length discrepancy, posture, Scheuermann's disease, congenital anomalies, spondylolisthesis and low education (Nachemson and Vingard 2000). There was a striking variability and inconsistency of results when all studies were considered – overall more studies indicated negative or no association between that factor and back pain rather than a positive association. They conclude that none of the variables considered in this review are strong predictors of future back pain.

Biomechanical risk factors

Assessing the role of physical factors in the aetiology of back pain is not straightforward, and as a consequence there have been conflicting reports over its importance. Various problems exist in the studies that have been done (Bombardier *et al.* 1994; Dolan 1998; Frank *et al.* 1996; Burdorf 1992). Much of the literature in this area is cross-sectional in nature; that is, risk factors and prognostic factors are measured at the same time as noting the presence or absence of back pain. This means that it is often difficult to determine if a factor contributed towards onset or towards prognosis. It also means that although a factor may be associated with back pain, we cannot be sure that it caused it. Prospective studies are better at identifying causation.

Furthermore, the measurement of exposure to a possible risk factor, such as frequent lifting, may be imprecise if based on self-report or job title rather than direct, objective measurement. There is also the 'healthy worker' effect, when those who have survived in an occupation without developing back pain will always be over-represented compared to those who had to leave the job because of back pain (Hartvigsen *et al.* 2001). This will tend to downplay the importance of mechanical factors.

In general there has been a failure to measure the different dimensions of exposure to a physical factor – degree of exposure, frequency and duration; thus invalid exposure assessment may fail to expose a relationship between mechanical factors and symptoms (Winkel and Mathiassen 1994).

These methodological problems with the literature on biomechanical risk factors for back pain have probably led to an under-reporting of their role, such that the association between these factors and back pain may well be stronger than was previously imagined (Dolan 1998). Hoogendoorn *et al.* (2000a) conducted a high-quality study using a prospective design in which exposure levels were actually measured rather than estimated, and psychological variables and other physical risk factors were accounted for in the analysis. Their results showed a positive association between trunk flexion and rotation at work and back pain, with a greater risk of pain at greater levels of exposure.

Taken individually, the reports provide only weak evidence of causation, but the consistency of reporting of certain factors and the strength of association between these factors and back pain is supportive of a definite relationship between biomechanical exposures and the onset of back problems (Frank *et al.* 1996; Burdorf and Sorock 1997).

Individual studies have shown certain mechanical factors to be associated with back pain or disc prolapse:

- repeated bending and lifting at work (Damkot *et al.* 1984; Videman *et al.* 1984; Kelsey *et al.* 1984a; Frymoyer *et al.* 1983; Marras *et al.* 1993; Waters *et al.* 1999; Zwerling *et al.* 1993)

- repeated bending at home (Mundt *et al.* 1993)

- prolonged bending (Punnett *et al.* 1991; Hoogendoorn *et al.* 2000a)

- unexpected spinal loading (Magora 1973)

- driving (Kelsey 1975; Kelsey *et al.* 1984b; Frymoyer *et al.* 1983; Damkot *et al.* 1984; Krause *et al.* 1997; Masset and Malchaire 1994)

- sedentary jobs (Kelsey 1975)

- a high incidence of back pain has been found in those who spend a lot of their working day either sitting or standing, but was much less common in those who were able to vary their working positions regularly during the day (Magora 1972).

Pheasant (1998) summarised the work done by Magora, which identified two distinct groups of people most at risk of back pain. In those whose jobs were physically very demanding and those whose jobs were essentially sedentary, about 20% of individuals experienced back pain. Those whose jobs entailed varied postures, some sitting and some standing, and were moderately physically active were at a much lower risk, with only about 2% of this group experiencing back pain.

Several large-scale reviews of the relevant literature have been conducted (Frank *et al.* 1996; Bombardier *et al.* 1994; Burdorf and

Sorock 1997; Ferguson and Marras 1997; Hoogendoorn *et al.* 1999; Vingard and Nachemson 2000). Ferguson and Marras (1997) included fifty-seven studies investigating risk factors; Burdorf and Sorock (1997) included thirty-five publications. Occupational physical stresses that have been found to be consistently and in general strongly associated with the occurrence of back pain across multiple systematic reviews are as follows:

• heavy or frequent lifting

• whole body vibration (as when driving)

• prolonged or frequent bending or twisting

• postural stresses (high spinal load or awkward postures).

Frank *et al.* (1996) estimated the relative risk of back pain associated with heavy lifting and whole body vibration to be three to four times normal, and that of spinal loading, postural stresses and dynamic trunk motion to be more than five times normal.

Psychosocial risk factors

The role of psychological and social dimensions as prognostic factors for chronic back pain and disability is now well known and is considered later in the chapter. Epidemiological studies addressing psychosocial risk factors as a cause of back pain are far fewer than those investigating physical factors. Low job satisfaction, relationships at work, including social support, high job demand, monotony or lack of control at work, stress and anxiety are factors that have an association with back pain in several studies, although the evidence for these factors is often weak or contradictory (Burdorf and Sorock 1997; Ferguson and Marras 1997). There are equal numbers of studies that are negative and show no relation between these psychosocial variables and back pain (Vingard and Nachemson 2000).

The role of low job satisfaction as a risk factor for back pain may be partly a product of less rigorous study designs that have failed to account for other psychosocial factors and physical work load (Hoogendoorn *et al.* 2000b). One study found that while work dissatisfaction was associated with a history of back pain, it was not related to the onset of back pain (Skovron *et al.* 1994). Two prospective studies indicate that low levels of perception of general health are predictors of new episodes of back pain (Croft *et al.* 1996, 1999).

Severe back pain has been found to be less prevalent among those with a higher socio-economic status, after physical work factors have been accounted for (Latza *et al.* 2000).

A review of psychosocial factors at work concluded that due to methodological difficulties in measuring variables, there is no conclusive evidence for psychosocial variables as risk factors for back pain, but that monotonous work, high perceived work load and time pressure are related to musculoskeletal symptoms in general (Bongers *et al.* 1993).

Frank *et al.* (1996) estimate that psychosocial factors have a weak relative risk for the occurrence of back pain, one to two times more likely than normal. Linton (2000b) made a thorough review of psychological risk factors for neck and back pain. He concluded that there was strong evidence that these factors may be associated with the *reporting* of back pain, and that attitudes, cognitions, fear–avoidance and depression are strongly related to pain and disability; however, there is no evidence to support the idea of a 'pain-prone' personality.

All risk factors

The evidence would suggest that individual, physical and psychosocial factors all could have an influence upon back pain onset. Studies that have included different factors have found that back pain is best predicted by a combination of individual, physical and psychosocial variables (Burton *et al.* 1989; Thorbjornsson *et al.* 2000). One prospective study found that physical and psychosocial factors could independently predict back pain (Krause *et al.* 1998), while another found that distress, previous trivial back pain and reduced lumbar lordosis were all consistent predictors of any back pain (Adams *et al.* 1999).

Most studies, however, have investigated a limited set of risk factors and have not assessed the relative importance of different variables. If risk estimates are not adjusted for other relevant risk factors, the overall effect may be to under- or over-estimate the role of particular variables (Burdorf and Sorock 1997). Research has only recently begun to address the relative contribution to back pain onset of individual, biomechanical and psychosocial factors together.

In terms of the relative importance of these different factors, several studies have shown that a history of trivial or previous back pain is a much stronger predictor of serious or future back pain than job satisfaction or psychological distress (van Poppel *et al.* 1998; Papageorgiou *et al.* 1996; Mannion *et al.* 1996; Smedley *et al.* 1997). After adjusting for earlier history, one study found that risk of back pain in nurses was still higher in those reporting heavier physical workload (Smedley *et al.* 1997). In a review of risk factors for occupational back pain, it was concluded that biomechanical factors are more significant factors of causation than psychosocial ones (Frank *et al.* 1996). In another review it was concluded that whereas the strength of psychosocial factors as risk indicators was strongly affected by sensitivity analysis, the role of physical load factors as risk indicators is more consistent and insensitive to slight changes in analysis (Hoogendoorn *et al.* 2000b).

If risk factors were clinically important, they would explain a large proportion of the predictive variables associated with back pain; however, even at best this is not so. The proportion of new episodes attributable to psychological factors at the most has been found to be 16% (Croft *et al.* 1996); another study found this to be only 3% (Mannion *et al.* 1996). While job dissatisfaction has been highlighted as a risk factor for back pain, in the original study that identified this, most of those who reported never enjoying their job did not in fact report back pain (Bigos *et al.* 1991). When all risk factors have been considered together, only between 5% and 12% of back pain has been explained (Mannion *et al.* 1996; Adams *et al.* 1999).

It is apparent that there are no simple causal explanations for back pain and that individual, physical and psychosocial factors may, to varying degrees, all have a role in aetiology. However, at most these factors, individually or combined, can only explain a small proportion of back pain. A past history of back pain is the factor most consistently associated with future back pain.

Onset

Although mechanical factors are associated with back pain and can therefore be seen as predisposing factors, onset is not always related to a specific event. Patients often report the precipitating factor involved flexion activities, such as lifting and bending. Generally, however, more patients report back pain that commenced for no apparent reason (Kramer 1990; Videman *et al.* 1989; Kelsey 1975; Laslett and Michaelsen 1991; McKenzie 1979). Both Kramer (1990) and Waddell (1998) found that about 60% of patients in their clinics developed pain insidiously.

Hall *et al.* (1998) examined the spontaneous onset of back pain in a study group of over 4,500 – and 67% could not identify a specific event that triggered their symptoms. By contrast, in a group that was required to report a specific causal event for compensation purposes only, 10% failed to attribute their pain to an incident. The authors considered spontaneous onset to be part of the natural history of back pain. The rate of spontaneous onset was greater in the sedentary employment group (69%) than the heavy occupation group (57%). McKenzie's clinic records also demonstrated the effect of compensation requirements on causal attribution. In 1973, in 60% of patients the onset of back pain was reported as 'no apparent reason'. After the introduction of a national compensation scheme in New Zealand, onset was related to an accident by 60% of patients (unpublished data). Whenever the patient is unable to recollect a cause for the onset of their symptoms, which clearly is common, the role of normal, everyday activities in precipitating the onset of symptoms should be considered.

The degree to which contemporary lifestyles are dominated by activities that involve flexion should thus be borne in mind; this may be sustained as in sitting or often-repeated motions such as bending. From the moment we wake and put on our socks, clean our teeth, go to the toilet, dry ourselves after a shower, sit down to eat breakfast, drive to work, sit at the desk, stoop over a bench or sit to eat lunch until the time in the evening when we 'relax' – either sitting on the sofa to watch television or play computer games, read or sew – we are in flexed postures of varying degrees. It would appear that these normal activities not only predispose people to back pain, but also can precipitate symptoms with no additional strain and can perpetuate problems once they arise (McKenzie 1981).

"Sitting is the most common posture in today's workplace, particularly in industry and business. Three-quarters of all workers in industrial countries have sedentary jobs" (Pope *et al.* 2000, p. 70). About 45% of employed Americans work in offices. Many display poor posture

and report increased pain when sitting, which is more severe the less they are able to change positions. Occupational back pain has long been associated with sedentary work, especially the seated vibration environment when driving (Pope *et al.* 2000). However, the vibration studies fail to discriminate between the effects of vibration and the effects of the sustained seated posture.

Individual and clinical prognostic factors

History of previous back pain is both a risk factor for future back pain and a prognostic factor for prolonged symptoms. Reported leg pain at onset is associated with poor outcomes and a greater likelihood of developing chronic symptoms (Goertz 1990; Lanier and Stockton 1988; Chavannes *et al.* 1986; Cherkin *et al.* 1996a; Carey *et al.* 2000; Thomas *et al.* 1999). Centralisation of leg pain, which is discussed elsewhere, has been shown to be a predictor of good outcomes (Donelson *et al.* 1990; Sufka *et al.* 1998; Long 1995; Werneke *et al.* 1999; Karas *et al.* 1997). The value of centralisation compared to other demographic and psychosocial variables has not been evaluated until recently. Inability to centralise the pain was found to be the strongest predictor of chronicity, compared with a range of psychosocial, clinical and demographic factors (Werneke and Hart 2000, 2001).

Biomechanical prognostic factors

As is seen from the assessment of risk factors, the physical variables that have been analysed do not explain a substantial amount of back pain onset, nor has the ergonomic approach brought dramatic benefits (Hadler 1997). However, once back pain has started, the same physical tasks become difficult and painful to do and will frequently affect symptoms. Even if the role of mechanical factors in onset is obscure, the ability of physical loading strategies to aggravate and relieve symptoms is quite pronounced.

Biomechanical factors are important both in the causation of an episode of back pain and in its perpetuation and aggravation (McKenzie 1972, 1981; Kramer 1990; Adams and Dolan 1995; Dolan 1998). The majority of spinal pain is seen as varying in intensity with the patient's activity and is *almost always aggravated by mechanical factors* (Spitzer *et al.* 1987). Indeed, this important report referred to *activity-related spinal disorders*, with the clear assumption of the importance of day-to-day activities and postures that influence patients' pain.

Various reports have investigated the role of physical loading strategies in symptom response – these highlight the effect that normal mechanical loads, such as sitting, walking or lying, have on aggravating or relieving symptoms (Table 2.2).

Table 2.2   Aggravating and relieving mechanical factors in those with back pain

	McKenzie 1979	Painting and Chester 1996	Biering-Sorensen 1983b	Boisson-nault and Di Fabio 1996	Stankovic and Johnell 1990
1. Aggravating					
Sitting	82%	83%	30%	74%	46%
Rising from sitting					39%
Bending		83%	65%	79%	46%
Driving				55%	
Sedentary		79%			
Walking	16%	48%			18%
Standing		37%	26%		24%
Sneezing or Coughing			22%		
Lying		61%		49%	7%
2. Relieving					
Sitting					7%
Rising from sitting					0%
Bending					2%
Walking	79%	41%	36%	38%	32%
Standing		45%			17%
Changing position / on the move		71%		53%	
Lying		32%	53%	70%	83%

These studies illustrate the mechanical sensitivity that back pain displays to different loading strategies. They reveal a range of different responses to the same loads – either worsening or improving symptoms, or having no effect. However, a common picture is of symptoms aggravated in positions involving flexion (sitting, rising from sitting, bending, driving) and improvement when walking, or being generally active, which are postures of extension. Alternatively, a smaller group of patients have their pain aggravated by standing and walking.

Common identified physical risk factors that predispose to back pain involve flexion – lifting, bending, driving and sitting; the precipitating event, however, is frequently trivial and unrelated. Once back pain has been initiated, postures involving flexion frequently perpetuate the problem and prevent resolution. This is not the only pattern of response to mechanical loading strategies, but clinically it is extremely common. Several clinical studies have demonstrated the value of avoiding flexion activities and postures (Williams *et al.* 1991; Snook *et al.* 1998; Snook 2000) – see Chapter 11 for detail.

"Controlling early morning lumbar flexion is a form of self-care that can help develop a sense of control or mastery over low back pain, and thereby build confidence and improve outcome" (Snook *et al.* 1998, p. 2606). McKenzie (1981) had previously identified the morning as a time when patients were frequently worse and at risk of suffering a relapse or exacerbation.

Psychosocial prognostic factors

While the evidence implicating psychosocial factors in the onset of back pain is limited, there is considerably more evidence relating these factors to the transition from acute to chronic back pain.

A cutting-edge review on fear–avoidance and its consequences concluded that pain-related fear and avoidance appear to be an essential feature in the development of a chronic problem for a substantial number of patients with musculoskeletal pain (Vlaeyen and Linton 2000).

A systematic review of psychological risk factors in back and neck pain concluded that these factors play a significant role in the transition to chronic problems and also may have a role in the aetiology of acute problems (Linton 2000a). Fuller conclusions based on the evidence from thirty-seven studies and supported by two or more good-quality prospective trials were as follows:

- psychosocial variables are clearly linked to the transition from acute to chronic pain and disability

- psychosocial factors are associated with reported onset of pain

- psychosocial variables generally have more impact than biomedical or biomechanical factors on disability

- cognitive factors (attitudes, cognitive style, fear–avoidance beliefs) are related to the development of pain and disability – especially passive coping, catastrophising, and fear–avoidance

- depression, anxiety and distress are related to pain and disability

- self-perceived poor health is related to chronic pain and disability

- psychosocial factors may be used as predictors of the risk of developing long-term pain and disability.

Emotional, cognitive and behavioural dimensions were specifically identified as being important in these studies; nonetheless, these factors only account for a proportion of the variance. Other factors are known to be important and psychosocial factors must be seen as part of a complex multidimensional view of musculoskeletal problems. Although it is tempting to conclude a causal relationship between these factors and the outcomes, this may be incorrect. The reciprocal nature of psychological factors and spinal pain has created a 'which came first, the chicken or the egg' dilemma – did the individual's depressive nature predispose them to back pain or did the persistent back pain produce depression? Nonetheless, efforts should be made to incorporate this information into clinical practice to enhance assessment and management (Linton 2000a).

All prognostic factors

Numerous factors have been associated with chronic back pain and failure to return to work. Generally these relate to three different aspects of a patient's presentation – clinical, psychological and social factors. Psychosocial factors that may have a role in the development of chronic musculoskeletal pain and disability are known as 'yellow flags'.

Table 2.3 lists the factors that have been associated with chronic back pain, disability or failure to return to work (Abenhaim *et al.* 1995; Klenerman *et al.* 1995; Gatchel *et al.* 1995; Philips *et al.* 1991; Burton *et al.* 1995; Cherkin *et al.* 1996a; Deyo and Diehl 1988a;

Hasenbring *et al.* 1994; Potter and Jones 1992; Potter *et al.* 2000; Goertz 1990; Hellsing *et al.* 1994; Williams *et al.* 1998b; Lanier and Stockton 1988; Pedersen 1981; Chavannes *et al.* 1986; Carey *et al.* 2000; Weiser and Cedraschi 1992; van der Giezen *et al.* 2000; Werneke and Hart 2000).

Table 2.3   Factors associated with chronic back pain and disability

Clinical factors	Psychological factors	Social factors
Leg pain	Fear–avoidance behaviour	Lower educational level
Nerve root pain	Depression	Lower income
Previous history of back pain	Anxiety about pain	Heavy manual work
Disc herniation	Passive coping strategies	Sitting occupation
Specific diagnosis	Catastrophising	Lack of alternative work duties to return to
Higher levels of reported pain and disability	Low self-efficacy beliefs External health locus of control beliefs	Low job satisfaction
Lack of centralisation	Poor general health Higher levels of reported pain and disability	Over-protective spouse

Factors that cause acute pain to become chronic are clearly complex, multiple and heterogeneous between individuals. The more sophisticated studies, which include a range of potential risk factors, suggest that chronic symptoms are predicted more by psychological than by clinical factors, or a combination of both (Burton *et al.* 1995; Klenerman *et al.* 1995; Gatchel *et al.* 1995; Deyo and Diehl 1988a; Hasenbring *et al.* 1994; Thomas *et al.* 1999). These studies suggest that chronic back pain disability and persistent symptoms are associated with a combination of clinical, psychological and social factors.

It is now widely accepted that psychological and social factors play a role in the maintenance of illness as pain moves from the acute to the chronic stage. It is further proposed that the patient-clinician relationship also has a role to play in the patient's recovery, with inappropriate advice or management preventing or prolonging recovery. Likely iatrogenic factors leading to disability include overemphasis on pain, and over-prescription of rest and time off work (Weiser and Cedraschi 1992). Failure to achieve centralisation has been highlighted as an important clinical prognostic factor that could be more significant than psychosocial ones (Werneke and Hart 2000, 2001).

Conclusions

This chapter has looked at some of the individual, biomechanical and psychosocial factors involved with precipitating and perpetuating episodes of back pain. One of the strongest risk factors for a future episode of back pain is a past history of back pain – such patients need education and information to reduce this risk. Biomechanical variables are risk factors in back pain onset, but also are notable in the perpetuation and aggravation of symptoms. Many of these relate to postures of flexion; the ubiquitous nature of this common posture has been noted.

There are some recent suggestions that psychological factors may predispose to back pain onset in a few individuals, and there is stronger evidence for the role of these factors in perpetuating episodes of back pain. Such factors may confound the effects of treatment. Management strategies need to recognise the possible existence of these 'yellow flags' and develop appropriate responses. The need for active patient involvement in management would appear to be paramount. A thorough explanation of the problem and how they can best manage it, reducing fears about movement, improving control and self-efficacy and avoiding passive interventions help this to happen. See Chapter 18 on patient management for a fuller description.

3: Pain and Connective Tissue Properties

Introduction

Pain is usually the prime concern of the patient, and so some means of understanding and interpreting pain is important. This chapter reviews certain aspects of pain that are relevant to the lumbar spine. The distinction between nociception and the pain experience is made; the most common sources of pain in the lumbar spine are identified; the differences between pain of somatic and neural origin, between local and referred pain, and also between pains initiated by mechanical or chemical mechanisms are made. The distinction between these two mechanisms of pain is an important determinant of the appropriateness of mechanical therapy (McKenzie 1981, 1990). In musculoskeletal problems a common cause of inflammation follows soft tissue trauma; the healing process of inflammation, repair and remodelling is also described. Some consideration is also given to chronic pain.

Sections in this chapter are as follows:

- nociception and pain

- sources of back pain and sciatica

- types of pain

- activation of nociceptors

- mechanical nociception

- chemical nociception

- trauma as a cause of pain

- distinguishing chemical and mechanical pain

- tissue repair process

- failure to remodel repair tissue

- chronic pain states.

Nociception and pain

The means by which information concerning tissue damage is experienced and transmitted to the cortex is termed *nociception*. This has several components (Bogduk 1993):

- the detection of tissue damage (transduction)

- the transmission of nociceptive information along peripheral nerves

- its transmission up the spinal cord

- modulation of the nociceptive signals.

The nerve endings that detect pain are not specialised receptors. Normally they are involved with other sensory functions, but as the stimulus becomes noxious, the graded response of the receptors crosses the threshold from normal mechanical or thermal sensation and triggers the nociceptive process (Bogduk 1993). After tissue damage is detected, this information is transmitted via the peripheral and central nervous system to the cortex; however, en route the nociceptive message is modulated. In this way the central nervous system can exert an inhibitory or excitatory influence on the nociceptive input (Henry 1989; Walsh 1991; Charman 1989). Given the current understanding of pain, the classical concept of pain being a straightforward reflection of specific tissue damage is outmoded (Waddell 1998). Especially with patients who have chronic pain, the factors that influence the clinical presentation are more than simple nociception.

Pain has been defined as *"an unpleasant sensory and emotional experience associated with actual or potential tissue damage, or described in terms of such damage"* (Merskey 1975). This much-quoted and widely accepted definition recognises that the experience of pain is a cortical phenomenon (Bogduk 1993; Adams 1997) and is influenced by affective and cognitive factors as well as sensory ones (Henry 1989; Johnson 1997; LaRocca 1992; Waddell 1998).

It is important to recognise that the experience of pain involves patients' emotional and cognitive reactions to the process of nociception. Patients' anxieties, fears and beliefs can strongly determine their response to injury, pain and treatment. Fear of pain and re-injury may lead to avoidance of activities that are believed will do more harm. It may lead patients to restrict their actions and movements and to withdraw from their normal lifestyle. An exaggerated fear of pain coupled with a hypervigilance to every minor discomfort can lead the patient into a perpetual circle of disuse, depression, disability and persistent pain (Vlaeyen and Linton 2000). Such lack of understanding of their condition causes inappropriate action in the face of pain and produces feelings of limited ability to control or affect the condition. Such avoidance in the long term will have a deleterious effect on the patient's recovery (Philips 1987).

We can start to address these factors by providing patients with a thorough understanding of their problem and educating them in the appropriate use of activity and exercise to regain function and reduce pain. Facilitating patients' control over their problem, encouraging active coping strategies and helping them confront their fear of pain should all be part of management (Klaber Moffett and Richardson 1995). Strategies based upon education and patient activity are important as a means of addressing patient responses to a painful condition as well as the condition itself.

Sources of back pain and sciatica

Any structure that has a nerve supply is capable of triggering the nociceptive process. This means that possible sources of pain around the lumbar region are the capsules of the zygapophyseal and sacro-iliac joints (SIJ), the outer part of the intervertebral discs, the interspinous and longitudinal ligaments, the vertebral bodies, the dura mater, nerve root sleeve, connective tissue of nerves, blood vessels of the spinal canal and local muscles (Bogduk 1994a, 1997; Butler 1991; Bernard 1997). The wide distribution of nociceptors around the lumbar spine makes it impossible to devise testing procedures that selectively stress individual components of the spinal segment.

An interesting insight into the most common sources of back pain and sciatica is provided by the progressive local anaesthetic studies performed by Kuslich et al. (1991) in patients undergoing surgery for decompression operations for disc herniations or spinal stenosis. In 193 consecutive patients who were awake or lightly sedated, each successive tissue was stimulated prior to anaesthetisation and incision and the area of provoked pain was recorded.

Table 3.1   Pain production on tissue stimulation in 193 patients in order of significance

Tissue	Number tested	Number and % some pain	Significant pain	Area of provoked pain
Always painful				
Compressed nerve root	167	166 (99%)	90%	Buttock, leg, foot
Often painful				
AF/PLL* – central	183	135 (74%)	15%	Central back
AF – lateral	144	102 (71%)	30%	Lateral back (buttock)
Vertebral endplate	109	67 (61%)	9%	Back
Dura – posterior				
Anterior	92	21 (23%)	6%	Buttock, leg
	64	15 (23%)	5%	Back, buttock
Rarely painful				
Facet capsule	192	57 (30%)	2.5%	Back (buttock)
Supraspinous ligament	193	49 (25%)	0%	Back
Interspinous ligament	157	10 (6%)	0.5%	Back
Muscle	193	80 (41%)	0%	Back
Never painful				
Fascia	193	32 (17%)	0.5%	Back
Spinous process	193	21 (11%)	0%	Back
Lamina	193	2 (1%)	0%	Back
Ligamentum flavum	167	0	0%	
Facet synovium	186	0	0%	
Nucleus pulposus	176	0	0%	

*AF/PLL = annulus fibrosus / posterior longitudinal ligament

Source: Kuslich *et al.* 1991

This study identifies compressed nerve roots as *the* source of significant leg pain, and the outer annulus fibrosus as *the* source of significant back pain, while all other anatomical sources of pain appear to be much less relevant. Normal nerve roots were rarely painful; it is only once the root has become compressed, stretched or swollen that pain was reproduced. The findings of this study accord with earlier work involving pain provocation studies around the time of surgery that identified the nerve root as the source of patients' limb pain and the intervertebral disc as the source of their spinal pain (Fernstrom 1960; Smyth and Wright 1958; Falconer *et al.* 1948; Wiberg 1949; Cloward 1959).

More recent studies have also shown the major role of the intervertebral disc as a cause of back pain (Schwarzer *et al.* 1995d), while other structures, such as the zygapophyseal and sacro-iliac joints, have a more limited aetiological significance (Schwarzer 1994b, 1995a).

Types of pain

One proposed pain classification system has suggested the following broad categories of pain (Woolf *et al.* 1998):

- transient pain, which is of brief duration and little consequence

- tissue injury pain

- nervous system injury pain.

Tissue injury pain relates to somatic structures, while nervous system injury pain includes neurogenic or radicular and pain generated within the central nervous system. The other source of pain that occasionally must be considered in the differential diagnosis is visceral pain from organs.

Table 3.2   Basic pain types

Pain type	Structures involved
Somatic pain	Musculoskeletal tissue
Radicular pain	Nerve root / dorsal root ganglion / dura
Central pain	Central nervous system
Visceral pain	Visceral organs

Somatic pain

Somatic structures include the intervertebral disc, posterior longitudinal ligament, SIJ, zygapophyseal joint capsule, etc. Only pain that originates from cutaneous tissue is felt localised to the area; all pain that stems from deep somatic structures is referred pain to a greater or lesser extent (Bogduk 1993, 1994a). The deeper the structure, the more difficult it is to localise the pain source – therefore most musculoskeletal pain is referred pain to a varying degree. The brain is simply aware of pain signals emanating from those structures that are supplied by a certain segment of the spinal cord. The mechanism for this is known as convergence. Neurons in the central nervous system receive afferents from structures in the lumbar spine and from the lower limb. The brain is unable to determine the true source of nociceptor signals from the shared neuron (Oliver and Middleditch 1991; Bogduk 1997). The pain is perceived deeply in the area appropriate to the deep segmental innervation of the body. This is more closely related to myotomes, the segmental innervation of muscles, than to dermatomes (Table 3.3).

Table 3.3   The segmental innervation of the lower limb musculature

Major muscle groups	Segmental innervation
Anterior	
Hip flexors / adductors	L2, 3, 4
Knee extensors	L3, 4
Foot and ankle extensors / invertors	L4, 5
Posterior	
Hip extensors / abductors	L4, 5, S1
Knee flexors	L5, S1
Foot and ankle flexors / evertors	L5, S1, 2

Source: Bogduk 1993

However, the segmental distribution of referred pain patterns should not be rigidly interpreted. There is considerable overlap between different segments in one individual, and considerable variation between individuals, so these areas should not be thought of as universally consistent locations. Furthermore, dorsal horn cells have the ability to increase their receptive field following injury, a mechanism by which the sensation of pain can spill over segmental boundaries (Gifford 1998).

Referred pain simply reflects the lack of localising information available with nociceptor activity from deep structures. The quality of somatic referred pain is deep and aching in quality, vague and hard to localise. The deeper the structure the more vaguely distributed and widespread is the pain (Bogduk 1993, 1994a). The stronger the noxious stimulus, the further the pain spreads down the limb (Kellgren 1939; Inman and Saunders 1947; Mooney and Robertson 1976).

Somatic pain can originate from any innervated tissues, but unfortunately it is impossible to localise the source of pain by the pattern of referred symptoms. Symptomatic intervertebral discs, zygapophyseal joints and SIJ are all capable of referral below the knee, but there are no clear distinguishing characteristics of the pain pattern or clinical features that are pathognomonic of any of these conditions (Schwarzer *et al.* 1994b, 1995a, 1995b; Dreyfuss *et al.* 1996).

Radicular pain

Radicular or neurogenic pain is produced when the nerve root or dorsal root ganglia are involved in symptom production. This is the product of pressure on nerve roots that are already inflamed or irritated, not on normal nerve roots. Although sudden onset of sciatica does occur, experimentally tension or pressure has only reproduced radicular pain on sensitised, not normal nerve roots (Smyth and Wright 1958; Kuslich *et al.* 1991).

It is different in quality from somatic pain, and is frequently associated with other abnormalities of nerve conduction such as weakness or numbness and abnormal tension tests (Bogduk 1994a; Cavanaugh 1995). Radicular pain is severe and shooting in quality, felt along a narrow strip, and thus different in quality from the vague, dull aching associated with somatic-referred pain. All nerve root pain will be felt in the leg, and it is always referred pain; often the leg pain will be worse than any back pain that may be present. However, all leg pain is *not* nerve root pain (Rankine *et al.* 1998). Radicular pain tends to be distributed in dermatomal patterns, with the L4, L5 and S1 nerve roots most commonly affected. Typically pain from L4 is felt down the anterior aspect of the thigh and leg, L5 is down the lateral aspect and S1 down the posterior aspect – however, variety exists, and pain patterns are not rigid.

Pain may be distributed anywhere in the dermatome in patches, or in a continuous line. The distal pain is often worse. Motor and sensory abnormalities are not always present; root tension signs are earlier and more common than signs of root compression (Waddell 1998). Signs and symptoms of root compression present as muscle weakness or wasting, absent or reduced reflexes and areas of paraesthesia, pins and needles or numbness. Sensory disturbance, when present, is found in the distal part of the dermatome – thus on the medial shin for L4, the great toe for L5 and the lateral border of the foot for S1.

Combined states

Referred pain is thus either somatic or radicular in origin. These two states may be combined in one individual (Bogduk 1994a). For instance, a patient may have back pain of somatic origin, from pressure of the annulus fibrosus, and leg pain of radicular origin, which is caused by involvement of the nerve root.

Central pain

Another form of neurogenic pain may arise from cells within the central nervous system, known as central pain. Classic examples of this are phantom limb pain, post-herpetic neuralgia and the pain from a brachial plexus lesion. There is growingngpeculation that in some musculoskeletal pains, especially chronic conditions, central mechanisms may be more important in the maintenance of symptoms than peripheral nociception (Bogduk 1993). Pain in this instance would be the result of abnormalities within the central nervous system.

A barrage of nociceptive input from a peripheral source, either somatic or radicular, can lead to sensitisation of central neurones. This is characterised by reduced thresholds and increased responses to afferent input, heightened responses to repeated stimuli, expansion of receptive fields and spontaneous generation of neuronal activity. Normal mechanical pressure can be interpreted as pain, and pain can be perceived without any appropriate peripheral input (Cavanaugh 1995; Gifford 1998; Johnson 1997; Siddall and Cousins 1997; Dubner 1991).

Visceral pain

Viscera may also refer pain – for example, renal pain may be felt in the loin and inguinal region, and cardiac pain in the arm (Bogduk 1993; Oliver and Middleditch 1991).

Activation of nociceptors

Only three mechanisms are known that can activate nociceptors – thermal, mechanical and chemical (Bogduk 1993; Zimmerman 1992; Cavanaugh 1995; Weinstein 1992). It is the latter two that are our concern here.

Mechanical nociception

Pain may be produced in the absence of actual tissue damage by excessive mechanical strain or tension upon collagen fibres. This is thought to be the result of the deformation of collagen networks so that nerve endings are squeezed between the collagen fibres with the excessive pressure perceived as pain (Bogduk 1993). No damage to the tissues need have occurred, and when the stress is removed the pain will abate. Mechanical pain can ensue from normal stresses upon weakened, damaged or abnormal tissues. If the excessive strain is so great as to produce actual tissue damage the inflammatory process will be provoked.

A simple example of mechanical articular pain is readily at hand. Bend your left forefinger backwards, using your right forefinger to apply overpressure. Keep applying this pressure until the nociceptive receptor system indicates its enhanced active state by the arrival of pain. This is simple mechanical deformation of pain sensitive structures. If you bend the finger backwards further, the intensity of the pain will increase; and if you maintain the painful position longer, the pain will become more diffuse, widespread and difficult to define. Thus, pain alters with increasing and prolonged mechanical deformation. If you now slowly return the finger to its normal resting position, the pain will disappear. This example has one significant implication: the finger is obviously being moved in one direction as the pain increases, and in another direction as the pain decreases.

Once the finger is returned to its normal position, the pain ceases. In this instance the sensation of pain does not depend on the existence of pathology. Mechanical forces sufficient to stress or deform local nociceptors produced the intermittent pain. The nociceptor system was activated by the application of mechanical pressure, and as soon as this was withdrawn, the nociceptors returned to their normal quiescent state. Intermittent low back pain can be caused in this same manner, by end-range mechanical stress. No chemical treatment will rectify or prevent pain arising from mechanical deformation. When intermittent mechanical pain is the main presenting symptom, drugs should never be the treatment of choice (McKenzie 1981).

"There are no drugs available that can inhibit the transduction of mechanical nociception. It is therefore futile to attempt to treat mechanical nociception with peripherally acting drugs. Mechanical transduction can only be treated by correcting the mechanical abnormality triggering nociception" (Bogduk 1993, p. 80).

Chemical nociception

In this situation pain is produced by the irritation of free nerve endings in the presence of certain chemicals, such as histamine, serotonin, hydrogen ions, substance p and bradykinin. These chemicals are released as a result of cell damage or by cells associated with the inflammatory process. Therefore, except in the case of inflammatory or infective diseases and certain degenerative conditions, chemical pain only occurs following trauma and actual tissue damage.

Trauma as a cause of pain

Pain due to trauma is produced by a combination of mechanical deformation and chemical irritation. Initially, mechanical deformation causes damage to soft tissues, and pain of mechanical origin will be felt. In most instances this is a sharp pain. Shortly after injury chemical substances accumulate in the damaged tissues. As soon as the concentration of these chemical irritants is sufficient to enhance the activity of the nociceptive receptor system in the surrounding tissues, pain will be felt.

In most instances pain of chemical origin will be experienced as a persistent discomfort or dull aching as long as the chemicals are present in sufficient quantities. In addition, the chemical irritants excite the nociceptive receptor system in such a way that the application of relatively minor stress causes increased pain that under normal circumstances would not occur. Thus, at this stage there is a constant pain, possibly a mild aching only, which may be enhanced but will never reduce or cease due to positioning or movement. As the concentration of chemical irritants falls below the critical threshold, this may be replaced by tenderness and increased sensitivity to mechanical stimulation, with intermittent pain with normal stress or periods of constant pain following excessive activity (Bogduk 1993; Saal 1995).

Distinguishing chemical and mechanical pain

As the cause of pain is an important determinant of the appropriateness of mechanical therapy, it is vital to distinguish between mechanical and chemical sources of nociception (McKenzie 1981, 1990). We can begin to distinguish between these types of pain by certain factors gained during the history-taking and largely confirm this impression during the physical examination. A key characteristic that indicates the possibility of pain of chemical origin is constant pain. Not all constant pain is inflammatory in nature, but chemical pain is always constant. The term *constant pain* indicates that the patient is *never* without an ache or discomfort from the moment they wake until the moment they fall asleep. The ache may be exacerbated by movements and be less at times, but the dull, relentless ache never goes away entirely. Constant pain may result from chemical or mechanical causes or be due to the changes associated with chronic pain.

Key factors in the identification of pain of an inflammatory nature:

* constant pain

* shortly after onset (traumatic or possibly insidious)

* cardinal signs may be present – swelling, redness, heat, tenderness

* lasting aggravation of pain by all repeated movement testing

* no movement found that reduces, abolishes or centralises pain.

Key factors in identifying constant pain of mechanical origin:

* certain repeated movements cause a lasting reduction, abolition or centralisation of pain

* movements in one direction worsens symptoms, whereas movements in the other direction improves them

* the mechanical presentation improves with the symptoms.

Intermittent pain is almost certainly mechanical in origin and is generally easier to treat than constant pain. During normal daily activities the patient is causing sufficient mechanical stresses to trigger nociceptive signals, which may persist after that activity has ceased. They may also be performing certain activities or sustaining certain postures that reduce mechanical deformation sufficiently to abolish their symptoms temporarily. This sensitivity to mechanical forces, in which different activities and postures both aggravate and reduce symptoms, is a notable characteristic of most back pain – consequently the terms *mechanical backache* (CSAG 1994) and *activity-related spinal disorders* (Spitzer *et al.* 1987).

Tissue repair process

Following tissue injury, the process that in principle leads to recovery is divided into three overlapping phases – inflammation, repair and remodelling (Evans 1980; Hardy 1989; Enwemeka 1989; Barlow and Willoughby 1992). *"No inflammation / no repair is a valid dictum"* (Carrico *et al.* 1984). In fact, each part of this process is essential to the structure of the final result. Connective tissue and muscle do not regenerate if damaged, but are replaced by inferior fibrous scar tissue (Evans 1980; Hardy 1989). To produce optimal repair tissue, all phases of this process need to be completed in the appropriate time.

Stages of Healing:

1. Inflammation

2. Tissue repair

3. Remodelling

Inflammation

In response to tissue damage, a host of inflammatory cells with specialist functions are released and attracted to the damaged area. There is increased local blood supply, leaking of plasma proteins and leukocytes from the blood vessels, and accumulation of white cells at the site of the injury (Enwemeka 1989; Evans 1980). These cells will be involved in the clearance of dead and dying cells and any foreign matter prior to the regrowth of new vascular channels and nerves into the damaged area. The cardinal signs of inflammation, heat, redness, pain, swelling and lack of function may be displayed (Evans 1980) and are a result of the inflammatory exudate. Swelling, heat and redness are products of the vascular activity; the pain results from the presence of noxious inflammatory chemicals and heightened mechanical sensitivity.

Just as tissue damage always causes inflammation, so inflammation always causes the tissues to become hypersensitive (Levine and Taiwo 1994). The inflammatory irritants sensitise the local pain receptor system and lower the thresholds at which the system is triggered, creating a state of 'peripheral sensitisation' (Cousins 1994; Woolf 1991). In this situation, the application of relatively minor mechanical stresses causes pain that under normal circumstances would not occur – allodynia; noxious stimuli create exaggerated responses – primary hyperalgesia; and there may be a spread of hyper-responsiveness to non-injured tissue – secondary hyperalgesia (Cousins 1994; Levine and Taiwo 1994). At this stage, there will be aching at rest, tenderness and exaggerated pain on touch and movement (Levine and Taiwo 1994). Movement can superimpose mechanical forces on an existing chemical pain and increase it, but it will never reduce or abolish chemical pain. This is significant in the differentiation between chemical and mechanical pain. Repeated movements will cause a lasting worsening of symptoms (McKenzie 1981).

Because of this heightened sensitivity, there is a lack of correlation between mechanical stimuli and the intensity of the pain response – it hurts much more than it should (Woolf 1991). When acute, this response is normal and it encourages protective, immobilising actions that are appropriate immediately after injury and during the inflammatory stage. Rest at this point has the important effect of reducing exudate and protecting the injured tissue from further damage. The same response at a later stage of the healing process does not serve any useful purpose, and is in fact detrimental. Only during the inflammatory period are rest and relative rest required; this must be followed by early mobilisation to optimise tissue healing. It is at this stage, however, when individuals learn the habit of avoiding activities because they hurt. If this habit is prolonged and individuals develop the habit of avoidance of painful movements, the repair process will be retarded, remodelling will not occur, normal function will not be restored and persistent symptoms are likely.

The aching will progressively lessen and healing and repair begin during the first seven to ten days after injury. Inflammatory cells, which are the source of chemically mediated pain, decrease in numbers until by the third week after injury none are present (Enwemeka 1989). *The patient will experience constant pain and tenderness until such time as the healing process has sufficiently reduced the concentration of noxious irritants.* The situation can occur during healing in which the level of chemicals falls below the threshold that triggers nociception, although tenderness would still be present. Normal mechanical loads may sufficiently irritate the tissues so as to re-trigger a constant chemical ache. Thus aching that abates, but is easily reproduced, represents an interface between mechanics and a resolving inflammatory state. If this is the case, tenderness should still be present. By two to three weeks, the constant pain due to chemical irritation should have abated and be replaced by a pain felt intermittently only when the repair itself is stressed.

In this initial stage a mesh of fibrin forms from the protein fibrinogen in the inflammatory exudate and seals the injury. During this time the application of ice, compression, elevation and gentle muscle movements are indicated to reduce the inflammatory exudate (Evans 1980). The greater the amount of exudate, the more fibrin will be formed and the more inextensible will be the repair. Ice, if applied in the first few days following injury, can reduce pain and oedema. Ice is of little value after the fifth day as the inflammatory cells are replaced by fibroblasts. These soon begin to lay down fibrils of collagen.

Tissue repair

The fibroplastic or repair stage commences as the acute inflammatory stage subsides and lasts about three weeks (Enwemeka 1989). It is during this phase that the collagen and glycosaminoglycans that will replace the dead and damaged tissue are laid down. There is cellular proliferation, which results in a rapid increase in the amount of collagen, and damaged nerve endings and capillaries 'sprout' and infiltrate the area (Cousins 1994). The cellular activity is stimulated by the physical stresses to the tissue. With inactivity, collagen turnover occurs and new collagen is made, but it is not oriented according to stress lines. At the end of this phase fibrous repair should be established, collagen mass is maximal, but the tensile strength of the new tissue is only 15% of normal (Hardy 1989).

To encourage good quality repair with collagen fibres oriented according to stress lines, gentle natural tension should be applied to recent injuries, commencing at about the fifth day (Evans 1980). Gentle tension applied early in the healing process promotes greater tensile strength in the long-term. From the first week a progressive increase in movement should be encouraged so that full range is possible by the third or fourth week. *It is within this period that appropriate education and movement provides the optimal climate for uncomplicated repair.* An experimental animal model showed that the application of stress during this repair phase was able to change the length of scar tissue and thus remodel it according to function. The same stresses applied to scar tissue that was three months old had little effect on its length (Arem and Madden 1976).

It should be noted, however, that at this stage if an over-enthusiastic approach to treatment is adopted the repair process can be delayed or disrupted, and the presence of inflammatory chemical irritants and exudate will be prolonged or re-stimulated. During this early stage of healing, movements should be just into stiffness and pain and entirely under the patient's control. Any discomfort provoked by the movement should abate as soon as the movement is released. If lasting pain is provoked, it is likely that re-injury has occurred, the inflammatory phase has been re-triggered and resolution of the problem will be further delayed.

Remodelling

Wound repair is only optimal if remodelling of the scar tissue occurs. This involves increases in strength and flexibility of the scar tissue through progressive increased normal usage and specific loading. Remodelling is the process of turning weak, immature and disorganised scar tissue into a functional structure able to perform normal tasks. The repair is unlikely to achieve the strength of the original tissue, but progressive loading and mechanical stimulation enhances the tensile strength and improves the quality of the repair. This occurs over several months after the original injury. Tensile strength is increased by stabilisation of the fibres through cross-linking, alignment of the fibres along the lines of stress and synthesis of type I collagen (Barlow and Willoughby 1992; Witte and Barbul 1997).

An animal model of healing following an induced rupture of a medial collateral ligament illustrates the role of scarring in tissue repair (Frank *et al.* 1983). All ligaments healed by scar tissue bridging the gap; this healing occurred quickly, with granulation tissue filling the rupture by ten days and signs of remodelling being noted after three weeks. Histologically collagen cross-links were significantly abnormal in the scar area, with increasing cross-links between ten days and six weeks, and return to normal values only seen at forty weeks. The scar started to contract three weeks after injury. At forty weeks scarring was still obvious to the naked eye; local hypertrophy and adhesions between the injury site and surrounding tissues were still present, but less than previously. Scar tissue was mechanically inferior to normal tissue, with lower failure properties, and persisting changes in quantitative and qualitative collagen and non-collagen matrix.

Several factors can operate to promote a less than optimal repair. The granulation tissue, which repaired the damage, can now act as glue to prevent movement between tissue interfaces. During the period when collagen turnover is accelerated, there is also increased molecular cross-linkage – these processes can produce adhesion formation and impair collagen gliding (Hunter 1994; Donatelli and

Owens-Burkhart 1981). Newly synthesised collagen will tend to contract after three weeks; this naturally occurring shrinkage is said to continue for at least six months (Evans 1980). Thus, recently formed scar tissue commences shortening unless it is repeatedly stretched. Provided the stretching process is commenced in the early stages following injury and continued well after full recovery, no soft tissue shortening is likely to develop. Low load regular application of stress also helps to increase the tensile strength of the repair tissue (Hardy 1989). Failure to perform the appropriate tissue loading will leave the repair process complete, but the remodelling stage incomplete – the individual may still be bothered by pain and limited function and the tissue weak and prone to re-injury. The nerves, which infiltrated the tissue during repair, can now be sourcas of pain each time the scar is stretched or loaded. This is a common cause of persistent symptoms in many patients.

The regular application of *intermittent* stress or loading to bone and normal soft tissue enhances structural integrity through the process of remodelling. During the healing process, loading for *prolonged* periods must be avoided as this may disrupt the repair process. *Prolonged stress damages, intermittent stress strengthens* (McKenzie 1981). Thus the proper rehabilitation of tissue damage involves progressive, incremental loading and activity to restore the structure to full function and to restore the patient's confidence to use it. This is the essential management strategy during the repair and remodelling stages.

In summary, no injury can be made to heal faster than its natural rate; whenever there has been tissue damage, the processes of inflammation, repair and remodelling have to occur to allow full restoration of normal function. *"Failure of any of these processes may result in inadequate or ineffectual repair leading to either chronic pathological changes in the tissue or to repeated structural failure"* (Barlow and Willoughby 1992). These processes are essentially the same in tendons, muscles, ligaments and all soft tissues; however, intrinsic factors may be more likely to impair the recovery process in tendon injuries, especially if the onset is through overuse rather than trauma (Barlow and Willoughby 1992). Early, progressive, active rehabilitation is essential to optimise repair and function. No passive modality used within physiotherapy has yet been shown to reduce the time for the completion of natural healing. We can avoid delay to the healing process and ensure that the climate for repair is favourable (Evans 1980). Strenuous mechanical therapy applied when the pain from the injury is essentially chemical will delay recovery. The integrity of the repair must be established before more vigorous procedures are applied. However, of equal importance is the use of a progressive, controlled programme of loading the tissues at the appropriate time during the repair process in order to promote a fully functional structure *that the patient is confident to use.*

Figure 3.1   Matching the stage of the condition to management

Week 1

Injury and   Protect from further damage.
Inflammation   Prevent excessive inflammatory exudate.
                        Reduce swelling.

Weeks 2–4

Repair and Healing   Gentle tension and loading without lasting pain.
                        Progressive return to normal loads and tension.

Week 5 onwards

Remodelling   Prevent contractures.
                        Normal loading and tension to increase strength
                        and flexibility.

Failure to remodel repair tissue

Following tissue damage, an important factor in the physiology of repair is the phenomenon of contracture of connective tissues. A characteristic of collagen repair is that it will contract over time. Recently formed scar tissue will always shorten unless it is repeatedly stretched, this contracture occurring from the third week to the sixth month after the beginning of the inflammation stage. Contracture of old scar tissue may in fact occur for years after the problem originated (Evans 1980; Hunter 1994). Cross-linkage between newly synthesised collagen fibres, at the time of repair, can act to prevent full movement. Nerve endings infiltrate this area during the repair process and thus can make the scar tissue a sensitised nodule of abnormal tissue (Cousins 1994).

In some patients contracture resulting from previous injury can now prevent the performance of full range of motion. These patients will have been unwilling to stretch the recent injury, perceiving the 'stretch' pain as denoting further damage, and they will not have received appropriate rehabilitation advice around the time of the injury. They will present later with restricted range of movement and pain provoked by stressing the scar tissue. The tissue will become progressively more sensitised and deconditioned for normal function with lack of use. A similar functional impairment may affect contractile tissues, and although this may restrict end-range flexibility, it is most commonly exposed with resisted movements that stress the muscle or tendon.

In such cases the remodelling of collagen by applying a long-term structured exercise programme will be necessary. By applying regular stress sufficient to provide tension without damage, collagen undergoes chemical and structural changes that allow elongation and strengthening of the affected tissue. Because tissue turnover is slow, one must recognise it may be a slow process. If the contracture has been present for some time, the remodelling programme will have to be followed for several months; Evans (1980) reports that some patients may have to exercise for the remaining years of their life. Applying tension to old injuries should be routinely practised, especially prior to participation in sporting activities (Hunter 1994). The animal experiment of Arem and Madden (1976) showed that 'old' scar tissue might be unresponsive to a remodelling programme. Well-established contractures, especially where the original healing process has been interrupted by repeated re-injury, causing the production of more inflammatory exudate, can be resistant to improvement.

Chronic pain states

Chronic pain is different in quality, as well as time, from acute pain. In the latter, biomechanical and biochemical factors may be the dominant influences on the pain experience and there is a more straightforward relationship between pain and nociception. With the passage of time, neurophysiological, psychological and social factors may come to dominate the maintenance of pain, and the link to the original tissue damage may become minimal (Waddell 1998; Adams 1997). The plasticity of the central nervous system following a barrage of peripheral input can cause pathological changes that maintain the pain state in the absence of peripheral pathology (Johnson 1997; Siddall and Cousins 1997). Psychological and behavioural attitudes and responses, as well as the process of nociception, shape individuals' experience of pain (Waddell 1998).

The acute and sub-acute model of tissue injury and healing described earlier is not an appropriate model for an understanding of chronic pain. If pain persists beyond the normal healing time, other factors can exist that complicate the picture (Johnson 1997). Persistent peripheral nociceptive input can induce changes in the central nervous system (Woolf 1991; Melzack 1988). This can lead to the sensitisation of neurones in the dorsal horn – a state characterised by reduced thresholds and increased responses to afferent input, such that normal mechanical stimuli is interpreted as pain. As well, there may be heightened responses to repeated stimuli, expansion of receptor fields, and spontaneous generation of neuronal activity (Johnson 1997; Siddall and Cousins 1997; Dubner 1991; Cousins 1994). This is known as *central sensitisation*.

Nociceptive signals can also be initiated in altered parts of the peripheral or central nervous system, which can produce the effect of localised 'phantom' pain in a part of the periphery where tissue damage no longer exists (Bogduk 1993). Pain can radiate to be felt in uninjured areas adjacent to the original problem (secondary hyperalgesia), normal movement can be painful (allodynia), repeated movements can exaggerate pain responses and pain signals can fire off without any appropriate stimulus (ectopic pain signals).

Psychosocial factors certainly have a role in peoples' response to a painful experience and can also be important in maintaining chronic pain (Bogduk 1993; Johnson 1997). Factors affecting pain responses are cultural, learned behaviour, meaning of pain, fear and anxiety, neurotocism, lack of control of events, passive coping style and focus on the pain (Cousins 1994). A recent systematic review of psychological risk factors in back and neck pain concluded that these factors play a significant role in the transition to chronic problems and can also have a role in the aetiology of acute problems (Linton 2000b). Psychosocial and cognitive factors are closely related to the development of chronic back disability. Depression, anxiety, passive coping and attitudes about pain are related to pain and disability. Catastrophising, hyper-vigilance about symptoms and fear–avoidance behaviour are attitudes and beliefs that have been highlighted as being particularly significant in this context. These psychosocial factors, which can have prognostic significance, are termed 'yellow flags'.

These psychological characteristics are thought to be key factors in the chronic pain experience. Chronic pain patients often feel little or no control over the pain, a helplessness that tends towards anxiety and depression, which in its turn can make people more concerned about symptoms (Adams 1997). The fear–avoidance model proposes that some individuals react to a pain experience by continued avoidance of any activity that they think might hurt, long after rest is of any therapeutic value, leading ultimately to disability and exaggerated pain behaviour (Lethem *et al.* 1983). The value of this model in predicting chronicity in back pain patients has been demonstrated (Klenerman *et al.* 1995; Waddell *et al.* 1993). It is proposed that this avoidance of pain is driven by a concept that pain equals further damage, leading the patient to further rest and avoidance of activity (Hill 1998).

There are thus neurophysiological and psychological reasons that are capable of maintaining painful states beyond the normal time-scale (Meyer *et al.* 1994; Cousins 1994). The patient with a chronic condition can not only be experiencing persistent pain, but also be distressed, inactive, deconditioned and have unhelpful beliefs about pain. They can be overly passive and reliant on others and possibly suffering economic and social deprivations due to the impact of the condition on their lifestyle (Nicholas 1996). The prevalence of this chronic pain syndrome is unknown; it possibly is a factor in those whose pain has persisted for months or years (Johnson 1997). Such a state may cloud the diagnostic and therapeutic usefulness of mechanically produced symptom responses (Zusman 1994). Therefore, there exist in some patients with chronic pain conditions various factors that can confound attempts to resolve the problem and can muddy the waters of diagnosis and symptom response.

Although these complicating factors can undermine treatment attempts, many patients with persistent symptoms will respond to mechanical therapy and a mechanical assessment should never be denied patients according to the duration of their symptoms. However, in patients with persistent symptoms there is a need to recognise the possible importance of non-mec`anical pain behaviour. This can involve peripheral sensitisation, central sensitisation or psychosocially mediated pain behaviour, or any combination of these factors, which will obscure or complicate any purely mechanical approach. The causes of chronic pain are different from the causes of acute pain. Although both problems can encourage reduction of normal activities and produce disability, in the acute stage this can be proportionate and appropriate whereas in the chronic stage this is inappropriate and irrelevant.

Clinicians' behaviour towards patients at all stages of a condition should guard against encouraging any passive responses to pain – especially so in the chronic patient. It is hardly surprising that patients get depressed, anxious, fearful and focussed on their persistent pain. Often health professionals seem unable to deal with it, some of whom imply it is primarily 'in their heads', as the pain is *"apparently discordant with discernible abnormalities"* (Awerbuch 1995). Maladaptive or inappropriate behaviour in the face of ongoing pain states does not represent malingering; it should be remembered that on the whole, the emotional disturbance is more likely to be a consequence of chronic pain rather than its cause (Gamsa 1990).

Although only a very small proportion of back pain patients develop chronic intractable pain (Waddell 1998), given the complexity of the pain experience, treatment in the acute stage should defend against chronic disability and in the chronic stage should be cognisant of psychological and behavioural dysfunction.

Conclusions

This chapter has considered aspects of pain that are relevant to a consideration of musculoskeletal pathology. It must be recognised that pain and nociception are different entities and that an individual's pain experience can be affected by cognitive, emotional or cultural as well as somatic factors. The multiplicity of factors that can affect the pain experience is especially relevant in chronic pain states when psychosocial and/or neurophysiological factors can dominate the patient's pain experience and militate against easy resolution of the problem.

In terms of pathology, the source of most back and radiating pain is one of the various innervated structures in or around the lumbar spine, with the intervertebral disc probably the most important. Less frequently, radicular pain is the product of nerve root involvement also. Nociceptors are activated by mechanical and/or chemical mechanisms, a differentiation between which is crucial in the use of mechanical diagnosis and therapy. An understanding of the stages of the repair process that follows tissue trauma is essential. When patients present with painful musculoskeletal problems, this can be due to different conditions in peripheral or central structures, with the pain maintained by different mechanisms (Table 3.4). Within several states a distinction can be made between pains of somatic or radicular origin.

Table 3.4   Pain-generating mechanisms

State of tissues	Pain mechanism
Normal	Abnormal stress – mechanical
Inflamed (acute)	Predominantly chemical – somatic and/or radicular
Healing (sub-acute)	Chemical / mechanical interface
Abnormal (contracted / scar tissue)	Mechanical – somatic and/or radicular
Abnormal (derangement)	Mechanical – somatic and/or radicular
Persisting hypersensitivity (chronic)	Peripheral / central sensitisation
Barriers to recovery (acute to chronic)	Psychosocial factors

An understanding of the different pain mechanisms that can pertain in different patients allows a broader perspective of the different factors that might need to be addressed in management.

4: The Intervertebral Disc

Introduction

This chapter presents aspects of anatomy and pathology that are relevant to an understanding of discogenic pain. It examines morphological changes that occur in the intervertebral disc and their relevance to back pain. This focuses chiefly on radial fissures through the annulus and disc herniations. The study of *biomechanics*, a term introduced by Breig (1961), is closely related to functional anatomy; it means the study of changes in anatomical structures occurring during movements of the body. Of most relevance to the concept presented here are the biomechanics of the intervertebral disc, the effects that abnormal morphology have on these biomechanics and the combined role that biomechanics and structural disruptions have in the creation of pathology.

The chapter is divided into the following sections:

- structural changes

- innervation

- mechanical or chemical pain

- diagnosing a painful disc

- the mobile disc

- discogenic pain

- radial fissures

- disc herniation

- stress profilometry.

Structural changes

As ageing occurs, the morphology of the intervertebral disc undergoes certain normal structural changes that make the disc more vulnerable to symptomatic pathology (Kramer 1990). Biochemical changes in the disc start early and continue throughout life – these changes involve the drying out of the disc, an increase in collagen and decrease in elastin. The net result is that the disc as a whole becomes more fibrous. Cells exhibiting necrosis increase; the distinction between the annulus fibrosus and the nucleus pulposus becomes blurred. The nucleus functions less efficiently at distributing radial pressure evenly to the annulus. In turn, the annulus fibrosus comes to bear increasing vertical loads. This has an effect on the structural integrity of the disc (Bogduk 1997). Distortion, disruption and fissuring occur in the layers of the annulus fibrosus. Three types of fissures (Figure 4.1) are commonly found in the annulus fibrosus (Hirsch and Schajowicz 1953; Yu *et al.* 1988a; Osti *et al.* 1992):

- transverse tears or rim lesions, with rupture of Sharpey's fibres in the periphery of the annulus near the ring apophysis, or in the outer wall of the annulus

- circumferential tears between the lamellae of the annulus

- radial fissures cutting across the layers of the annulus.

Figure 4.1   Commonly found fissures of the annulus fibrosus

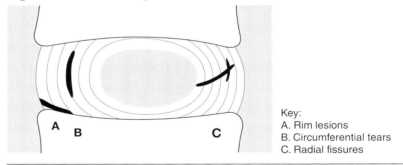

Key:
A. Rim lesions
B. Circumferential tears
C. Radial fissures

There is desiccation and loss of coherence in the nucleus pulposus (Yu *et al.* 1989). The homogenous structure of the disc may be disrupted as the nucleus becomes more fibrous, desiccated and disintegrated, and discrete fibrous lumps of nucleus or annulus may appear (Adams *et al.* 1986; Brinckmann and Porter 1994; Yu *et al.* 1988b; Kramer 1990). The degenerative changes are frequently visible in both parts of the disc together, with the drying out and disintegration of the nucleus pulposus often associated with radial fissures and disruption of the annulus fibrosus (Yu *et al.* 1989).

Much of this altered morphology, including quite gross changes in structure, will be asymptomatic as the inner two-thirds of the annulus fibrosus and the whole of the nucleus pulposus is without innervation.

Innervation

There is ample evidence going back many years that the intervertebral disc is innervated; this is reviewed by Bogduk (1994b, 1997). In general it has been found that the nucleus pulposus and the inner two-thirds of the annulus fibrosus are without nerve endings, which only exist in the outer third, or less, of the annulus. For instance, in samples obtained from patients undergoing back operations, receptors have been found in the outer half and the outer 3mm of the annulus (Yoshizawa *et al.* 1980; Ashton *et al.* 1994). Nerve endings are present in all aspects of the outer annulus, but not uniformly – nerve endings are found most frequently in the lateral region of the disc, a smaller number in the posterior region and the least number anteriorly (Bogduk 1997). Nerve endings are also found in the anterior and posterior longitudinal ligaments (Bogduk 1997).

There is evidence that in painful and degenerated discs the innervation can be much more extensive (Coppes *et al.* 1997; Freemont *et al.* 1997). In eight out of ten severely degenerated and painful discs, the innervation extended into the inner two-thirds of the annulus, and in two out of ten to the periphery of the nucleus pulposus (Coppes *et al.* 1997). Freemont *et al.* (1997) found considerable variety in the extent of innervation of the discs they studied, which were from patients with chronic back pain. Nerves extended into the inner third of the annulus in nearly half and into the nucleus pulposus in nearly a quarter.

Mechanical or chemical pain

It has been suggested that either mechanical or chemical mechanisms could initiate discogenic pain (Bogduk 1997). Plenty of evidence exists for mechanical disc problems; two possible means by which pain is produced are discussed below. These relate to radial fissures and internal disc derangements. In the presence of radial fissures, with or without a displacement, excessive mechanical stress would be placed upon the remaining intact portions of the annulus. The fissures would disrupt the normal even distribution of load-bearing on the annulus fibrosus and disproportionate loads would be borne by the residual, innervated outer lamellae. The stress peaks recorded by stress profilometry (see later section) could be examining the same phenomenon. Alternatively, internal displacements of discal material, whose position could be influenced by spinal postures, could exert pressure on the intact outer, innervated part of the annulus. Such displacements if unchecked could progress to full-blown disc herniations. In both instances pain is the result of excessive mechanical loads on weakened tissue.

An alternative model suggests a chemical rather than a mechanical mechanism of disc pain (Derby *et al.* 1999; Bogduk 1997). Chemical nociception may occur if nerve endings in the annulus are exposed to inflammatory cells. With severe back pain, patients' cells associated with chronic inflammation have been found in the anterior annulus (Jaffray and O'Brien 1986). It is proposed that chemical discogenic pain can be detected when concordant pain is provoked at very low pressures on discography (Derby *et al.* 1999). In seventy-eight chronic back pain patients undergoing discography and surgical fusion, a chemical mechanism detected in this way was believed to be responsible for symptoms in about half of the sample.

Pain from a nerve root may also be caused by mechanical or chemical mechanisms, or a combination (Garfin *et al.* 1995; Olmarker and Rydevik 1991; Rydevik *et al.* 1984). Disc herniations or stenosis may cause compression or tension leading to oedema, impairment of nutritional transport and subsequent intraneural damage and functional changes in nerve roots. This may result in inflammation of the nerve or produce nutritional compromise and ischaemia. In patients undergoing surgery for disc herniations, inflammatory cells have been harvested from around the nerve root (Gronblad *et al.* 1994; Spiliopoulou *et al.* 1994; Doita *et al.* 1996; Takahashi *et al.* 1996). Experiments using animal models have indicated the inflammatory effect of nucleus pulposus beyond the annular wall (McCarron *et al.* 1987; Olmarker *et al.* 1993).

However, the presence of inflammatory cells is variable. In patients investigated at surgery, such cells were found abundantly in about 60 – 70% of individuals (Gronblad *et al.* 1994; Doita *et al.* 1996) and a complete absence of inflammatory cells at surgery has also been noted (Cooper *et al.* 1995). Furthermore, animal experiments using only mechanical factors have been shown to produce histological and physiological abnormalities consistent with radicular pain following compression of the nerve root and dorsal root ganglion (Howe *et al.* 1977; Triano and Luttges 1982; Rydevik *et al.* 1989; Hanai *et al.* 1996; Yoshizawa *et al.* 1995), the dorsal root ganglion being especially sensitive to abnormal loads, which rapidly induce heightened mechanical sensitivity.

Another mechanism that may explain whether radicular pain is mechanical or chemical in origin relates to the type of disc herniation. One study found some inflammatory cells were present in up to 50% of patients with sequestrations. In patients with extrusions and protrusions, about 30% and 25%, respectively, had some inflammatory cells (Virri *et al.* 2001). Inflammatory cells were also more common when a positive straight leg raise was present, especially if bilaterally positive.

The literature would thus suggest that either mechanical or chemical mechanisms might be the source of patients' symptoms. The prevalence of each at present is unknown. These different mechanisms will respond differently to therapeutic loading strategies. An appropriate mechanical evaluation in the presence of a mechanical problem should generate a favourable response, while in the presence of a chemically maintained problem symptomatic response will be unfavourable.

Diagnosing a painful disc

It is not entirely clear why discs become painful; there are several models that have been used to describe the cause of internal disc pain (Bogduk 1997; Kramer 1990; McNally *et al.* 1996; Crock 1970, 1986). One of the key confounding factors in the debate about the cause of back pain is the existence of morphological abnormality in asymptomatic populations.

A systematic review of studies about radiographs and back pain concluded that although radiographic findings indicating disc degeneration are associated with back pain, this does not indicate a causal relationship (van Tulder *et al.* 1997c). More detailed imaging studies with magnetic resonance imaging (MRI), found 'abnormal discs' (bulging or herniated) in 20 – 76% of asymptomatic populations that were studied (Boden *et al.* 1990; Jensen *et al.* 1994; Weinreb *et al.* 1989; Boos *et al.* 1995). Patterns of disc disruption, including fissures and herniations, have been seen as commonly in volunteers as in patients with back pain (Buirski and Silberstein 1993). In a particularly thorough study, in which patients with sciatica were matched with volunteers without back pain by age, sex and physical risk factor, 76% of those with no symptoms had a disc herniation and 22% had one that involved the nerve root (Boos *et al.* 1995). However, the proportion of patients with symptoms who had nerve root compression was significantly greater – this was 83%.

In fact, MRI is often not particularly good at determining what is a painful disc when compared to invasive methods such as discography. This actually seeks to reproduce the patient's pain by injecting into the disc (Horton and Daftari 1992; Brightbill *et al.* 1994; Ricketson *et al.* 1996; Simmons *et al.* 1991). Discography involves physical stimulation of the disc through needle placement, which is correlated with morphological abnormalities and pain response (Sachs *et al.* 1987). In volunteers without back pain, discography is not particularly painful (Walsh *et al.* 1990). It has been an essential tool in revealing the significance of radial fissures in the annulus fibrosus as a cause of chronic back pain (Vanharanta *et al.* 1987; Moneta *et al.* 1994). However, extensive radial fissures, which are strongly associated with back pain, are also found not to be a cause of pain in some individuals and at some segmental levels (Smith *et al.* 1998).

Despite continuing controversy, discography is still seen by many authorities to be the only certain way of identifying symptomatic discogenic pain as long as stimulation of a control disc at an adjacent level does not reproduce their pain (Bogduk 1997; Schwarzer *et al.* 1995d).

The study by Donelson *et al.* (1997) has shown the reliability of a mechanical assessment of patients' pain response to predict the presence of discogenic pain and the competency of the annular wall. The assessment process was superior to MRI scanning in distinguishing painful from non-painful discs – this study is described in more detail later.

The mobile disc

Asymmetrical loading of the disc tends to displace the nucleus pulposus to the area of least pressure (McKenzie 1981; Kramer 1990; Bogduk 1997). Thus the anterior compression caused by flexion 'squeezes' the nucleus backwards, and conversely extension forces it forwards. This effect has been confirmed in cadaveric experiments (Shah *et al.* 1978; Krag *et al.* 1987; Shepperd *et al.* 1990; Shepperd

1995) and in living subjects using various imaging techniques (Schnebel *et al.* 1988; Beattie *et al.* 1994; Fennell *et al.* 1996; Brault *et al.* 1997; Edmondston *et al.* 2000). All these studies have shown a posterior displacement of the nucleus pulposus with flexion and an anterior displacement accompanying extension of the lumbar spine. In vivo experiments have been almost entirely conducted in asymptomatic volunteers. In the one attempt to study nuclear movement in a symptomatic population, pain changes were not found to correlate with movement of the nucleus (Vanharanta *et al.* 1988). It would seem that movement of the nucleus becomes less predictable when the disc becomes more degenerated (Schnebel *et al.* 1988; Beattie *et al.* 1994).

Based on experimental work carried out by his team, and clinical experience, Kramer (1990) has written in some detail about the mobile disc. Displacement occurs most rapidly in the first three minutes of asymmetrical loading, but will continue for several hours at a slower rate if the asymmetrical compression is maintained. Because of the more fibrous nature of the nucleus pulposus with advancing age, it is displaced less easily in older individuals. The nucleus pulposus that has been displaced by asymmetrical loading returns to its original position once the loading is released. If the loading on the disc is sustained, the displaced nucleus has a tendency to remain in its abnormal position, but its return can be facilitated by *compression in the other direction*.

"Postures of the spine which result in decentralization of the nucleus pulposus due to asymmetrical loading of the intervertebral segment play an important role in the pathogenesis and in the prophylaxis of intervertebral disc diseases" (Kramer 1990, p. 29).

There may come a point when the natural resilience of the disc to recover from asymmetrical loading is undermined by structural changes within the disc. *"The intervertebral disc becomes vulnerable when tears and attritional changes cause the annulus fibrosus to lose its elasticity and allow the central gel-like tissue of the nucleus pulposus to be displaced beyond its physiological limits"* (Kramer 1990, p. 29).

If the internal architecture of the disc is intact, displacement is soon reversed on returning to a symmetrical posture. However, the changes that occur during ageing make the disc more vulnerable to symptomatic pathology (Kramer 1990). In the presence of radial fissures, displacements can exert pressure on the outer annulus, which is innervated. As long as this holds, the displacement can be reversed, but if it weakens sufficiently or ruptures, the displacement herniates through the outer annulus. An intact hydrostatic mechanism in the disc is thus essential to influence any displaced tissue. If the outer annular wall is intact, the hydrostatic mechanism is also intact and displaced tissue can be affected by loading. However, once the outer wall is ruptured or so attenuated as to be incompetent, then movements and positions will have no lasting effect on displaced discal tissue.

Discogenic pain

As an innervated structure, the intervertebral disc is capable of being a source of pain in its own right. Studies involving discography have shown that internal disc disruption, with intact outer annular walls and no mass effect beyond the disc wall, can be a painful entity (Bernard 1990; Park *et al.* 1979; Milette *et al.* 1995, 1999; McFadden 1988; Schellhas *et al.* 1996; Grubb *et al.* 1987; Horton and Daftari 1992; Fernstrom 1960; Wiley *et al.* 1968; Wetzel *et al.* 1994; Colhoun *et al.* 1988; Ohnmeiss *et al.* 1997). These studies show that discogenic pain, without nerve root involvement, can be the cause of back and leg pain.

Direct stimulation of the disc carried out during surgical procedures also demonstrates the entity of discogenic pain (Wiberg 1949; Kuslich *et al.* 1991; Smyth and Wright 1958). In these studies, back pain only was produced; sciatic leg pain could only be reproduced by stimulation of swollen, stretched or compressed nerves. Buttock pain was reproduced, with difficulty, on simultaneous stimulation of the nerve root and annulus (Kuslich *et al.* 1991). However, other studies involving mechanical stimulation of discs have been able to reproduce leg pain (Fernstrom 1960; Murphey 1968), although only in a minority (Fernstrom 1960).

The site of the referred pain depended on the site where the annulus was being stimulated. The central annulus and posterior longitudinal ligament produced central back pain, while stimulation off centre produced lateral pain to the side being stimulated (Kuslich *et al.* 1991). Cloward (1959) found the same direct correlation between the site of stimulus and the site of referred pain, central or lateral, in his experiments with cervical disc patients. Murphey (1968) found that on stimulation of the lateral part of the disc, patients reported leg pain.

Kuslich *et al.* (1991) found considerable variability in the sensitivity of the annulus. Although they were unable to explain why, they suggested this could be the result of differing innervation or levels of chemical irritants. One-third of patients were exquisitely tender upon stimulation of the annulus, one-third were moderately tender and one-third were insensitive. Various other tissues were stimulated in this study involving 193 sedated but awake patients, from which the authors concluded that the intervertebral disc is *the* cause of back pain (see Table 3.1 for more detail). Fernstrom (1960), also found disc sensitivity to be variable with just over half of 193 discs responding painfully to pressure. A possible cause of this symptomatic variability is the inconsistency that is present relative to the extent and presence of innervation in the disc.

Radial fissures

When discography is combined with computerised axial tomography (CAT) scans, it permits four separate categories of information (Sachs *et al.* 1987). These relate to generalised degeneration, annular disruption, pain response (pressure sensation, dissimilar pain, similar pain or exact reproduction of pain), volume of contrast medium injected into the disc and other comments. The extent of fissures in the annulus is gauged from the spread of the contrast medium, which is assessed by CAT scans. Originally four grades of ruptures or fissuring were listed (Sachs *et al.* 1987); later authors have suggested additions (Table 4.1, Figure 4.2).

Table 4.1 Grading of radial fissures in annulus fibrosus

Grade	Description	Pain status
0	None	No
1	Into inner annulus	No
2	Into outer annulus	Yes / No
3	To outer annulus	Yes / No
4	3 + circumferential spread between lamellae in both directions (Aprill and Bogduk 1992)	Yes / No
5	Complete tear with leakage beyond annulus (Schellhas *et al.* 1996)	Yes / No

Some discrepancy exists over the definition of grade 3 fissures. Some authors state that this is when the annular disruption extends *beyond* the outer annulus (Sachs *et al.* 1987; Ninomiya and Muro 1992), while others believe that this is a radial fissure that extends *into* the outer annulus (Schellhas *et al.* 1996; Aprill and Bogduk 1992).

Figure 4.2   Grades of radial fissures according to discography

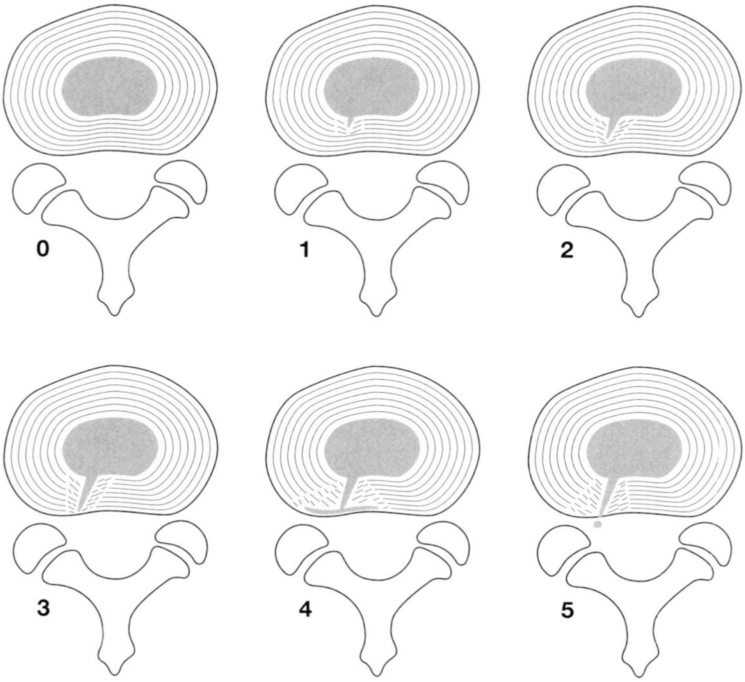

Key:
0. None
1. Inner annulus
2. Outer annulus
3. To outer annulus

It is the presence of radial fissures into the outer third of the annulus that are most closely associated with painful discs, rather than general degeneration of the disc (Vanharanta *et al.* 1987; Moneta *et al.* 1994). Although the higher grade radial tears are found in asymptomatic individuals, the correlation between grade 3 and 4 fissures and back pain is very strong, and these are commonly found in chronic back pain populations that receive invasive imaging (Vanharanta *et al.* 1987; Moneta *et al.* 1997; Aprill and Bogduk 1992; Smith *et al.* 1998; Ricketson *et al.* 1996; Milette *et al.* 1999; Ohnmeiss *et al.* 1997). Indeed, so strong is the association between grade 3/4 fissures and exact reproduction of patient's pain that *"no other demonstrable morphological abnormality has been shown to correlate so well with back pain"* (Bogduk 1997, p. 205).

The studies of Milette *et al.* (1999) and Ohnmeiss *et al.* (1997) make clear that grade 2 radial fissures are as potent a source of symptoms as grade 3 fissures and even protrusions. In one sample of patients with chronic back and leg pain, the presence of radial fissures into the outer annulus was shown to be a more important predictor of symptomatic discs than the outer contour of the annular wall; that is, disc bulges and protrusions (Milette *et al.* 1999).

Grade 4 radial fissures with circumferential spread of contrast medium are strongly correlated with an MRI feature known as a *high-intensity zone* (HIZ). This was recognised by Aprill and Bogduk (1992) who, along with others (Schellhas *et al.* 1996), found it highly predictive of painful discs. However, other authors have found it to be a poor predictor of painful discs (Ricketson *et al.* 1996; Smith *et al.* 1998). It is suggested that the HIZ represent an irritated or inflamed outer annular fissure, which is different from a disc herniation (Aprill and Bogduk 1992; Schellhas *et al.* 1996).

Disc herniation

Although radial fissures can be a source of pain in their own right, the fissure may also act as a conduit for displaced discal material (Porter 1993; Bogduk 1997). These displacements are termed disc herniations.

Definitions

There has been a lack of standardisation of terminology used to describe disc herniations, and synonyms are many and varied. There have been recent attempts to standardise the nomenclature and classification of lumbar disc pathology (Milette 1997; Fardon *et al.* 2001). This distinguishes annular fissures, herniations and degenerative changes, as well as disc infections and neoplasia. Different types of herniation are further delineated as protrusion, extrusion and sequestration, and intravertebral, when aspects of size, containment, continuity and location are considered. In relation to mechanical therapy, a key consideration is the state of containment – when *contained* the outer annular wall is intact, when *non-contained* disc material is displaced beyond the annular covering.

Kramer (1990) distinguishes four stages of discal displacement (Figure 4.3):

- intradiscal mass displacement – non-physiological displacement of tissue within the disc

- protrusion – the displaced material causes a bulge in the intact wall of the annulus

- extrusion – the disc material is displaced through the ruptured annular wall

- sequestration – a discrete fragment of disc material is forced through the ruptured annular wall into the spinal canal.

Figure 4.3   Four stages of disc herniations – in reality there will be many sub-stages

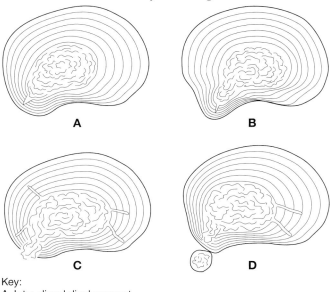

Key:
A. Intra-discal displacement
B. Protrusion
C. Extrusion
D. Sequestration

In this text the term *disc herniation* is used as a non-specific term that includes any of the more specific terms that carry with them clear-cut pathological and prognostic meaning (Table 4.2). If the hydrostatic mechanism is intact and the herniation is contained, then forces exerted on it can affect a displacement – it is reducible. If the hydrostatic mechanism is no longer intact, the outer wall is breached or incompetent and the herniation is non-contained, then the displacement cannot be affected by forces – the displacement is now irreducible.

Table 4.2   Disc herniations: terms and pathology used in this text

Term	Pathology	Hydrostatic mechanism
Herniation	Non-specific term including any of below	Non-specific term
Protrusion	Intact and competent annular wall	Intact
Protrusion	Intact annular wall, but so attenuated as to be incompetent	Not intact
Extrusion	Annular wall breached by intra-discal mass that protrudes through, but remains in contact with disc	Not intact
Sequestration	Annular wall breached by intra-discal mass that has separated from disc	Not intact

Routes and sites of herniations

The majority of fissures and herniations occur posteriorly or postero-laterally, the direction that causes greater symptoms, as displacement beyond the annular wall can involve the nerve root. A smaller proportion of herniations are directly lateral or anterior, and some go in a cephalic or caudad direction into the endplate of the vertebral body above or below. Lateral or far-lateral herniations may also involve the nerve root, as these can extrude into or lateral to the intervertebral foramen. The clinical importance of anterior and vertebral herniations, or Schmorl's nodes, is less well established.

An understanding of the pathogenesis of displacements can suggest movements and positions that could be utilised in their treatment. Some studies (Bernard 1990; Fries et al. 1982; Maezawa and Muro 1992; Ninomiya and Muro 1992; Fuchioka et al. 1993) have described the routes of displacements or existing fissures and the final point of herniation (see Table 4.3 and Figure 4.4). The findings from these different studies, involving over 2,000 patients who were surgical candidates, are striking in their similarities. Because they were so similar, and for simplicity, the mean from the four studies is shown.

Table 4.3   Herniation routes/fissures and sites of final herniation*

Site	Fissures	Protrusions	Extrusions
Central	57%	28%	14%
Postero-lateral	20%	59%	79%
Far lateral	11%	8%	4%
Multiple	19%	9%	

* % shown = mean from four studies with over 2,000 patients

Source: calculated from original data in Bernard 1990; Fries et al. 1982; Maezawa and Muro 1992; Ninomiya and Muro 1992; Fuchioka et al. 1993

Over half of all displacements and fissures appear to start centrally in the disc, while about a quarter start postero-laterally. However, well over half end up herniating postero-laterally on the dura and/or nerve root, with another quarter herniating centrally. The majority of all displacements thus occur in the sagittal plane, implicating flexion/extension movements both in their pathogenesis and treatment (Ninomiya and Muro 1992). Less than 10% of all displacements commence and herniate far laterally into, or lateral to, the intervertebral foramen. These run obliquely to the sagittal plane and implicate torsional or lateral forces both in their pathogenesis and their treatment. Herniation routes, however, do not follow straight lines and on occasion underwent complex twists and turns, even crossing the mid-line.

Figure 4.4   Routes and extrusion points of herniations
(see Table 4.2 for detail and references)

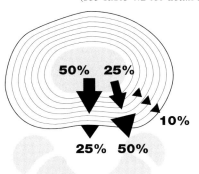

The prevalence of lateral disc herniations, known as extreme or far lateral, varies from 6% to 12% of all surgically treated herniations in different studies (Abdullah *et al.* 1988; Kunogi and Hasue 1991; Jackson and Glah 1987; Patrick 1975; O'Hara and Marshall 1997; Postacchini *et al.* 1998). These tend to occur at slightly higher segmental levels than the more common postero-lateral herniation, about 75% occurring at L3 – L4 and L4 – L5, and nearly 10% occurring at L2 – L3. This compares with 98% of postero-lateral herniations occurring at L4 – L5 and L5 – S1.

Postero-lateral herniations involve the descending nerve root, which is situated nearer the mid-line. Far lateral disc herniations affect the nerve root exiting at that segmental level, which is the nerve above. Thus, an L4 – L5 lateral herniation would affect the L4 nerve, while a postero-lateral herniation would affect the L5 nerve root (see Figure 4.5). Therefore, lateral herniations are more likely to be involved when signs and symptoms point to upper lumbar nerve root compression (Abdullah *et al.* 1988).

Figure 4.5   At L4 – L5, a lateral disc herniation (left) affects the exiting nerve root (L4); a postero-lateral disc herniation (right) affects the descending nerve root (L5)

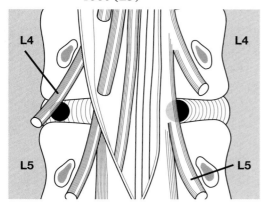

Reports of anterior herniations are much less frequent, but do appear in the literature as case reports and MRI studies (Buirski 1992; Jinkins *et al.* 1989; Brooks *et al.* 1983; Cloward 1952). Jinkins *et al.* (1989), in a retrospective review of 250 MRI examinations, listed the directional differentiation of disc extrusions, the clinical significance of which is unproven (see table). Just as posterior herniations are frequently found in asymptomatic populations (Boden *et al.* 1990; Jensen *et al.* 1994; Weinreb *et al.* 1989; Boos *et al.* 1995), it is likely that anterior and vertebral herniations are also frequently incidental findings of unknown clinical significance.

Table 4.4   Directional differentiation of disc extrusions on MRI

Type of extrusion	*Proportion*
Posterior/ Postero-lateral	57%
Anterior	29%
Vertebral	14%

Source: Jinkins *et al.* 1989

Of the anterior herniations, about half were in the mid-line and the rest were antero-lateral or directly lateral. Both anterior and vertebral herniations were much more common at upper lumbar levels (L1 – L2 to L3 – L4). Anterior and vertebral disc herniations are reported to cause back and diffuse non-specific limb pain, and non-specific paraesthesia (Jinkins *et al.* 1989; Cloward 1952; Brooks *et al.* 1983). Straight leg raise and neurological examination are negative.

Intravertebral disc herniation, also known as Schmorl's nodes, can be an asymptomatic and incidental finding (Bogduk 1997). They have been reported with varying frequencies in several studies of cadaveric spines with greater occurrence in the thoracic and upper lumbar spines (Resnick and Niwayama 1978; Hilton *et al.* 1976). The incidence of Schmorl's nodes in back pain patients in one study was found to be 19% compared to 9% in a control group, with a particularly high incidence in those between 10 and 40 years old (Hamanishi *et al.* 1994). Cadaveric experimental studies have shown that endplate damage can unleash a chain of disc degeneration affecting the whole disc (Adams *et al.* 2000b). The damage leads to reduced pressure in the nucleus pulposus and increased peaks of compressive stress in the annulus fibrosus. Buckling and fissuring of the annulus and displacement of the nucleus can follow. An increased density of sensory nerve endings has been found in the endplates of patients with severe back pain and disc degeneration (Brown *et al.* 1997).

Schmorl's nodes are reported to occur acutely with significant trauma such as motorcycle accidents and falls, particularly in adolescents and young adults, and can be associated with severe back pain and significant disability (McCall *et al.* 1985; Fahey *et al.* 1998). One study using discography noted leakage of contrast material into the vertebral body in fourteen of 692 discs injected (Hsu *et al.* 1988). Pain on injection was concordant with the patient's pain and severe or moderately severe in thirteen of the fourteen (93%), compared to 42% in the remaining discs. This statistically significant difference suggests that endplate disruptions can be a source of symptoms.

In summary, the primary source of symptomatic disc herniations is posterior or postero-lateral. Postero-lateral and the much less common lateral disc herniations are the cause of radicular pain. However, anterior or antero-lateral herniations may also be a more unusual cause of symptoms. The role of intravertebral disc herniations or Schorl's nodes in symptom production is less well established, but they appear capable of producing back pain and possibly unleashing a degenerative process leading to degradation of the whole disc (Bogduk 1997).

Herniated material

When discs do actually herniate, there is no consensus about the material that is involved in this pathological process. Histological analysis of disc herniations from different studies shows that extrusions can consist predominantly of nucleus pulposus, endplate or annulus fibrosus (Brock *et al.* 1992; Yasuma *et al.* 1986, 1990; Gronblad *et al.* 1994). Combinations of the different material are also found – although 34% of extrusions in one study were nucleus only, the rest were mixtures of nucleus, annulus and endplate (Moore *et al.* 1996). Harada and Nakahara (1989) also found combinations of the three different tissues, and occasionally bone, in their samples, with fragments of annulus or annulus and endplate being the most common finding. Takahashi *et al.* (1996) suggested that most of the herniated material was nucleus and/or annulus, but that distinguishing between the two was difficult. It is suggested that herniations comprising predominantly nucleus pulposus are common in younger patients, whereas in older patients the extruded material is more likely to be annular and endplate (Yasuma *et al.* 1986, 1990; Harada and Nakahara 1989). Clearly the herniated material is variable.

Stress profilometry

In this procedure a stress transducer is drawn through the disc, monitoring the vertical and horizontal stress profiles through the whole disc. It was developed and tested on cadavers, which revealed distinct patterns of stress associated with degenerative changes (McNally and Adams 1992; McNally *et al.* 1993; Adams *et al.* 1996a, 1996b). Comparing degenerated to non-degenerated discs, there is a 50% reduction in the diameter of the 'functional nucleus' and a 30% fall in its pressure. This is accompanied by an 80% increase in the width of the 'functional annulus', and an increase of 160% in compression 'stress peaks' in the annulus (Adams *et al.* 1996a). In degenerated discs, greater loads fall on the annulus.

These measurements reveal the increased stresses that fall on the annulus fibrosus as a consequence of the degenerative changes that affect the nucleus. These stresses were most marked at lower lumbar levels and in the posterior annulus. Stress peaks in the posterior annulus were exaggerated after creep loading (Adams *et al.* 1996b) and may predispose to annular failure or disc prolapse (McNally *et al.* 1993). High peaks of compressive stress may predispose to further damage and may elicit pain from innervated parts of the annulus or from the vertebral endplates (Adams *et al.* 1996a). It is suggested that multiple stress peaks may represent an early painful stage of disc pathology, when the annulus is failing, but still functioning (Adams *et al.* 1996a). This is consistent with the concept of discogenic pain from grade 2 annular fissures.

Stress peaks also vary according to the posture of the motion segment being tested. In 'degenerated discs' exposed to extension, there was a generalised increase in stress peaks in the posterior annulus, while flexion tended to equalise the compressive stress. However, in seven of the nineteen motion segments tested, lumbar extension decreased maximum compressive stress in the posterior annulus by a considerable amount (Adams *et al.* 2000a).

McNally *et al.* (1996) investigated stress profilometry and discography in a small group of patients. Patterns of stress distribution varied widely between discs, but anomalous loading of the posterolateral annulus was highly predictive of a painful disc. Discogenic pain was most associated with single and multiple stress peaks in the annulus, broadening of the 'functional annulus' and depressurisation of the nucleus.

Conclusions

In summary, the intervertebral disc is a common source of pain in its own right. It undergoes certain morphological changes that make it susceptible to becoming symptomatic. Considerable degeneration of an asymptomatic nature can occur. It has nerve endings in its outer layers, and in the diseased state this innervation can be much deeper in the disc. Even radial fissures and disc herniations can be found in asymptomatic populations, but these findings are frequently symptomatic. By direct stimulation at surgery and by exerting pressure with injection using discography, patients' familiar back and leg pain has been reproduced.

The structural abnormality that appears most closely linked to discogenic pain is the radial fissure. Numerous studies have shown that it is this particular disruption of the outer lamellae of the annulus that correlates closest with painful discs. Indeed, no other morphological abnormality is so clearly associated with back pain. Pain may be the result of excessive mechanical loads on innervated, weakened tissue. Alternatively, the fissure may act as a conduit for displaced tissue, which is affected by positions and movements.

Additionally, but much less commonly, the disc can be a source of radicular pain by causing tension or compression of lumbar nerve roots. In this pathology, a radial fissure and displaced discal tissue are necessary to exert pressure on the outer annular wall. If the annulus remains intact, movements or positions can influence the displacement. If the outer annular wall is ruptured or weakened sufficiently, then the displacement may herniate through it, and loading is no longer able to affect its location. The clinical presentations of these different entities are examined in the next chapter.

5: Disc Pathology – Clinical Features

Introduction

The intervertebral disc is a common cause of back pain and the most common cause of radiculopathy or sciatica (Schwarzer *et al.* 1995d; Spitzer *et al.* 1987; AHCPR 1994). It has been proven that the disc is innervated. Although this may be partial and variable between individuals, it is a potential source of pain in its own right (Bogduk 1994b). Schwarzer *et al.* (1995d) found the disc to be the source of pain in 39% of a sample of chronic back pain patients. However, the gross and most renowned representation of discal pathology, the 'disc herniation' causing sciatica, is by most estimates comparatively rare – occurring in less than 5% of the back pain population (CSAG 1994) – although in one population survey 12% of those with back pain described symptoms of sciatica (Deyo and Tsui-Wu 1987). The clinical presentation of discogenic pain and of sciatica will be outlined.

Sections in this chapter are as follows:

- discogenic pain – prevalence
- discogenic pain – clinical features
- sciatica – prevalence
- sciatica – clinical features
- state of the annular wall
- natural history of disc herniation.

Discogenic pain – prevalence

Schwarzer *et al.* (1995d) found in a sample of ninety-two consecutive chronic back pain patients undergoing invasive imaging in tertiary care that, according to their strict criteria, 39% could be diagnosed as suffering from *internal disc disruption*. Pain and guarded movements are present; there is normal radiology and computer tomography (CT) imaging. The definitive diagnosis relies on two tests: the reproduction of the patient's pain with discography and the use of CT discography to reveal internal disc disruption. As a control, stimulation of at least one other disc should fail to reproduce pain, and to prove disruption a grade 3 radial fissure should be present on CT discography.

Using discography to reproduce patients' symptoms has resulted in the classification of 75%, 57% and 33% respectively of the populations studied as having discogenic symptoms (Ohnmeiss *et al.* 1997; Donelson *et al.* 1997; Antti-Poika *et al.* 1990). It will only ever be a select group who receive this invasive imaging, namely chronic back pain patients in hospital settings who have failed to improve with previous conservative care and in whom clear indications for surgery have not been found – that is, no definite nerve root involvement. Nonetheless, these studies suggest that the intervertebral disc is the most common single source of back pain.

Discogenic pain – clinical features

In patients who have nerve root involvement, direct stimulation of the annulus fibrosus has either been unable to provoke leg pain (Kuslich *et al.* 1991) or has done so in only a minority (Fernstrom 1960). However, in patients who have not had clear signs or symptoms of nerve root involvement, leg pain has been commonly provoked by discographic stimulation (Park *et al.* 1979; McFadden 1988; Milette *et al.* 1995; Donelson *et al.* 1997; Ohnmeiss *et al.* 1997; Colhoun *et al.* 1988; Schellhas *et al.* 1996). Ohnmeiss *et al.* (1997) found that pain referred into the thigh or calf was as common in those patients with a grade 2 disruption of the annulus as a grade 3 disruption. In their sample, those without internal disc disruption were significantly less likely to have lower limb pain than those who had a discogenic source of symptoms. Referral of pain into the leg can clearly be a feature of discogenic pain; in those with nerve root involvement, it appears that the leg pain is primarily a result of nerve root compression.

Schwarzer *et al.* (1995d) compared those who had the diagnosis of internal disc disruption to those who did not, according to various aspects of their clinical presentation. There was no statistically significant association between historical or examination findings and whether patients had a positive discography. Sitting, standing, walking, flexion, extension, rotation and straight leg raise were neither more likely to aggravate nor relieve pain in patients who had discogenic pain than in those whose pain was non-discogenic, nor could pain patterns distinguish the two groups, both having buttock, groin, thigh, calf and foot pain. Those with bilateral or unilateral pain distribution were more likely to have discogenic pain than those with central symptoms.

Rankine *et al.* (1999) examined the clinical features of patients with an HIZ with no evidence of neural compromise. On simple history-taking and clinical examination, they were unable to differentiate those with this sign from those without it. Features examined were pain referral above or below the knee, aggravation of pain by standing, walking, sitting, bending, lying, lifting and coughing, and neurological symptoms and signs. None of these variables were more common in those with an HIZ, and so they could not define particular clinical features that predicted this outer annular disruption.

A dynamic mechanical examination is much more successful at detecting symptomatic discs and determining the state of the outer annular wall (Donelson *et al.* 1997). Sixty-three chronic patients, the majority experiencing pain below the knee with no neurological deficits and no clear surgical indications on MRI, underwent discography and a McKenzie mechanical evaluation. The experienced McKenzie clinicians who conducted the examination were blinded to the outcomes from the discography. The clinicians used the movement of pain proximally or distally during the examination to classify the patients as centralisers, peripheralisers or no symptomatic change. Their classification was then correlated with the outcomes from discography. The criteria for a positive discogram were exact pain reproduction and an abnormal image, as long as no pain was reproduced at an adjacent level.

Thirty-one patients were classified as centralisers, sixteen as peripheralisers and sixteen as 'no change'. About 70% of centralisers and peripheralisers had a positive discogram, whereas only two patients (12.5%) in the 'no change' group had a positive discogram. Among the centralisers with a positive discogram, 91% had a competent annular wall on discography, whereas among peripheralisers with a positive discogram, only 54% had a competent annular wall. All these differences were significant ($P < 0.05$).

Thus most centralisers had discogenic pain with a competent annular wall, and most peripheralisers also had discogenic pain with a much higher prevalence of outer annular disruption. Symptoms that did not change during the mechanical assessment were very unlikely to be discogenic in origin. The authors conclude *"a non-invasive, low-tech, relatively inexpensive clinical assessment using repeated end-range lumbar test movements can provide considerably more relevant information than non-invasive imaging studies. Namely, it can distinguish between discogenic and nondiscogenic pain and provides considerable help in distinguishing between a competent and incompetent annulus"* (Donelson *et al.* 1997, p. 1121).

According to this study, if pain centralises or peripheralises, the probability of discogenic pain is 72%, while if pain remains unchanged the probability of non-discogenic pain is 87% (positive and negative predictive values recalculated from original data). Centralisation of pain has been recorded in about 50 – 90% of populations studied (Donelson *et al.* 1990, 1991, 1997; Long 1995; Delitto *et al.* 1993; Erhard *et al.* 1994; Werneke *et al.* 1999; Sufka *et al.* 1998). It is a very common occurrence in acute and chronic backs, and strongly suggests diagnostic implications.

Sciatica – prevalence

Disc herniations are the most common cause of nerve root involvement in back pain, commonly known as sciatica (Spitzer *et al.* 1987; AHCPR 1994). It has been estimated that this involves less than 5% of all those who have back pain (CSAG 1994; Heliovaara *et al.* 1987); some studies give higher estimates. When a definition was used of pain that radiated to the legs and that increased with cough, sneeze or deep breathing, 12% of those with back pain fit into this category (Deyo and Tsui-Wu 1987). A study conducted in Jersey in the Channel Islands recorded the frequency of diagnoses given by physicians for absences from work because of back pain (Watson *et al.* 1998). In this group, over 7% were diagnosed as having sciatica and a further 5% as having a prolapsed intervertebral disc. Dutch GPs diagnosed 14% of over 1,500 patients with radicular pain, and most of the rest (72%) with non-specific back pain (Schers *et al.* 2000). In tertiary care, the prevalence of neurological symptoms is greater; in a study of nearly 2,000 patients, 21% were found to have neurological signs and a further 41% had distal leg pain (Ben Debba *et al.* 2000).

Sciatica – clinical features

The classical criteria that need to be present to make the diagnosis of a symptomatic disc herniation with nerve root involvement are shown in Table 5.1 (Porter 1989; Porter and Miller 1986; Kramer 1990).

Table 5.1	Criteria for identifying symptomatic disc herniation with nerve root involvement

- unilateral leg pain in a typical sciatic root distribution below the knee
- specific neurological symptoms incriminating a single nerve
- limitation of straight leg raising by at least 50% of normal, with reproduction of leg pain
- segmental motor deficit
- segmental sensory change
- hyporeflexia
- kyphotic and/or scoliotic deformity
- imaging evidence of a disc protrusion at the relevant level.

Lumbar disc herniations occur most commonly among young adults between the ages of 30 and 40 (Deyo *et al.* 1990). However, it is reported that 1 – 3% of operations for lumbar disc herniations are performed on patients who are under 21 years of age (Silvers *et al.* 1994), and 4% on those over sixty (Maistrelli *et al.* 1987).

Typically the imaging study is done on suspicion of a disc herniation because of the clinical presentation of a patient. Variability of signs and symptoms is considerable. Over 95% of disc herniations occur at the L4 – L5 and L5 – S1 levels, thus the nerves most commonly affected are L5 and S1 (Andersson and Deyo 1996). Kramer (1990) states that about 50% of all herniations may be clearly assigned to a single segmental level, predominantly L5 and S1. The other cases are either not specific enough to be assigned a definite level or else more than one root is involved. Another study locates over 97% of just over 400 disc herniations at L4 – L5 and L5 – S1 interspaces (Kortelainen *et al.* 1985) (see Table 5.2).

Table 5.2   Distribution of single nerve root involvement in disc herniations

Segmental level	Proportion of single nerve root involvement	Interspace	Disc herniations (%)
L2	0.5%		
L3	0.5%	L2 – L3	<1%
L4	1.0%	L3 – L4	<2%
L5	44%	L4 – L5	57%
S1	54%	L5 – S1	41%

Source: Kramer 1990; Kortelainen *et al.* 1985

Typically the pain is referred down the lateral (L5) or posterior (S1) aspect of the thigh and leg below the knee into the dorsum of the foot and the big toe (L5), or the heel and outer aspect of the foot (S1) (see Table 5.3 and Figure 15.1). Nerve root tension signs are present – if L4, L5 or S1 are involved, this is the straight leg raise test; if upper lumbar (L1 – L3), this is the femoral nerve stretch test. Weakness may be present and is found in tibialis anterior (L4/L5), extensor hallucis longus (L5) or the calf muscles (S1/S2). If sensory deficit occurs, this is most common in the big toe (L5) or the outer border of the foot (S1). However, the radicular pain pattern or location of sensory deficit is not a definite means of identifying the nerve root involved. A disc herniation at L4 – L5, although more likely to produce symptoms of an L5 lesion, may also produce symptoms of an S1 lesion. Likewise, a disc herniation at L5 – S1, although more likely to produce symptoms of an S1 lesion, may produce symptoms of an L5 lesion (Kortelainen *et al.* 1985). Herniations at both levels may affect both nerve roots.

Table 5.3   Typical signs and symptoms associated with L4 – S1 nerve roots

	L4	L5	S1
Distribution of pain and *sensory loss*	(Anterior thigh) Anterior / *medial leg* (Great toe)	(Lateral thigh) Lateral leg Dorsum of foot *Great toe*	Posterior thigh Posterior leg *Lateral border of foot* Sole
Motor weakness	Quadriceps *Dorsiflexion*	*Big toe extension Extension of the toes*	*Plantarflexion* Eversion
Reflex	Knee		Ankle

Source: Waddell 1998; Nitta *et al.* 1993; Smyth and Wright 1958; Butler 1991; Kramer 1990

Some patients may present with small, isolated patches of distal pain rather than the typical dermatomal pattern. Root tension signs, due to irritation of the nerve root, occur earlier and more commonly than motor, sensory and reflex signs, which only occur once the function of the root is disturbed. These findings are variable. Flexion in standing, as described in this book, is also a form of root tension sign.

Flexion increases the compressive force acting on the nerve root complex and aggravates symptoms (Kramer 1990; Schnebel et al. 1989). *Patients will generally be made worse in positions of flexion.* However, sometimes temporary relief may be gained during sitting, while the intervertebral foramina are enlarged, but upon returning to an upright position symptoms return to their former intensity or are worse. Disc-related symptoms are also affected by other activities that increase intra-discal pressure, such as coughing, sneezing or straining (Kramer 1990).

Unfortunately, none of the questions or tests that are part of the history and physical examination has a high diagnostic accuracy by itself (Andersson and Deyo 1996; Deyo et al. 1992; van den Hoogen et al. 1995; Deville et al. 2000). The history-taking and physical examination in patients with suspected lumbar nerve root involvement have been shown to involve considerable disagreement – Kappa value 0.40 after the history and 0.66 after the examination (Vroomen et al. 2000).

The presence of sciatica has a high sensitivity (0.95) and specificity (0.88), but poor diagnostic accuracy in identifying disc herniations (Andersson and Deyo 1996; van den Hoogen et al. 1995). The straight leg raise test has a high sensitivity, but low specificity, while the crossed straight leg raising test is less sensitive, but much more specific (Andersson and Deyo 1996; van den Hoogen et al. 1995; Deyo et al. 1992; Deville et al 2000). The sensitivity of other neurological signs tends to be less good, while the specificity is somewhat better. In particular, muscle weakness tests have a higher specificity. Patients with disc herniations have significantly less range of forward flexion compared to patients with no positive findings, and also significantly more pain distributed in to the legs on extension in standing (Stankovic et al. 1999).

Most of the studies that these papers review involve surgical cases at the severe end of the pathological spectrum, and so their results are based on biased samples that do not correspond to the true range of patients; those with definite disc herniations will tend to be over-represented. When the prevalence of a disease in a population is high as in these studies, the predictive value of tests will be over-inflated. In the back pain population as a whole, in which the prevalence of disc herniations is much lower, the predictive value of these tests will be poorer. This means a substantial probability of false-positive test results (Andersson and Deyo 1996; Deville *et al.* 2000). The accuracy of individual tests is likely to be improved by considering combinations of responses and tests.

Upper lumbar disc herniations are relatively rare compared to herniations in the low lumbar spine, but they do occur. One series of about 1,400 patients identified 73 with herniations that affected L1, L2, and L3 nerve roots (Aronson and Dunsmore 1963). This represented only 5% of the total, of whom 70% had involvement of L3, 25% involvement of L2 and 5% involvement of L1. Radiation of pain was primarily over the lateral and anterior aspect of the thigh, and some cutaneous sensory loss was present in about 50% of patients in the same area. Muscle weakness mostly affected quadriceps or psoas, but extensor hallucis longus was occasionally affected. The knee jerk was reduced or absent in 50% of patients.

Part of the clinical presentation of acute back pain patients may be a deformity of kyphosis and/or scoliosis or lateral shift. The aetiology of the shift for a long time has been thought to relate to disc herniations (O'Connell 1943, 1951; Spurling and Grantham 1940; Falconer *et al.* 1948). Conceptually it was imagined that the shift occurred to avoid pressure on the nerve root. The widely quoted theory suggested that a contralateral shift was an attempt to reduce pressure on a nerve root from a disc herniation that was lateral to the root, while an ipsilateral shift was an attempt to reduce pressure on a nerve root from a herniation that was medial to it (Kramer 1990; Weitz 1981). These theories have now been disproved. Although it is described in the literature, clear-cut definitions and standardised terminology have not been used. Lateral shifts are still generally believed to relate to disc pathology (see Chapter 9).

State of the annular wall

Displacement great enough to cause significant deformity can with further displacement cause rupture of the annulus and perhaps even extrusion of disc material. Deformity is a sign of major displacement, as are the other criteria of a significant disc lesion such as constant radicular pain, constant numbness or myotomal weakness. If no position or movement can provide *lasting* improvement of symptoms, we can surmise an incompetent annular wall in which the hydrostatic mechanism of the disc has been lost. The annular wall may have been breached by herniated discal material (extrusion or sequestration), or else the outer annular wall has become so attenuated and weakened as to be incompetent (protrusion). This presentation is associated with a poor chance of rapid improvement under conservative care as it is at the extreme end of the pathological continuum.

However, displacements develop from an embryonic stage when only minor symptoms of spinal pain will be experienced. Being well contained by a relatively healthy annulus, minor displacements are short-lived and rapidly reversible, being at the minor end of the continuum. A less extreme clinical presentation on the continuum is intermittent leg pain and neurological symptoms that are influenced by movements and positions. In this instance we may surmise an intact annular wall, a functioning hydrostatic mechanism, and a displacement which loading can either push to the periphery or to the centre of the disc. Positions and movements may be found that have an effect on the displacement with a consequent increase or decrease of pressure on the symptom-generating annulus and/or nerve root.

"The symptoms caused by a disk protrusion vary because the protruding disk tissue is still part of an intact osmotic system and participates in the pressure-dependent changes of volume and consistency of the disk. As long as the protruding tissue is covered by strong intact lamellae of the annulus fibrosus, the displaced fragment can relocate back into the center of the disk.... In some cases the protruded tissue can displace further and rupture the annulus fibrosus as a disc extrusion" (Kramer 1990, p. 128).

Disc herniations thus represent a continuum, at the severe end of which the annulus is ruptured and breached by an extrusion or a sequestrum is extruded from the disc into the spinal or vertebral canal. In such a case recovery will only occur slowly with the passage of time if treated conservatively or else the patient is a likely case for surgery. At the less extreme end of the continuum a protrusion may be the source of symptoms, held in place by a competent annulus. The hydrostatic mechanism of the disc is still intact, and with the use of repeated movements and sustained postures the displacement may be reduced and the symptoms resolved. Therefore a key clinical decision arises as to whether the annulus is competent and the displacement still responds to mechanical forces, or it is incompetent or ruptured and no longer amenable to lasting changes. Pathologically and clinically, the distinction is between a protrusion with a competent annular wall and an extrusion/sequestration (Table 5.4). It is those with an incompetent or ruptured annular wall who are possible surgical candidates – see next section.

Table 5.4   Differences between sciatica due to a protrusion or an extrusion/sequestration

Disc protrusion	*Disc extrusion/sequestration*
LBP =/> thigh / leg pain	Leg pain >> LBP / No LBP Distal pain ++
Gradual onset leg pain	Sudden onset leg pain
Onset leg pain LBP remains the same	Onset leg pain LBP eases or goes
Postural variation ++	Less postural variation
Intermittent / constant pain	Constant pain
Intermittent / constant tingling	Constant numbness
Variable deformity	Constant deformity
Variable weakness	Motor deficits
Moderate / variable tension signs	Major, constant tension signs Crossed straight leg raise positive
Movements able to decrease, abolish or centralise symptoms	Movement increases distal symptoms No movement able to decrease, abolish or centralise symptoms in a lasting way
	Severe restriction walking capacity
Possible neck pain	

LBP = low back pain

Source: Kramer 1990; Brismar *et al.* 1996; Beattie *et al.* 2000; Pople and Griffith 1994; Vucetic *et al.* 1995; Uden and Landin 1987; McKenzie 1981; Jonsson *et al.* 1998; Jonsson and Stromqvist 1996b

Natural history of disc herniation

Given the difficulties of case definition, heterogeneity of pathology and presentation, recruitment bias, inadequate follow-up and variable interventions, identifying the natural history of disc herniations is difficult. Considerable variability in the history of those with disc herniations will be seen. Some will make a speedy and spontaneous recovery, while others will run a protracted course despite multiple conservative treatment interventions. Just as the underlying pathology varies, so too does the potential for easy resolution.

It should also be borne in mind that the correlation between the morphological abnormality and symptoms is not straightforward. Disc herniations may exist in the asymptomatic population (Boos *et al.* 1995), symptoms may resolve with little regression of a herniation and symptoms may show little change with a substantial reduction in herniation size (Matsubara *et al.* 1995).

Nonetheless, it is generally considered that the natural history of disc herniation if left untreated is positive, if rather protracted (Saal 1996; Kramer 1995; Weber 1994). The worst pain from discogenic sciatica is in the first three weeks, when any inflammatory response is most intense and the mechanical effect of the extruded disc material is greatest (Kramer 1995). It is recommended, because of the positive natural history within the first three months, that surgery is rarely indicated before six to twelve weeks (Saal 1996). It is also suggested that neither the failure of passive conservative care nor imaging test results and the presence of neurological deficit should be used as sole criterion for proceeding with surgical intervention. The only specific indicators for early surgery are (Saal 1996):

- cauda equina syndrome

- progressive neurological deficit

- profound neurological deficit (e.g. foot drop) showing no improvement over six weeks.

A trial evaluating the effect of NSAIDs in the management of sciatica used a placebo control group, which allows a reasonably true assessment of natural history. Weber *et al.* (1993) compared piroxicam to a placebo in over 200 patients with acute sciatica; there was no difference in outcomes between the two groups. Over the first four weeks, average pain on the visual analogue scale improved from about five and a half out of ten to two out of ten, function improved markedly and 60% were back to work. There was no further improvement in leg symptoms at three months or one year, while back pain was reported to be worse at three months but the same at one year as at four weeks. About 40% of patients still complained of back and/or leg pain, and 20% were still out of work at one year. Previous episodes of sciatica were associated with poorer prognosis.

The natural history and clinical course of patients with nerve root signs and symptoms may be poor. Of eighty-two consecutive patients followed for a year following in-patient conservative therapy, only 29% were fully recovered and 33% had come to surgery (Balague *et al.* 1999). Most recovery occurred in the first three months, after which there was little further improvement (Figure 5.1). A positive neurological examination was associated with failure to recover at one year. However, surgery is not a simple panacea; 5 – 15% of surgical candidates have poor outcomes and further operations (Hoffman *et al.* 1993). In a Finnish study, 67% of 202 patients, whether having had surgery or not, continued to have significant problems as long as thirteen years after the onset of severe sciatica (Nykvist *et al.* 1995).

Figure 5.1   Recovery from severe sciatica

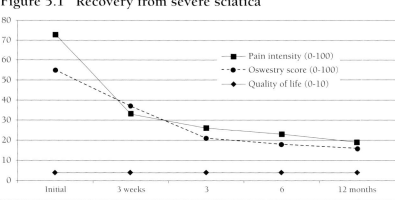

Source: Balague *et al.* 1999

Bed-rest has been shown to be no more effective than 'watchful waiting' in acute sciatica (Vroomen *et al.* 1999). The latter group was instructed to be up and about whenever possible, but to avoid straining the back or provoking pain, and were allowed to go to work. Both groups used NSAIDs and analgesics. In both groups at two weeks about 70% reported some improvement and 35% a great improvement; on the visual analogue scale average pain in the leg was reduced from sixty-five to forty, and average pain in the back from forty-seven to thirty. At twelve weeks, 87% of both groups reported improvement and pain scores had fallen to fifteen in the leg and twenty in the back. The leg pain was worse initially, but overall improved more than the back pain (Figure 5.2). About 18% of both groups received surgery ultimately.

Figure 5.2   Recovery from sciatica in first three months

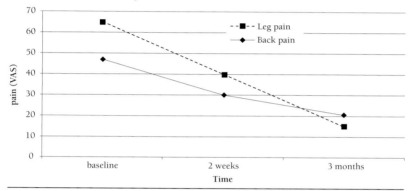

Source: Vroomen *et al.* 1999

Numerous studies have noted the regression of disc herniation when patients have been exposed to repeat imaging studies and conservative treatment. Unfortunately these studies are unable to define the time-scale of recovery, only its occurrence. Regression of herniation and improvement or resolution of symptoms usually occurred within six months or a year, although some follow-up studies were done up to two years after initial assessment. Maigne *et al.* (1992) performed repeat CT scans on forty-eight patients, all of whom showed a reduction in herniation, in eight of which this was between and 50% and 75% and in thirty-one between 75% and 100% reduction in size. Regression was seen in fourteen out of twenty-one patients on repeat CT scans (Delauche-Cavallier *et al.* 1992), and twenty-five out of thirty-six herniations (Ahn *et al.* 2000b). Larger herniations, and extrusions or sequestrations rather than protrusions, have repeatedly shown a greater tendency to decrease in size (Maigne *et al.* 1992; Matsubara *et al.* 1995; Delauche-Cavallier *et al.* 1992; Ahn *et al.* 2000b; Bozzao *et al.* 1992; Komori *et al.* 1996).

Regression of the disc herniation is generally associated with an improvement in symptoms, although not always exactly. In thirteen patients whose leg symptoms resolved with conservative treatment, eleven demonstrated resolution or improvement in the disc herniation, but in two the size of herniation was unchanged (Ellenberg *et al.* 1993). The absolute area and sagittal and transverse measurements of the disc herniation have been shown to correlate with symptoms (Thelander *et al.* 1994). Constant symptoms were associated with larger herniations than intermittent symptoms, which were associated with larger herniation compared to those with no pain. The area of herniation decreased markedly over time, mirroring an improvement in symptoms. Teplick and Haskin (1985) reported on eleven patients with regression or disappearance of herniation, in nine of whom the associated radicular symptoms resolved. Bush *et al.* (1992) followed up over a hundred patients treated with epidural injections. At one year 14% had undergone surgery, and in the remaining patients pain was reduced by 94%. Complete or partial regression had occurred in 75% of the disc extrusions and 26% of the disc protrusions. Eleven patients with extrusions who had a repeat MRI at a median time of twenty-five months all had a regression of the herniation and resolution of their sciatica (Saal *et al.* 1990).

It is suggested that recovery from neurological deficit is variable, again depending upon the initial insult to the nerve root (Saal 1996) (see Table 27.2). Spontaneous recovery, when likely to occur, will generally show initial signs of improvement in the first three to six weeks.

Table 5.5   Recovery from neurological deficit

Possible pathology	Degree of nerve damage	Presentation	Pattern of recovery
Neurapraxia	Mild	Mild sensory loss, with/without mild motor deficit	Recovers in 6 – 12 weeks
Axonotmesis	Moderate	Absent reflex, moderate motor deficit, numbness	Recovers in 3 – 6 months
Axonotmesis	Severe	Absent reflex, Severe motor deficit, numbness	May take up to one year to improve, or may not recover fully at all

Source: Saal 1996

The natural history of disc herniations is generally good. Major improvements in symptoms and function happen in the first three or four weeks, while recovery from neurological deficit occur more slowly. After three months further recovery is less certain, so patients who still have symptoms at this point are not guaranteed the normal good natural history. Patients who have more severe pathology, such as extrusions and sequestrations, are as likely to have a good recovery, and may in fact do better than those with protrusions. However, despite the generally good prognosis, a substantial minority will have persistent symptoms at one year, and many will improve but not become fully symptom-free.

Conclusions

Recognition of symptomatic discogenic pain is problematic, as no specific signs or symptoms exist. However, a mechanical evaluation may accurately detect discogenic pain from assessment of symptom location change or lack of it. The signs and symptoms denoting sciatica include pain patterns, paraesthesia, muscle weakness and tension signs; these are variably present. Lateral shifts may be present and may be associated with poor prognosis if correction is not possible. Definite and proven sciatica due to an irreducible disc herniation is one of the few indicators for possible surgical intervention.

The primary source of symptomatic disc herniations is posterior or postero-lateral, with the latter being the most important cause of radicular pain. Anterior and vertebral herniations have a much more limited role in symptoms. The first key clinical decision concerns the postural loading that may reduce the disc displacement: should the patient be flexed or extended, or moved laterally? The second clinical decision concerns the ability to affect the disc displacement in a lasting way: is this a contained lesion with the hydrostatic mechanism intact, or has the annular wall been breached or become incompetent? Factors in the history may help us to determine these issues, which should be confirmed by the patient's response to a full mechanical evaluation.

6: Biomechanics

Introduction

Certain principle movements are available at the lumbar vertebrae. Range of movement varies considerably between individuals and may be affected by age and by the presence of back pain. Postures alter the sagittal angle of the lumbar vertebrae. Different movements and positions have various mechanical effects on the spine. Sustained movements have a different effect to single movements. Due to the biomechanical properties of collagenous tissue, the loading history on the spine may be significant. Experimental studies provide in vitro information about the effects of loading strategies.

This chapter considers some of the effects and characteristics of common postures and movements as revealed by physiological, clinical and experimental data. For a more detailed consideration of biomechanics, it is recommended that a clinical anatomy text be consulted (Bogduk 1997; Oliver and Middleditch 1991; Twomey and Taylor 1994a, 1994b; Adams 1994).

Sections in this chapter are as follows:

- movements at the lumbar spine

- range of movement

- lumbar lordosis

- loading strategies and symptoms

- effect of postures on lumbar curve

- biomechanics of the lumbar spine

- time factor and creep loading

- creep in the lumbar spine

- optimal sitting posture

- effect of time of day on movements and biomechanics

- effect of posture on internal intervertebral disc stresses.

Movements at the lumbar spine

The principal movements available at the lumbar spine as a whole and its individual motion segments are axial compression and distraction, flexion, extension, axial rotation and lateral flexion. Horizontal translation does not occur as an isolated or pure movement, but is involved in axial rotation (Bogduk 1997). There is considerably more sagittal movement available in the lumbar spine than rotation or lateral flexion, especially at the lowest segments. Flexion is substantially greater than extension.

Range of movement

Mobility of the lumbar spine varies considerably between different individuals. It may also be influenced by the following factors: age, sex, ligamentous laxity, genetics and pathology (Oliver and Middleditch 1991). In individuals, age and back pain are the most significant causes of variable movement patterns over time.

Age

Age causes increased stiffness of the motion segment and a decline in total range. From childhood to 60-year-olds there is nearly a halving of sagittal and frontal plane movements. During adulthood the change is less marked, but still it declines by about a quarter (Twomey and Taylor 1994a, 1994b). However, standard deviation accounts for up to 23% of the mean range of movement – there is a considerable range of what is 'normal'. This means a stiff and sedentary 40-year-old may display less mobility than a flexible and active 60-year-old.

Back pain

In general, patients with back pain are less mobile than asymptomatic individuals; however, there is such a wide spectrum of mobility that assigning people to diagnostic groups on the strength of movement loss is very difficult (Adams and Dolan 1995). Several studies have found differences in the range of movement between back pain patients and controls. Patients with back pain have been found to have significantly less flexion than control groups without pain (Pearcy *et al.* 1985; McGregor *et al.* 1995), and patients with tension signs showed significantly less flexion and extension (Pearcy *et al.* 1985). Groups with back pain have been found to have a significantly diminished range of spinal extension compared to controls without back pain (Pope *et al.* 1985; Beattie *et al.* 1987).

Thomas *et al.* (1998) found a statistically significant reduction in all planes of movement in a back pain group compared to a control group. About 90% of patients had at least one restriction of the seven tested, while 40% of controls had at least one restriction. The presence of three or more restrictions was found in 50% of patients, but only in 3% of those without symptoms. The largest differences between back patients and asymptomatic controls were in standing extension (12 degree difference) and finger-to-floor flexion (10 centimetre difference). Waddell *et al.* (1992) found measures of total flexion and extension, among other measurements, to successfully discriminate patients from controls.

Range of movement has also been shown to improve with patient recovery (Pearcy *et al.* 1985; Magnusson *et al.* 1998a). Improvements in impairment and disability can clearly discriminate those who are successfully treated and those who fail treatment (Waddell and Main 1984).

Because of the high degree of variability between individuals, detecting impairment due to back pain is problematic (Sullivan *et al.* 1994). For example, if an individual's normal range was above average, a loss of movement due to back pain may go undetected. Another individual, whose mobility is well below average, may give the appearance of impairment but be asymptomatic. The key contrasts are between the patient's present ability to move compared to normal and how this changes over time.

Time of day
Time of day affects an individual's flexibility, with increased range later in the day. Other aspects of spinal mechanics also change (see later section – *Effect of time of day on range of movement and biomechanics*).

Lumbar lordosis

The relationship between back pain and the lumbar lordosis has been evaluated in several studies with contradictory findings. Several studies have found that the lumbar lordosis of back pain subjects was significantly less than a control group without back pain (Jackson and McManus 1994; Simpson 1989; Magora 1975; Magora and Schwartz 1976). However, other studies have found no differences between symptomatic and asymptomatic groups and did not correlate loss of lordosis with back pain (Hansson *et al.* 1985; Pope *et al.* 1985; Torgerson and Dotter 1976; Frymoyer *et al.* 1984).

Burgin *et al.* (2000) undertook a systematic literature review of postural variations and back pain, for which they identified six further studies. These demonstrated an association between an increased or decreased lumbar lordosis and back pain. However, as no study used a longitudinal prospective study design, a cause-and-effect relationship could not be established.

The range of what should be considered a normal lumbar lordosis is considerable (Torgerson and Dotter 1976; Jackson and McManus 1994; Hansson *et al.* 1985; Dolan *et al.* 1988). In a study in which measurements were made in 973 pain-free individuals, the mean lumbar lordotic angle was 45 degrees, with most of the sample falling somewhere in the range 23 – 68 degrees (Fernand and Fox 1985).

Given that the range of normal lordosis is so wide, identification of abnormality by observation only, as in the radiography studies above, is clearly difficult, if not impossible. An individual may have always had a small lordotic angle but no back pain; alternatively, in an individual who normally has a large lordotic angle, the advent of back pain may be accompanied by a reduced but still normal angle. Simply using observation, only very severe alterations should be given clinical significance. For instance, a recent onset inability to extend and absent lordosis is clinically relevant. Ultimately, the only way to test the correlation between the lumbar angle and symptoms is to alter the posture and record the symptomatic response. Most studies that have observed the role of posture in spinal problems have failed to make a direct correlation between posture and symptoms *at the same time*.

Loading strategies and symptoms

A few studies have made direct correlations between postures assumed and symptoms. Some studies have looked at the effect of different seating positions and comfort in asymptomatic populations. These studies are mentioned in more detail in the chapter on postural syndrome. The consistent finding is that seating that helps maintain the lumbar lordosis is generally found to be most comfortable, while more flexed postures were much more likely to produce discomfort or pain (Harms 1990; Eklund and Corlett 1987; Mandal 1984; Knutsson *et al.* 1966).

The study of Harms-Ringdahl (1986) of healthy volunteers has shown the effect of sustained loading in the cervical spine. They maintained a protruded head posture and began to feel pain within two to fifteen minutes, which increased with time until they were eventually forced to discontinue the posture.

Mechanical diagnosis and therapy uses the concept that sustained postures and movements cause symptoms to decrease, abolish, centralise, produce, worsen or peripheralise. Certain therapeutic loading will have a favourable effect on symptoms and should be encouraged, while other loading has an unfavourable effect on symptoms and should be temporarily avoided. The next chapter discusses the phenomenon of centralisation at length. In the subsequent chapter, which reviews relevant literature, a section looks at studies that have investigated directional preference. This is the concept that patients with symptoms find their pain worsens with certain postures or movements, often but not always with flexion, and improves with the opposite posture or movement, often but not always with extension.

This is illustrated in the study by Williams *et al.* (1991) that compared the effects of two sitting postures on back and referred pain over a twenty-four- to forty-eight-hour period. There was a significant reduction in back and leg pain at all test points in the group that had been encouraged to maintain their lordosis and were provided with a lumbar roll. There was no change in severity of leg symptoms, but there was a worsening of back pain in the group who had been instructed to maintain a flexed posture when sitting. Centralisation above the knee occurred in over half the lordotic group, while peripheralisation occurred in 6%. Centralisation was reported in 10% of the flexion group, and peripheralisation in a quarter of the group.

The role of posture in predisposing to back pain incidence and then in perpetuating or aggravating it once present is considered in Chapter 2, and studies into directional preference are referred to in Chapter 11. Different postures clearly have different effects on symptoms, and consequently a good understanding of the biomechanics of posture on the lumbar spine is important.

Effect of postures on lumbar curve

Everyday positions, movements and activities affect the lumbar spinal curve. These positions, whose physiological effect is well known, are the ones asked about during the patient interview. In the sagittal plane certain activities are fundamentally activities of flexion, some activities of extension and some may be either (Table 6.1 and Figure 6.1).

Table 6.1   Effect of different postures on the spinal curve

Postures of flexion	Postures of extension	Variable postures
Sitting	Standing	Side lying
Bending	Walking	
	Supine lying (legs extended)	
	Prone lying	

Standing / walking

Upright postures, such as standing and walking, are primarily activities of extension. When standing straight the lumbar lordosis is emphasised; comparatively, when sitting it is reduced considerably, and the spine becomes more flexed (Lord *et al.* 1997; Andersson *et al.* 1979; Dolan *et al.* 1988; Keegan 1953). Walking increases extension as the hind leg anteriorly rotates the pelvis, accentuating the lordosis (McKenzie 1981).

Figure 6.1   The effect of different postures on the lumbar curve

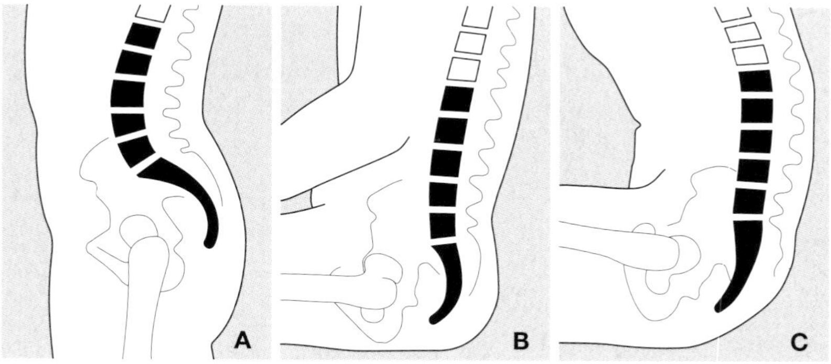

Key:
A. Standing – lordosis and anterior pelvic rotation
B. Sitting upright – reduced lordosis
C. Sitting slouched – kyphosis and posterior pelvic rotation

Sitting

When moving from standing to unsupported sitting, the lumbar lordosis decreases by on average 38 degrees, most of this movement occurring with the rotation of the pelvis, which on average accounts for 28 degrees (Andersson *et al.* 1979). Sitting is primarily an activity of flexion; however, the amount is dependent upon numerous other factors. Sitting relaxed produces the most lumbar flexion, crossing the legs flexes the spine and sitting erect produces less extension than upright standing (Dolan *et al.* 1988). Thus, although sitting is a more flexed posture than standing, several factors may influence the degree of flexion that is attained (Table 6.2).

A backrest has some affect on lessening flexion in sitting, but a lumbar support has a more significant influence with increased support causing increasing lordosis, although the exact position of the support is less important (Andersson *et al.* 1979). A significant factor in the angle of the lumbar spine when sitting is the rotation that occurs at the pelvis. As the pelvis rotates posteriorly, as in slumped sitting, the lumbar spine is made to flex; as it rotates anteriorly, as in erect sitting, the lumbar spine is made to extend (Black *et al.* 1996; Andersson *et al.* 1979; Majeske and Buchanan 1984). The use of a lumbar roll facilitates a direct increase in the lordosis as well as ensuring a more anteriorly rotated pelvis (Andersson *et al.* 1979; Majeske and Buchanan 1984).

The angle between the thighs and the trunk has an effect on the lumbar curvature due to tension in the posterior thigh muscles (Harms 1990). Increasing hip flexion rotates the pelvis posteriorly and has the effect of flattening or flexing the spine (Keegan 1953). Thus, sitting with the knees above the hips, as is common on many settees/lounge chairs or car seats, flattens the spine.

Table 6.2   Factors that affect the spinal curve in sitting

Factors that accentuate the lordosis	*Factors that increase flexion*
Anterior rotation of pelvis	Posterior rotation of pelvis
Hip extension	Hip/knee flexion
Backrest inclined backwards	Crossing legs
Lumbar support/roll	

Bending
Leaning forward is obviously an activity of flexion. Bending fully causes more flexion of the lumbar spine than sitting (Keegan 1953). Flexion moments are exerted on the lumbar spine when a person leans forward; the further they lean, the greater the resulting moment. The magnitude of the flexion moment is a product of the weight of the trunk above the spine and the distance from the spine to the line

of gravity acting through the trunk, known as the *moment arm*. The greater the moment arm, for instance if a person were to lean forward and hold a weight in outstretched hands, the greater the force acting on the spine (Bogduk 1997). Lowering one's height by squatting produces less flexion of the spine than purely bending forward.

Lying

The shape of the spinal curve in lying is dependent upon the position adopted. Three basic postures are available: side, prone or supine. In side lying the spine may be either flexed or extended depending on the position of the legs. Increasing hip flexion, with its concomitant posterior rotation of the pelvis, flattens the lordosis, while increasing amounts of hip extension accentuate it. Lying in the foetal position is one of extreme flexion, while lying with hip or hips extended tends to extend the spine. Side lying also causes a degree of lateral translation towards the side the individual is lying on (McKenzie 1981). In supine lying, the spinal curve is dependent upon the position of the legs. With knees and hips extended, the anterior thigh muscles anteriorly rotate the pelvis and increase the lordosis, while with hip and knee flexion the pelvis rotates posteriorly and the spine flattens. Prone lying for most people is a position of relative lumbar extension.

Biomechanics of the lumbar spine

Biomechanics (Breig 1961) is the study of changes in anatomical structures occurring during movements of the body. Flexion and extension involve two components – sagittal rotation and sagittal translation. For instance, in flexion there is a combination of anterior sagittal rotation and anterior translation of the lumbar vertebrae (Oliver and Middleditch 1991).

With flexion, the intervertebral disc is compressed anteriorly and the posterior annulus is stretched. Flexion causes a posterior displacement of the nucleus pulposus (Shah *et al.* 1978; Krag *et al.* 1987; Shepperd *et al.* 1990; Shepperd 1995; Schnebel *et al.* 1988; Beattie *et al.* 1994; Fennell *et al.* 1996; Brault *et al.* 1997; Edmondston *et al.* 2000). The movement causes a lengthening of the vertebral canal and places tension on the spinal cord and the peripheral nervous system. Intradiscal pressure, measured in the nucleus pulposus, increases by up to 80% in full flexion (Adams 1994).

With extension, the intervertebral disc is compressed posteriorly and the anterior annulus is stretched. The movement is associated with impacting of the spinous processes, or the inferior articular processes, on the lamina below. Loading may be concentrated in the area of the pars interarticularis (Oliver and Middleditch 1991). Extension causes an anterior displacement of the nucleus pulposus (Shah *et al.* 1978; Krag *et al.* 1987; Shepperd *et al.* 1990; Shepperd 1995; Schnebel *et al.* 1988; Beattie *et al.* 1994; Fennell *et al.* 1996; Brault *et al.* 1997; Edmondston *et al.* 2000). Extension reduces the size of the vertebral canal and intervertebral foramen. Nuclear pressure is reduced by up to 35% in extension (Adams 1994).

For a detailed analysis of movement, coupled movements, the control and restraint of movement and the effects of testing spinal segments to failure, readers are referred to clinical anatomy texts (Bogduk 1997; Oliver and Middleditch 1991; Twomey and Taylor 1994a, 1994b; Adams 1994).

Time factor and creep loading

Various studies in asymptomatic volunteers have demonstrated the role of sustained loading in the generation of spinal pain (Harms 1990; Harms-Ringdahl 1986; Eklund and Corlett 1987). It is not the act of slouched sitting or, in the cervical spine, protrusion of the head that causes the ache to appear, but rather the maintenance of this end-range position for a sustained period. With muscular activity reduced, the mechanical stress falls mostly on non-contractile articular and peri-articular structures such as ligaments, joint capsules and the intervertebral disc. The effect of sustained or repeated loading on collagenous structures has an important role in the pathogenesis and maintenance of musculoskeletal problems.

Insidious onset back pain is more common in life than sudden injury. Experimental findings offer supportive evidence that explain this phenomenon by fatigue damage, which occurs at low loads with accumulative stress (Dolan 1998; Adams and Dolan 1995; Wilder *et al.* 1988). This highlights the role of loading history in spinal mechanics and the aetiology of back pain – for instance, sustained loading generates stress concentrations in the posterior annular fibres (Adams *et al.* 1996b), which may be a cause of pain in vivo (McNally *et al.* 1996). As the largest avascular structure in the body, the intervertebral disc is particularly prone to fatigue failure as it has a very limited capacity for repair or remodelling (Adams and Dolan 1995, 1997). Creep loading in flexion, together with anterior translation with time, may be a cause of distortion or structural damage to any collagenous spinal structure. Attenuation and fissuring in the lamellae of the annulus, or weakening of ligaments and joint capsule, are all possible with sustained loading (Adams *et al.* 1980; Twomey *et al.* 1988).

Creep, hysteresis and set

If a constant force is left applied to a collagenous structure for a prolonged period of time, further movement occurs. This movement is very slight; it happens slowly, is imperceptible and is known as *creep* (Bogduk 1997). Creep is the result of rearrangement of collagen fibres and proteoglycans and of water being squeezed from the tissue. Brief stress does not act long enough on the tissue to cause creep, whereas sustained force allows displacement to occur so that elongation of the structure occurs.

Upon release from the force, as long as this has not been excessive, the structure begins to recover. However, restoration of the initial shape of the structure occurs more slowly and to a lesser extent than the initial deformation. The rate at which recovery happens between loading and unloading is known as *hysteresis* (Bogduk 1997). Initially the structure may not return to its original length, but remain slightly longer. This difference between initial and final length is known as *set*. This often occurs after creep, but if the interval between creep loading is sufficient, full recovery may occur and the structure eventually returns to its original shape. Depending upon the tissues and the forces applied, structures may be temporarily lengthened if loading is tensile or compacted if loading is compressive.

However, if the collagen fibres are not given enough time to recover before creep loading occurs again, or if creep loading has caused the bonds between and within collagen fibres to be broken, the set may persist indefinitely. Thus normal forces applied over lengthy and repeated periods of time may cause an alteration of the mechanical properties of collagenous structures. Not only may ligaments, capsules or parts of the disc become lengthened and less capable of fulfilling their normal mechanical functions, but also the structure may become vulnerable to injury. In this way tissues may become susceptible to fatigue failure.

After sustained or repetitive normal mechanical stresses, structures may fail at loads that are substantially less than that needed to cause damage with a single application of force. While one loading has no deleterious affect upon the tissue, the same loading, within normal bounds, prolonged or frequently applied may eventually lead to disruption of the tissue. *"The clinical importance of fatigue failure is that damage to tissues may occur without a history of major or obvious trauma"* (Bogduk 1997, p. 77); hence 'no apparent reason' for the onset of musculoskeletal problems is so common.

Creep in the lumbar spine

Flexion creep loading

Creep has a profound effect on the mechanical properties of the motion segment (Adams 1994). Experimentally the effects of creep in the lumbar spine have been studied relative to flexion, extension and axial loading (reviewed by Twomey and Taylor 1994a, 1994b). During creep loading, in flexion the anterior part of the disc is compressed, the posterior part is stretched and the zygapophyseal joint surfaces are compressed. Fluid is expressed from the soft tissues so that there is relative deprivation of nutrients. There is progressive anterior movement, so that the range of flexion increases. During sustained flexion, creep causes an increase in the flexion angle of 10% in twenty minutes (McGill and Brown 1992). Sustained flexed postures also have the effect of reducing the resistance of the spinal ligaments, therefore making the spine weaker and more susceptible to injury – holding a flexed posture for five minutes reduces resistance by 42%, holding it for an hour reduces resistance by 67% (Bogduk 1997).

"If the amount of 'creep' involved after prolonged load bearing in flexion is considerable, then recovery back to the original starting posture (hysteresis) is extremely slow. It takes considerable time for the soft tissues to imbibe fluid after it has been expressed during prolonged flexion loading. Many occupational groups (e.g. stonemasons, bricklayers, roofing carpenters and the like) regularly submit their lumbar spines to this category of insult. They work with their lumbar column fully flexed and under load for considerable periods of time. There is often little movement away from the fully flexed position once it has been reached, and little opportunity for recovery between episodes of work in this position" (Twomey and Taylor 1994a, p. 144).

Sustained loading in flexion causes creep deformation of the lumbar vertebral column that progresses with time, and from which there is not immediate recovery, especially in older specimens. This predisposes the spine to be more susceptible to flexion injuries (Twomey and Taylor 1982; Twomey et al. 1988). Disc mechanics depend upon loading history as well as the load that is applied (Adams et al. 1996b). Flexion and fatigue loading to simulate a vigorous day's activity (Adams and Hutton 1983) and one hour of sitting (Wilder et al. 1988) have been shown to produce distortions, weakening and radial fissures in the lamellae of the annulus. Static loading to simulate extended and flexed sitting postures found that the latter generated considerably greater tensile force in the region of the posterior annulus (Hedman and Fernie 1997).

The role of repeated and sustained flexion postures in the aetiology of structural damage to spinal tissues has been explored experimentally. A modelling experiment has shown that bending may cause annular failure as the strain is highly localised in the posterior disc and if increases in fibre length exceed 4%, the annulus would be damaged (Hickey and Hukins 1980). Computer-generated disc models predict posterior annular fissuring will occur with flexion and compression (Natarajan and Andersson 1994; Shirazi-Adl 1989, 1994; Lu et al. 1996). Sustained flexion loading may lead to distortion and rupture of the annulus, which may be followed by extrusion of disc material (Adams and Hutton 1983, 1985a; Gordan et al. 1991; Wilder et al. 1988). Flexion and compression, with or without lateral bending or rotation, may cause disc prolapse, which may be sudden or gradual (Adams and Hutton 1982, 1985a; McNally et al. 1993; Gordan et al. 1991). However, these events are not easily produced and structural failure in the intervertebral disc may involve internal damage to the annulus rather than prolapse of disc material (Adams and Dolan 1995).

In contrast to the above effects, flexed postures have several physiological and mechanical advantages. Flexion is said to improve the transport of metabolites in the intervertebral disc and reduce the stress on the zygapophyseal joints and on the posterior half of the annulus fibrosus. It gives the spine a high compressive strength and reduces the stress peaks in the posterior annulus fibrosus (Adams and Hutton 1985b; Adams et al. 1994).

Extension creep loading

Compared to flexion, prolonged maintenance of an extended posture when working is unusual, although prolonged standing tends to increase the lordosis. However, high peaks of repetitive extension loading occur in certain sports, such as fast bowlers in cricket, gymnasts and high jumpers. The forces involved are considerable as the inferior articular process impacts on the lamina of the vertebrae below – with the highest concentration on the pars interarticularis. Repetition of extension and flexion movements may cause fatigue fractures of the pars interarticularis – which is the site at which spondylolysis occurs (Twomey and Taylor 1994b) (see section in Chapter 13 for more detailed consideration).

Axial creep loading

Axial creep loading occurs each day after the recumbent posture during sleep. The pressure sustained by the intervertebral discs causes a loss of fluid, amounting to a 10% loss in disc height. The fluid loss means that the individual is 1 – 2% shorter at the end of the day, and the loss is made up during sleep when the discs are rehydrated due to the osmotic pressure of the proteoglycans. Rehydration occurs more rapidly in the flexed than in the extended position (Bogduk 1997). The average change in human stature throughout the day is about 19mm (Adams *et al.* 1990). In effect, the disc swells during the night and is compressed during the day. The changes in disc height occur rapidly: 26% of the loss over eight hours upright occurs in the first hour and 41% of recovery over four hours occurs in the first hour of rest (Krag *et al.* 1990).

Optimal sitting posture

Two recent studies (Harrison *et al.* 1999, 2000; Pynt *et al.* 2001) have reviewed the evidence relating to the optimal sitting and driving posture. Harrison *et al.* (1999), in a thorough review of the biomechanical and clinical literature, concluded that the consensus on the optimal sitting position included maintenance of the lordosis with a lumbar support, seat inclination backwards, arm rests and seating that allowed freedom of movement. Flexion in sitting was shown to cause several disadvantages, and the consensus was in favour of a lordosis when sitting.

Pynt *et al.* (2001) reviewed the advantages and disadvantages of the lordotic and kyphotic sitting posture, drawing mostly on cadaveric and a few clinical studies. They summarise the main arguments of proponents of both postures (Table 6.3). They found many of the arguments previously used by those who advocate the flexed posture to be flawed and unsubstantiated, and some of the data they re-evaluated. They conclude that the lordotic sitting posture, if regularly interrupted with movement, is the optimal seating position for spinal health and for preventing low back pain.

"In summary, then, a sustained lordosed sitting posture decreases disc pressure and thereby disc degeneration, exhibits less injurious levels of ligament tension, and although it increases zygapophyseal loading, this is not of itself considered hazardous to spinal health. A sustained kyphosed sitting posture, on the other hand, increases intradiscal pressure leading to increased fluid loss, decreased nutrition, and altered cell synthesis and biomechanics of the disc, appearing to culminate ultimately in disc degeneration that is a cause of low back pain" (Pynt et al. 2001, p. 14).

Table 6.3   Proposed advantages and disadvantages of kyphotic and lordotic sitting postures

Advantages of flexed position	*Disadvantages of flexed position*
Unload ZJ, but increase loading on IVD	Increase intradiscal pressure
	Increase tensile stress posterior AF
	Increase compressive load posterior AF
	Compressive force born entirely by IVD, ZJ only resists shear
	Poor position to resist creep
	Increased creep
	Dehydrates IVD
	Decreased nutrition

Advantages of lordotic position	*Disadvantages of lordotic position*
Decrease intradiscal pressure	
Reduce compressive forces on IVD	Increase compressive load posterior AF
Balance of forces acting on ZJ	Increases load on ZJ

AF = annulus fibrosus
IVD = intervertebral disc
ZJ = zygapophyseal joint

Source: Pynt *et al.* 2001

Effect of time of day on range of movement and biomechanics

Time of day affects not only the water content of the disc, and thus disc height, but this in turn affects range of movement and spinal biomechanics. Range of motion increases during the day (Ensink *et al.* 1996; Adams *et al.* 1987). There is a significant change in flexion and a smaller change in extension. From morning to evening one study found an average gain of eleven degrees of flexion, but only three degrees of extension (Ensink *et al.* 1996).

The axial creep loading that occurs during the day causes the disc to lose height, bulge more, and become stiffer in compression and more flexible in bending. Disc tissue becomes more elastic as the water content is reduced and disc prolapse becomes less likely. Maximal stress is thus exerted on the disc and posterior longitudinal ligament in the morning (Adams *et al.* 1990). Creep causes an increased stress on the annulus, a reduction of pressure on the nucleus pulposus and closer contact between the zygapophyseal joints (Adams 1994).

Because of the increased fluid content of the disc in the early morning, it is more resistant to flexion. Compared to later in the day, the stresses caused by forward bending are about 300% greater on the disc and 80% greater on the ligaments of the neural arch (Adams *et al.* 1987). Consequently, it is concluded that there is an increased risk of damage occurring to the disc when bending in the early morning. An experimental model using bovine discs has demonstrated that both flexion loading and high hydration rates were key factors in causing the break up and displacement of fragments of nucleus (Simunic *et al.* 2001).

Effect of posture on internal intervertebral disc stresses

Nachemson and colleagues in the 1960s (Nachemson and Morris 1964; Nachemson and Elfstrom 1970) performed the earliest measurements of disc pressures in vivo in a variety of normal postures (reviewed in Nachemson 1992). A needle attached to a miniature pressure transducer was placed in the nucleus pulposus of the L3 disc and measurements made in some common static positions, as well as some dynamic activities.

If the pressure in upright standing was 100%, in lying it was about 20 – 50%, and in sitting upright or leaning forward was about 150%. When sitting, the pressure in the disc is reduced by an inclined backrest, a low lumbar support, and the use of arm rests. Bending forward and lifting weights, whether sitting or standing, causes substantial increases in pressure – for instance, from 500 Newtons when standing at ease to 1700N when standing bending forward, weights in each hand, arms extended (Nachemson 1992).

Nachemson (1992) refers to six other reports that generally verified their preliminary findings. Quinnell and Stockdale (1983) confirmed the same relative disc pressures in lying, sitting and standing; however, the absolute values they recorded were less. Since these earlier studies of intradiscal pressure little new work has been done until recently. Wilke *et al.* (1999) performed a single case study of an individual with a non-degenerated L4 – L5 disc with pressure recordings over a twenty-four-hour period in a range of different activities. Their results generally correlated with Nachemson's data, except in one critical area. While the pressure in lying was 20% of relaxed standing, sitting slouched in a chair was also less, about 60% of standing. Turning over in bed, bending forward in sitting or standing, lifting and standing up from a chair all had the effect of causing substantial increases in pressure. Lifting with a rounded back caused considerably more pressure than lifting with knees bent and a straight back. Over a period of seven hours rest at night, pressure increased 240%.

On the finding that the intradiscal pressure in relaxed sitting may in fact be less than that in relaxed standing, the authors comment that both muscle activity and lumbar curvature affect the pressure. Slouched sitting may reduce pressure due to minimal muscle activity. The finding contradicts most other work that has been done in this field.

Another recent intradiscal pressure study reported findings from a group of patients and volunteers (Sato *et al.* 1999). Again, the pressure in lying was found to be much less than that in standing or sitting, and although the pressure in sitting was more than in standing, the difference was not substantial. Lying was about 20% of standing, sitting was about 20% more than standing, and the angles of flexion/extension had a considerable affect. While bending backwards in sitting or standing increased pressure by 10 – 20%, bending forward increased it by 100 –150%. The degree of disc degeneration correlated linearly with reduced intradiscal pressure – more degeneration, less pressure.

In summary, the magnitude of pressure in the disc is influenced by various factors, such as trunk muscle activity, posture, body weight, size of disc, disc degeneration and externally applied loads (Sato *et al.* 1999). Posture is only one component in the equation; however, these studies show that it has a potent affect upon the pressure within the disc. All the studies report a substantial decrease in intradiscal pressure when non-weight bearing. Sitting is generally, but not universally, found to cause a higher intradiscal pressure than standing. Extension raises intradiscal pressure, but considerably less than does flexion.

Nachemson's original findings were used to justify ergonomic concepts used in back school. Before extrapolating these findings to the clinical situation, some limitations ought to be recognised. If the intervertebral disc is severely degenerated, the hydrostatic property is lost; therefore all pressure measurements can only be done in individuals with relatively normal discs (Nachemson 1992). Painful discs are likely to be morphologically abnormal, in which instance pressures may be substantially different. Most of the early studies were done at L3 disc, while the majority of symptomatic pathology occurs at the lower two discs. Perhaps most importantly, these measurements are made in the nucleus pulposus, which is not the site of discogenic pain. This most commonly is in the outer annulus (Moneta *et al.* 1994).

A more recent technique, stress profilometry, has sought to evaluate stresses in the intervertebral disc in both the nucleus and the annulus. To date, most work on stress profilometry has been conducted in vitro, with only one in vivo study. Stress peaks vary according to the posture of the motion segment being tested. In a cadaver study, 'degenerated discs' exposed to extension showed a generalised increase in stress peaks in the posterior annulus, while flexion tended to equalise the compressive stress. However, in seven of the nineteen motion segments tested, lumbar extension decreased maximum compressive stress in the posterior annulus by a considerable amount (Adams *et al.* 2000a). See Chapter 4 on intervertebral disc for more detail.

Conclusions

The chief movements available at the lumbar spine are flexion and extension. Over time, an individual's mobility may vary because of the ageing process and because of back pain. Because there is a considerable range of normal values in mobility between people, movement loss must be judged against the individual's normal range and be correlated with pain response. Movement cannot be solely judged against some theoretical normative database.

With the use of everyday positions, the spine adopts movements of flexion, extension, and so on. These commonly adopted postures have clear effects on the lumbar curve, and patients' symptomatic responses to these loading strategies help us to understand their directional preference or lack of it. This understanding has important diagnostic and management implications.

Movements have different physiological affects on the lumbar spine, and in particular on the intervertebral disc. Some of this data comes from cadaveric studies, and extrapolation from in vitro studies to real life should not be taken too far. Nonetheless, it is apparent that different postures and movements influence internal disc dynamics and disc pressures. The role of loading history in causing fatigue damage to collagenous structures, such as the disc, is clearly significant in morphological change and in back pain. The frequency with which patients report that their musculoskeletal pain developed for 'no apparent reason' becomes understandable in this context.

7: Diagnosis and Classification

Introduction

Despite the technological advances that have been made in recent years, we are still unable to identify the origin of back pain in the majority of patients. Even with the advent of advanced imaging technology, such as computerised axial tomography (CAT) scanning and magnetic resonance imaging (MRI), our ability to identify the precise structure that generates symptoms and the exact nature of the pathology affecting it remains extremely limited.

Fordyce *et al.* (1995) lists the following as known causes of specific back pain with our present state of knowledge:

- disc herniation

- spondylolisthesis, usually in the young

- spinal stenosis, usually in the older age group

- definite instability, exceeding 4 – 5mm on flexion-extension radiographs

- vertebral fractures, tumours, infections and inflammatory diseases.

He goes on to state: *"The best evidence suggests that fewer than 15% of persons with back pain can be assigned to one of these categories of specific low back pain"* (Spitzer *et al.* 1987). However, ambiguities exist even about some of these conditions – in middle-aged patients the association between spondylolisthesis and back pain is weak and only found in women (Virta and Ronnemaa 1993). *"There is lack of scientific agreement on how to define spinal instability"* (AHCPR 1994), and sagittal translation exceeding 4mm is found in those without back pain (Woody *et al.* 1983; Hayes *et al.* 1989). Furthermore, even within these groups, the most efficacious treatment has not been clearly defined. The vast majority of the back pain population, the other 85% at least, belong in the realm of non-specific back pain where the ambiguity of their diagnosis rests on the particular 'expert' that they consult (Deyo 1993).

While both clinicians and patients await the elucidation of this diagnostic ambiguity, management must be offered to those who seek health care for the problem of back pain. If a diagnosis cannot be clearly made, classification systems may be a clinically useful way to characterise different sub-groups and their management strategies.

This chapter considers some of the issues concerning diagnosis and back pain. It describes the most widely adopted classification systems in use, those described by the Quebec Task Force (Spitzer *et al.* 1987), and the US and UK guidelines for back care (AHCPR 1994; CSAG 1994). The categories within these systems will be used to indicate those patients who are contraindicated for mechanical diagnosis and therapy and those who may be selected for a mechanical evaluation.

Sections in this chapter are as follows:

* identification of specific pathology

* classification of back pain

* Quebec Task Force classification

* classification by pain pattern

* other classification systems

* diagnostic triage

* indications for mechanical diagnosis and therapy

* factors in history that suggest a good response

* contraindications for mechanical diagnosis and therapy.

Identification of specific pathology

Although some specific diagnoses such as spinal stenosis or disc herniation may be suspected from clinical examination, to confirm such a diagnosis requires paraclinical investigations. Sophisticated imaging studies, blood tests or biopsies are examples of tests used to confirm a diagnosis. One way of interpreting clinical tests is their ability to relate an abnormal finding to the presence of disease. *Sensitivity* is the term used to describe those who have the 'disease' that are correctly identified as 'disease positive' by the test. *Specificity* is the term used to describe those who do not have the 'disease' that are correctly identified as 'disease negative' by the test (Altman 1991). A key failing of many types of spinal imaging, however sophisticated, is their inability to relate pathology to symptoms. Abnormal morphology may be found in individuals who have no symptoms, thus the specificity of that test is poor. In effect, many people may be told, for instance, that they have degenerative disease of the lumbar spine, when in fact these radiographic findings are not related to their symptoms – these are false-positive findings. To base diagnosis and management upon these findings alone is seriously questionable.

A recent systematic review of studies looking at the association between radiographic findings and non-specific back pain concluded that there was no firm evidence for a causal relationship between the two (van Tulder *et al.* 1997c). Spondylolysis, spondylolisthesis, spina bifida, transitional vertebrae, spondylosis and Scheuermann's disease did not appear to be associated with back pain. Degeneration, defined by the presence of disc space narrowing, osteophytes and sclerosis, appears to be associated with back pain, but not in any causal way (van Tulder *et al.* 1997c). When any of these abnormalities are found on radiography, 40 – 50% will be false-positive findings; that is, found in those with no back pain (Roland and van Tulder 1998). The authors suggest that a finding of advanced disc degeneration on radiography should have this information inserted in any report: *"Roughly 40% of patients with this finding do not have back pain, so finding may be unrelated"*. They advise similar caveats to accompany the reporting of any of the other morphological abnormalities listed above.

The more sophisticated imaging studies are also associated with poor specificity. Computer-assisted tomography (CAT) found abnormalities, mostly disc herniation, in about 20% of asymptomatic individuals younger than 40 and in 50% of asymptomatic individuals older than 40 (Wiesel *et al.* 1984).

Numerous studies have identified the very high rate of false-positive findings on magnetic resonance imaging (MRI) of the lumbar spine. Bulging or protruded discs have been found in over 50% of asymptomatic individuals (Jensen *et al.* 1994; Weinreb *et al.* 1989), and in those over 60 years 36% of subjects had a disc herniation and 21% had spinal stenosis (Boden *et al.* 1990). When patients were matched to controls by age, sex and physical risk factors, 76% of the asymptomatic controls had protrusions or extrusions of the disc, which in 22% even included neural compromise. In the patients, the respective proportions were 96% and 83% (Boos *et al.* 1995). Patterns of disc disruption have been seen as commonly in volunteers without back pain as in patients (Buirski and Silberstein 1993), and MRI has failed to reliably predict symptomatic discs that have been identified by discography (Brightbill *et al.* 1994; Horton and Daftari 1992).

These studies clearly show that imaging studies *by themselves* have very little value in identifying abnormal morphology of symptomatic significance, and thus should not be used to formulate diagnosis or treatment in isolation from the patient's clinical presentation. Imaging studies can identify abnormal morphology, but this may not be relevant. It is well recognised that in the case of disc herniations imaging studies should be used to confirm the findings of a clinical evaluation – the diagnosis can only be confirmed by MRI or CAT, but in the absence of the clinical presentation false-positive findings are likely (Deyo *et al.* 1990).

Some authors argue that with the use of intra-articular or disc stimulating injections, a source of pain may be found in over 60% of back pain patients (Bogduk *et al.* 1996). According to their criteria, the prevalence of discogenic pain is about 39%, the prevalence of zygapophyseal joint pain is about 15% and the prevalence of sacro-iliac joint pain is about 12%. These diagnoses, however, rely upon invasive procedures involving significant exposure to x-rays, which are costly and require high levels of skill – they are not a realistic alternative for the majority of back pain patients. Furthermore, while injections may identify these diagnostic groups, no clinical criteria have been revealed that would allow their identification by simpler means, and at this stage no effective treatments exist for such diagnoses.

Mechanical evaluation can identify and affect the mechanism of symptom generation. The McKenzie assessment process has been found to be superior to MRI in distinguishing painful from non-painful discs. *"A non-invasive, low-tech, relatively inexpensive clinical assessment using repeated end-range lumbar test movements can provide considerably more relevant information than non-invasive imaging studies"* (Donelson *et al.* 1997).

Our desire as clinicians to diagnose and label back pain should be circumspect with a natural humility in light of the above. Using unproven pathological labels may not only be a fraudulent attempt to augment our professional credibility, it may also lead to exaggerated illness behaviour by patients and abnormal treatment patterns by clinicians.

"We use unproven labels for the symptoms of back pain; our ability to diagnose 'facet syndrome' has been disproven in several randomised trials. 'Degenerative disc disease' is common among all of us above 30 years of age. 'Isolated disc resorption' is a common diagnosis presumed to require fusion operation on in some parts of the world. 'Segmental instability' is also generally undefined. These are diagnostic 'waste baskets' into which we sort our patients. Abnormal diagnostic behaviour leads some patients into sick role behaviour. Patients become afraid, they ask, 'Can you cure degenerative disc disease?' Ill-defined labels help to produce a person who cannot cope, leading to illness behaviour, which in turn might lead physicians and surgeons to perform 'abnormal' treatment" (Nachemson 1999a, p. 475).

Classification of back pain

In the absence of clear diagnoses, classification systems provide several advantages (Spitzer *et al.* 1987; Fairbank and Pynsent 1992; Delitto *et al.* 1995). They help in making clinical decisions, may aid in establishing a prognosis, and are likely to lead to more effective treatment if patients are treated with regard to classification. They aid communication between clinicians and offer an effective method of teaching students. Classification systems also further our understanding of different sub-groups and should be used in the conduct of audit and research.

Unfortunately, there exists a wide variety of back pain classifications from which to choose (Fairbank and Pynsent 1992; Riddle 1998), and more systems continue to appear. Three classification systems based on extensive research reviews will be briefly mentioned (Spitzer *et al.* 1987; AHCPR 1994; CSAG 1994). These highlight the fact that most back pain is non-specific, but also that we must be aware of certain specific pathologies that are far less common — nerve root pathology and serious spinal pathology.

Quebec Task Force classification

After an exhaustive review of the literature, the Quebec Task Force (QTF) reported on Activity-Related Spinal Disorders (Spitzer *et al.* 1987), within which they addressed the problem of diagnosis. They highlighted the fact that in the vast majority pain is the only symptom — which, although initially nociceptive in origin, can be influenced by psychological and social factors during the progression into chronicity. Although pain may develop due to irritation of bones, discs, joints, nerves, muscles and soft tissues, the identification of the precise origin of pain is difficult. Pain characteristics are generally non-specific for different structures, and clinical observations cannot easily be corroborated through objective methods. *"Non-specific ailments of back pain....with or without radiation of pain, comprise the vast majority of problems"* (Spitzer *et al.* 1987).

The QTF determined that their classification system must be compatible with present knowledge, universally applicable, involve mutually exclusive categories, be reliable between clinicians, be clinically useful and be simple to use. Using these criteria as a guide, the QTF recommended the following classification be universally adopted.

Table 7.1   QTF classification of back pain

1. Back pain without radiation
2. Back pain with radiation to proximal extremity
3. Back pain with radiation to distal extremity
4. Back pain with radiation to distal extremity and positive neurological signs (i.e. focal muscle weakness, asymmetry of reflexes, sensory loss in a dermatome, or loss of bladder, bowel or sexual function)
5. Presumptive compression of a spinal nerve root on radiographs (i.e. instability or fracture)
6. Compression of a spinal nerve root confirmed by special imaging techniques (i.e. as category 4 with moderate or severe findings on neuroradiological review at appropriate level)
7. Spinal stenosis
8. Post-surgical status, 1 – 6 months after intervention, asymptomatic (8.1) or symptomatic (8.2)
9. Post-surgical status, > 6 months after intervention, asymptomatic (9.1) or symptomatic (9.2)
10. Chronic pain syndrome
11. Other diagnoses (i.e. metastases, visceral disease and fracture).

Source: Spitzer *et al.* 1987

Their first four categories represent *most* cases and are determined by history-taking and clinical assessment, categories 5 – 7 depend upon paraclinical investigations and categories 8 – 10 on response to treatment. Each of the first four classifications is subdivided by a temporal division into acute (< 7 days), sub-acute (7 days – 7 weeks) and chronic (> 7 weeks), as well as work status (working or idle).

Categories 1, 2 and 3 describe disorders of somatic structures, while QTF 4 and 6 describe disorders affecting the nerve root as well. QTF 4 includes the classic radicular syndromes most frequently caused by disc herniations; if this is confirmed by an imaging study, this becomes QTF 6.

Classification by pain pattern

The QTF uses pain pattern as a means of classification of non-specific back pain. Pain pattern is certainly an indicator of severity. Patients with sciatica or referred symptoms are substantially more disabled (Leclaire *et al.* 1997) and have a more protracted rate of recovery and return to work than patients with back pain alone (Andersson *et al.* 1983; Hagen and Thune 1998). Leg or sciatic pain is a factor that is commonly recognised as having a poorer prognosis for recovery and a greater likelihood of developing chronic symptoms (Goertz 1990; Lanier and Stockton 1988; Chavannes *et al.* 1986; Cherkin *et al.* 1996a; Carey *et al.* 2000; Thomas *et al.* 1999), and as a risk factor for predicting future episodes of back pain (Smedley *et al.* 1998; Muller *et al.* 1999).

When the QTF classification system or a similar system has been used, higher categories are associated with increasing severity of symptoms and reduced functional ability (Atlas *et al.* 1996a; Selim *et al.* 1998; BenDebba *et al.* 2000). The hierarchical classification demonstrated progressive increases in the intensity of pain, associated disability, the use of medical services and a gradual reduction in health-related quality of life. *"Patients with equivocal evidence of radiculopathy tend to have intermediate impairment, compared with the impairment in those with sciatica and with the impairment in those with LBP alone"* (Selim *et al.* 1998). Patients with distal leg pain and positive neural tension signs were nine times more likely to receive an advanced imaging study than patients with back pain only, and thirteen times more likely to come to surgery (BenDebba *et al.* 2000). The natural history and clinical course of patients in QTF categories 4 and 6 is frequently poor. Of 82 consecutive patients followed for a year following in-patient conservative therapy, only 29% were fully recovered and 33% had come to surgery. Most recovery occurred in the first three months, after which there was little further improvement (Balague *et al.* 1999).

The QTF recommendations support the concept of classification of non-specific spinal disorders by utilising pain patterns. The first four categories of the QTF are very similar to the pain pattern classification first proposed by McKenzie (1981). The classification offers a way of monitoring deteriorating or improving spinal disorders. Movements or positions that produce increasing peripheral symptoms are to be avoided. The centralisation of pain results from a reduction in the deformation or compression of the nerve root and articular structures, and thus movements or positions that cause this abolition of peripheral symptoms are to be encouraged. By causing tingling in the outer toes to cease and pain felt below the knee to change location to the buttock and thigh, the severity of the condition is reduced and the classification changes from QTF 4 to QTF 2. *This simple way of monitoring symptoms provides clinicians with a reliable way to judge a worsening or improving clinical situation and thus the appropriateness of certain procedures.*

Rather than representing different categories within the back pain population, the different pain patterns actually represent stages of the same problem that commonly change during the natural history of the episode as it waxes and wanes. They represent a way of monitoring the status (improving, worsening or unchanging) of a condition and the response to therapeutic loading strategies. Any loading that reduces, abolishes or centralises distal pain should be pursued, just as alternatively any loading that produces, increases or peripheralises pain should be avoided. It is hoped that we will change a patient with QTF category 3 to QTF 1, prior to complete abolition of pain. *The value of pain pattern classification is thus not in representing distinct categories, but as a means of monitoring symptom severity and response to therapeutic loading strategies.*

Other classification systems

Two national guidelines published in the USA (AHCPR 1994) and the UK (CSAG 1994) have recommended an even simpler classification system based upon a hierarchy of pathological risk. After determining that it is a musculoskeletal problem, the initial focused assessment should classify patients into one of three groups:

- serious spinal pathology – cauda equina syndrome, cancer, neurological disorder, inflammatory disease, etc.

- nerve root problems – disc herniation, spinal stenosis

- mechanical backache – non-specific back and radiating leg pain representing the majority of patients, in which symptoms vary with different physical activities and time.

Diagnostic triage

Within this diagnostic triage, the majority of all patients will be in the 'simple backache' group, with true nerve root problems said to affect less than 5%, and less than 2% due to serious spinal disease (such as tumour or infection) and inflammatory conditions (CSAG 1994). There is some overlap between the three classification systems. Respectively these groups represent QTF categories 1, 2, 3 (mechanical backache), QTF categories 4, 5, 6, 7 (nerve root pathology) and QTF category 11 (serious spinal pathology).

The first category, mechanical backache, describes the patients most commonly referred for conservative physiotherapy treatment by physicians. The second category, nerve root pathology, describes a much smaller group who are also seen regularly and are often suitable for conservative treatment. The last category, serious spinal pathology, is unsuitable for conservative treatment. It is hoped that most patients attending physiotherapy will have been screened by medical practitioners and those with unsuitable pathologies excluded. However, in case unsuitable patients are referred, and as physioclinicians are more commonly becoming first-line practitioners in assessing back pain patients, *an awareness of the 'red flags' indicating serious spinal pathology is imperative*. The first task is to screen out patients who have 'red flags', which indicate serious spinal pathology.

Serious spinal pathology
These conditions are very unusual; in a cohort of over 400 patients with acute back pain in primary care, six (1.4%) had 'red flag' conditions (McGuirk *et al.* 2001). Three of these had fractures and three had carcinomas. A few key questions during the medical history could alert clinicians to 'red flag' pathology and ensure that serious underlying conditions, such as cancer, inflammatory diseases or significant neurological disorders are not missed (AHCPR 1994; CSAG 1994; Deyo *et al.* 1992):

Cauda equina syndrome/widespread neurological disorder:

- bladder dysfunction (usually urinary retention or overflow incontinence)

- loss of anal sphincter tone or faecal incontinence

- saddle anaesthesia about the anus, perineum or genitals

- global or progressive motor weakness in the lower limbs.

Possible serious spinal pathology (cancer, infection, fracture):

- age (>55)

- history of cancer

- unexplained weight loss

- constant, progressive, non-mechanical pain, worse at rest

- systemically unwell

- persisting severe restriction of lumbar flexion

- widespread neurology

- systemic steroids

- history of intravenous drug use

- history of significant trauma enough to cause fracture or dislocation (x-rays will not always detect fractures)

- history of trivial trauma and severe pain in potential osteoporotic individual

- no movement or position centralises, decreases or abolishes pain.

Possible inflammatory disorders:

- gradual onset

- marked morning stiffness

- persisting limitation of movements in all directions

- peripheral joint involvement

- iritis, psoriasis, colitis, uretheral discharge

- family history

- no movement or position centralises, decreases or abolishes pain.

Management

It is imperative (CSAG 1994) that patients with symptoms indicating spinal cord damage, cauda equina syndrome or a widespread neurological disorder are referred to a specialist immediately. *For these patients, mechanical therapy is absolutely contra-indicated*. If there is not a direct referral system to a specialist, you must send these patients directly to the emergency department. Although very rare, it is extremely important that patients who are suspected of having these conditions are sent to the appropriate specialist straight away.

Failure to react promptly to a patient who reports loss of bladder control can result in permanent loss of bladder, bowel and sexual function. A recent retrospective review of patients who had had surgery for cauda equina syndrome highlighted the need for urgency of referral in such cases (Shapiro 2000). Patients who had the diagnosis made and surgery performed within 48 hours of onset were compared to those who had surgery more than 48 hours after onset. Those who had delayed surgery were significantly more likely to have persistent bladder and bowel incontinence, severe motor deficit, sexual dysfunction and persistent pain.

Patients with other possible serious spinal pathology or inflammatory disorders should also be referred to the appropriate specialists. *For these patients, mechanical therapy is absolutely contra-indicated*. If there are suspicious clinical features or if acute pain has not settled in six weeks, an erythrocyte sedimentation rate test and plain radiograph should be considered (CSAG 1994).

Detailed descriptions of specific examples of serious spinal pathology are given in a Chapter 12. Assessment for 'red flag' pathology is also included in the chapter on history-taking (14).

Nerve root problems

The following aspects of the clinical presentation gained during the history-taking can indicate nerve root pain (CSAG 1994; AHCPR 1994):

•   unilateral leg pain > back pain

•   pain radiating to foot or toes, especially in dermatomal pattern

•   numbness or paraesthesia in the same distribution

•   history of weakness in the legs

- history of neurogenic claudication (limitation of walking distance due to leg pain).

The following signs, gathered during the physical examination, will heighten suspicion of neurological involvement (CSAG 1994; AHCPR 1994):

- weakness of ankle dorsiflexion, or great toe or calf and hamstring muscles, suggesting involvement of L4, or L5 or S1 nerve roots

- loss of ankle reflex, suggesting involvement of S1 nerve root

- loss of sensation in area of medial ankle, big toe or lateral foot, suggesting involvement of L4, or L5 or S1 nerve roots

- reduced straight leg raise

- cross straight leg raise (in which straight leg raising the opposite leg increases symptoms in the painful leg)

- in patients with irreducible disc herniations or spinal stenosis, no movement or position will be found that will centralise, decrease or abolish pain.

This abbreviated neurological examination will detect most clinically significant nerve root pathology at the lower lumbar levels (L4 – L5 and L5 – S1), where over 90% of all disc herniations occur (AHCPR 1994; Deyo *et al.* 1990). It will miss the much less common lesions involving upper lumbar levels. These may be suspected with anterior thigh pain and reduced sensation, quadriceps weakness and reduced quadriceps reflex – present in less than 5% of patients with proven disc herniations (Deyo *et al.* 1990). Patients with nerve root involvement usually do not display all the above signs and symptoms. Patients with stenosis generally present with fewer neurological signs, are much less likely to have the marked root tension signs found in those with disc herniation and complain of intermittent claudication.

Established musculoskeletal causes of nerve root problems, which may be suspected clinically but need paraclinical investigations to be confirmed, are:

- disc herniations

- spinal stenosis

- malignant and non-malignant tumours (rare).

Management

The two main causes of nerve root pathology are disc herniations and spinal stenosis. Disc disease is discussed in more detail in Chapter 4, and the clinical features of sciatica in Chapter 5. It is important to be aware that this diagnosis represents a continuum from reducible protrusions through to non-contained sequestrations, whose prognosis is very different. For many the prognoses with conservative management is reasonable, and this is the recommended approach at least in the first six weeks – during which period 50% are said to recover from the acute attack (CSAG 1994; Deyo *et al.* 1990), although this seems rather over-optimistic. A minority, with the more extreme pathology, may need surgery. Stenosis, although irreversible, is usually not progressive and is discussed in more detail later.

Management decisions must be made with awareness of the greater pain and disability often associated with nerve root problems compared to simple backache. As a consequence, these patients may respond more slowly, and some may not respond at all to conservative treatment. In pathological terms, the two entities of backache and nerve root problems represent different conditions affecting different structures with different natural histories. See Chapter 3 for a summary of somatic and radicular pain. *However, there is no reason to differentiate these groups as far as initial management is concerned.* These were the patients referred to previously (McKenzie 1981) as those with derangement 5 or 6. Greater caution should be exercised when testing patients with nerve root problems.

Simple or mechanical backache

The criteria for this group are as follows (CSAG 1994):

* mostly aged 20 – 55 years at onset

* lumbosacral region, buttocks and thighs

* 'mechanical' in nature; that is, the pain varies with physical activity and over time

* patient is generally well.

In essence, after those with specific serious pathology or nerve root involvement, this is all the rest – that is, the majority of those who have back problems.

This group includes those previously (McKenzie 1981) referred to as having derangement 1, 2, 3 and 4, dysfunction and postural syndrome and also those with other entities such as sacro-iliac joint, hip problems or those with symptomatic spondylolisthesis.

Management

The initial management pathway for both simple backache and nerve root problems should be the same. A mechanical evaluation should follow the history-taking, and details from both elements of data gathering should be used in patient classification. Following the mechanical evaluation, which is described later, many patients are classified as mechanical responders and management using extension, lateral, flexion, or some combination of forces can be instigated. Some patients with nerve root pathology display signs of non-contained disc lesions – that is, not amenable to conservative therapy – irreducible derangements. Other mechanical non-responders may belong in other categories such as stenosis, sacro-iliac joint (SIJ) problems, spondylolisthesis or chronic back pain.

Indications for mechanical diagnosis and therapy

The majority of back pain patients, with or without referred symptoms, thus include those ideally suitable for a mechanical evaluation either by repetitive end-range motion and/or static loading. The effect of repeated or static end-range loading on pain patterns can determine, often on day one, the potential of that patient to respond to mechanical therapy. Treatment response indicators are looked for during the mechanical evaluation when a directional preference or other consistent mechanical response is sought, thus indicating the presence of one of the three mechanical syndromes (derangement most commonly, followed by dysfunction and then posture). This will include the majority of patients with non-specific spinal pain. By using such an assessment, we can classify sub-groups within the non-specific spectrum of mechanical spinal disorders – that is derangement, dysfunction, or posture syndromes. Thus we are able to identify those patients who may be helped and, just as importantly, those who are unlikely to respond to mechanical therapy.

Some patients in QTF classifications 3 and 4 may turn out to have irreducible derangements or present clinically as spinal stenosis (QTF 7). Patients who fit into QTF category 4, with significant motor deficit and severe constant pain due to nerve root irritation, are less likely to respond because of the severity of their pathology. However, a trial of mechanical therapy is always valuable as there are exceptions, and those who have intermittent symptoms of nerve root interference should certainly be evaluated. Once nerve root compression has been confirmed with imaging studies (QTF 6), the likelihood of surgical intervention is much greater (Atlas *et al.* 1996a).

In others in whom a consistent mechanical response is not forthcoming when mechanical therapy has been tested for several days, other classifications may need to be considered. Chapter 13 gives descriptions of conditions not encompassed within the three mechanical syndromes described previously (McKenzie 1981). These may need to be considered in the differential diagnosis, *but only if the response is atypical to one of these syndromes*. The history and mechanical evaluation, which is described later, allows classification into one of the mechanical syndromes (derangement, dysfunction or posture). Classification is confirmed or questioned by the patient's response to mechanical therapy, which can involve testing over several days. If classification into a mechanical syndrome is not confirmed, differential diagnosis should be considered. It is thus essential to conduct a full mechanical evaluation in all suitable cases before proceeding to include non-mechanical differential diagnoses. *Secondary classifications should only be considered once the extended mechanical evaluation has ruled out a consistent mechanical response.*

Once this has been done, the specific and non-specific categories (see Chapter 13) are those commonly considered in the literature; this includes spinal stenosis, hip joint problems, SIJ, back pain in pregnancy, zygapophyseal joint problems, spondylolisthesis, instability, mechanically inconclusive, post-surgical and chronic pain syndromes. The descriptions given make clear that while the existence of some of these categories are both substantiated by the literature and putative recognition is clinically feasible, for other categories the evidence fails to endorse their existence as a clinical entity and/ or their recognition through physical examination.

The classification algorithm and the accompanying criteria and operational definitions are detailed in the appendix.

Factors in history that suggest a good response

An episodic history of back pain

Several aspects of history indicate factors that are frequently associated with a good response to mechanical diagnosis and therapy. Patients who have experienced recurring episodes of back and referred pain can do very well on the protocols outlined in this book. These patients describe long periods – weeks or months at a time – when they are completely symptom-free and can move fully and freely, and then unexpectedly they develop another episode of back pain. Patients with such a history can be very receptive to ideas on better self-management of their condition, especially if they have received passive or manipulative therapy in the past that has provided short-term relief, but given them no better long-term control. When taught appropriate exercises, these patients feel much more able to self-manage their problem by reducing the rate of recurrences and by resurrecting the exercises if symptoms return (Udermann *et al.* 2000, 2001; McKenzie 1979; Laslett and Michaelsen 1991). Not providing patients with the ability to manage their recurrent problem better is clearly poor practice.

Intermittent back pain

A second and perhaps more significant factor denoting those patients who will be most responsive is the group who feel their symptoms intermittently; that is, there are times during the day when, as a result of being in certain positions or performing certain activities or for no apparent reason, the patient has no pain. Even in those patients who have had symptoms for years and may be deemed chronic, intermittent symptoms indicate the likelihood of a good prognosis. Back pain that behaves in this way is demonstrating mechanically responsive pain – certain positions or movements are causing strain upon spinal tissues that generates pain, while other positions or movements reduce deformation of spinal tissues and relieve the pain. Frequently patients are very aware of postures that aggravate or relieve their symptoms, and educating them to temporarily avoid aggravating factors and make use of reductive factors is very straightforward.

If patients have pain and paraesthesia below the knee on an intermittent basis, they should respond well to the appropriate procedures. However, should they have constant pain below the knee, constant paraesthesia or numbness and motor or reflex deficit, rapid resolution is much less likely, and failure to respond to conservative care is common.

Variability in pain pattern

Another factor that can be a good predictor of a patient who responds well to mechanical therapy is when the patient reports that their pain changes location. It might be on the left sometimes, or at times on the right of their spine. Alternatively, a patient might report that the distal spread of their pain varies during the day and with different physical activities. Sometimes they only have back pain, and sometimes it radiates into their thigh or leg. They could report that in maintaining certain postures such as sitting they experience leg pain, but this is abolished when they walk about. This variability of pain pattern often indicates a patient who will do well with the management strategies outlined in this book.

A good indication of patient suitability for this approach to treatment is often obtained on day one during the mechanical assessment. If, during the initial testing procedures, pain centralisation or reduction of pain intensity occurs, this is invariably indicative of a good prognosis. However, it is sometimes necessary to conduct the mechanical evaluation over several days in order to ensure exposure of response.

Contraindications for mechanical diagnosis and therapy

Patients whose history suggests 'red flag' pathology are absolutely unsuitable for treatment. Those with suspected fractures, metastases, cauda equina, bone weakening disease or progressive neurological disease should be *immediately* referred on for further investigation (see Chapter 12). Usually a full mechanical evaluation is unnecessary as the relevant information can be gained during the initial interview. *A full mechanical assessment might be contraindicated in such individuals.* Patients with suspected but as yet undiagnosed inflammatory joint diseases, such as rheumatoid arthritis, ankylosing spondylitis, Reiter's syndrome, etc. should be referred for rheumatological assessment.

Conclusions

This chapter has described the initial algorithm for evaluation of those with back pain. In very general terms, patients either present with mechanical low back pain, nerve root pathology or serious spinal pathology. The latter, if detected, is unsuitable for mechanical diagnosis and therapy and any patient with the features outlined above should be referred on to a specialist – these are considered in more detail in the chapter on serious spinal pathology (Chapter 12).

Ninety-eight percent or more of patients with back pain are suitable for a mechanical evaluation, including those with and without signs of nerve root involvement. The full mechanical assessment, which is described later, seeks to identify those patients whose conditions are mechanically responsive and fit into one of the mechanical syndromes. These are described in the chapters on derangement, dysfunction and posture syndromes. Testing for them should be carried out over several days.

Not all patients fit neatly into one of the mechanical syndromes. During the period of mechanical evaluation, atypical or inconclusive responses may arise. In this instance one of the specific or non-specific categories described in Chapter 13 should be considered.

Table 7.2 gives an outline of initial clinical categories. The anatomical definitions for specific categories, their criteria and operational definitions are detailed in the appendix – *this is essential reading*. The clinical reasoning algorithm focusing on the mechanical syndromes is given in more detail in the next chapter. Descriptions of serious spinal pathology, the mechanical syndromes and other categories are given in later chapters.

Table 7.2   **Initial management pathway – key categories, estimated prevalence in back pain population**

Serious spinal pathology <2%	*Nerve root pathology <10%*	*Simple backache >90%*
Specialist referral	Mechanical evaluation	Mechanical evaluation
	Mechanical responders	Mechanical non-responders
		Irreducible derangements
		Other

Patients with either simple back pain or that involving nerve root signs or symptoms can be considered for initial mechanical evaluation. Most of these will prove to be positive mechanical responders. A few will be non-responders due to irreducible derangements or other pathology. A very small number of patients present with 'red flags' indicating serious spinal pathology – for such patients mechanical therapy is contraindicated and urgent appropriate referral is required.

8: Mechanical Diagnosis

Introduction

As discussed in the chapter on diagnosis and classification, specific diagnoses within the field of spine care are still largely illusory. For this reason non-specific classifications have been suggested, except in the instance of serious spinal pathology (Spitzer *et al.* 1987; CSAG 1994; AHCPR 1994). McKenzie (1981, 1990) proposed three non-specific mechanical syndromes – posture, dysfunction and derangement – which are now widely used in musculoskeletal care.

A syndrome is a characteristic group of symptoms and pattern of happenings typical of a particular problem (*Chambers Dictionary*). It describes an entity that is recognisable by its typical pattern of symptoms, which can be used to guide treatment as it also describes a distinguishing pattern of responses. Syndrome recognition is achieved through a mechanical evaluation – that is, a focused history-taking and physical examination.

The three separate mechanical syndromes can be recognised by certain features of the clinical presentation and by applying a structured sequence of loading. The characteristic of each in response to repeated and/or sustained end-range loading is completely different. Correct identification allows the application of the appropriate mechanical therapy. Within these syndromes can be found the vast majority of non-specific spinal problems.

The history-taking and physical examination that is required in order to explore each clinical presentation is given in later chapters. This chapter briefly defines the three mechanical syndromes and their accompanying conceptual models. Their clinical presentations and more detail will be given in the chapters relevant to each syndrome.

Sections in this chapter are as follows:

- derangement syndrome
- dysfunction syndrome
- postural syndrome

- the role of mechanical diagnosis and therapy in the management of back pain.

Derangement syndrome

This is the most common of the three mechanical syndromes encountered in spinal problems. The clinical pattern in derangement is much more variable than in the other two syndromes. Pain from derangement can arise gradually or suddenly. Pain can be constant or intermittent, it may move from side to side, and proximally and distally; repeated movements and sustained postures can rapidly and progressively worsen or improve the severity and spread of pain. Signs and symptoms may be either somatic, radicular or a combination of the two, depending on the severity of the condition. Derangement syndrome is also characterised by a mechanical presentation, which usually includes diminished range or obstruction of movement and may include temporary deformity and deviation of normal movement pathways. Because both the symptomatic and mechanical presentations are influenced by postural loading strategies during activities of daily living, they may vary during the day and over time. Inconsistency and change are characteristic of derangement.

Internal derangement causes a disturbance in the normal resting position of the affected joint surfaces. Internal displacement of articular tissue of whatever origin will cause pain to remain constant until such time as the displacement is reduced. Internal displacement of articular tissue obstructs movement.

The conceptual model that has been used to explain derangement syndrome relates the presentation to internal intervertebral disc displacements (McKenzie 1981, 1990). These may present in a variety of different ways, as derangements are a continuum. At its embryonic stage, individuals may suffer from brief bouts of back pain and minor limitations of function that last only a few days and resolve spontaneously. At its most extreme, the internally displaced tissue overcomes the restraining outer wall of the annulus fibrosus and extrudes into the spinal or intervertebral canal, causing predominantly radicular signs and symptoms. The conceptual model is discussed at length in Chapter 9.

The derangement syndrome is clearly distinguishable from the other mechanical syndromes, both by its presentation and its response to loading strategies. A unique characteristic of the derangement syndrome is the ability of therapeutic loading strategies to bring about lasting changes in the symptoms and mechanics of back pain. Certain loading patterns may cause pain to worsen or peripheralise, while opposite loading strategies cause a reduction, abolition or centralisation of symptoms and a recovery of movement. These types of changes are only found in derangement syndrome. Many derangements respond to extension and some to lateral or flexion loading – these would be the principles applied to reduce the derangement, restore mobility and improve the symptoms.

In some instances of more severe derangements, no loading strategy is able to exert a lasting change on symptoms. All treatment principles either have no effect or else only produce a worsening or peripheralisation of symptoms. In this instance the mechanical evaluation has detected an irreducible derangement. When related to the conceptual model, this concerns an incompetent or ruptured outer annular wall that is not amenable to resolution by loading strategies and is at the extreme end of the pathological continuum.

Derangement syndrome is characterised by a varied clinical presentation and typical responses to loading strategies. This includes worsening or peripheralisation of symptoms in response to certain postures and movements. It also includes the decrease, abolition or centralisation of symptoms and the restoration of normal movement in response to therapeutic loading strategies.

Dysfunction syndrome

In the dysfunction syndrome, pain is never constant and appears only as the affected structures are mechanically loaded. Pain will stop almost immediately on cessation of loading. When affecting articular structures, the dysfunction syndrome is always characterised by intermittent pain and a restriction of **end-range movement**. When affecting contractile structures, functional impairment is demonstrated when the muscle or tendon is loaded at any or certain points during the physiological range. Movements and positions consistently cause pain to be produced, but symptoms cease when the position or loading is ended.

It is relatively straightforward to distinguish these separate types of dysfunction in extremity problems, whereas in the spine the distinction is not so clear. In the spine the syndrome presents as articular dysfunction, with pain at limited end-range.

Pain from the dysfunction syndrome is caused by mechanical deformation of structurally impaired tissues. This abnormal tissue may be the product of previous trauma or inflammatory or degenerative processes. These events cause contraction, scarring, adherence, adaptive shortening or imperfect repair. Pain is felt when the abnormal tissue is loaded.

Dysfunction syndrome arises from a past history of some kind, such as trauma or a previous episode of back pain, or it can arise insidiously, resulting from years of poor posture or degenerative changes. There may have been a previous episode of back pain, the original cause of which has recovered by fibrous repair. Six to eight weeks later the individual is left with persistent symptoms each time they stretch the affected tissue, and full function does not return, or persisting poor postural habit could have the effect of overstretching ligamentous and capsular structures, causing minor but recurrent micro-trauma and repair. Eventually this may lead to a loss of elasticity, a restricted range of movement and pain when the affected tissues are stretched. Whatever the initial cause, adaptive shortening of tissues now causes a painful restricted end of range; pain is produced each time the affected tissue is stretched or compressed, but abates as soon as the position is released. In each instance tissues have gone through the repair process, but have not been adequately remodelled to return to full function.

When structural changes and or impairment affect joint capsules or adjacent supporting ligaments, painful *restriction* of *end-range* movements in one or more directions will be experienced. Pain from the dysfunction syndrome persists until remodelling of the affected structures occurs. Alternatively, abnormal tissue may persist f om an unreduced derangement, in which case there will be a painful *blockage* to *end-range* and symptoms are produced on compression of the joint.

Generally, the exact tissue at fault in dysfunction syndrome is not known. In spinal problems pain is always produced at end-range, when tissues are stretched and/or compressed. Thus in the spine dysfunction presents as articular, but involvement of contractile structures cannot be ruled out. In one instance, adherent nerve root, the source of symptoms is known. In this form of dysfunction a past derangement causing an episode of sciatica has resolved, but the repair process has left some tethering or adherence that now inhibits full movement of the nerve root/dural complex. The syndrome is also a common consequence of spinal surgery id appropriate rehabilitation is not instigated. In the case of an adherent nerve root, flexion is markedly restricted and each attempt to flex fully reproduces the patient's pain, which can be felt in the back or the leg. This is the only dysfunction that can produce peripheral pain; all other examples cause spinal pain only. Most commonly these are caused by dysfunctions affecting movements into extension and flexion.

Pain from dysfunction will not go away by itself, but persists as long as the adaptive shortening or blockage to movement exists, and is consistently reproduced every time the affected tissue is stressed. The only way to resolve dysfunction is a regular remodelling programme that repeatedly stresses the tissue in order to return it to full function.

It should be noted that the most common classification is derangement, and if this is suspected it is not possible at the outset to make a diagnosis also of 'underlying dysfunction'. The derangement is always treated first as the main source of symptoms, which can present with end-range pain, and it is not possible to know if there is an underlying dysfunction until the derangement is reduced. On most occasions, once the derangement is reduced there is no 'dysfunction' to treat.

Dysfunction is classified by the direction of impairment. For instance, if the patient lacks extension range and end-range extension produces symptoms, this is an extension dysfunction. If patients have a limited and painful range of flexion with end-range pain on repeated flexion, which is no worse on cessation of movement, this is a flexion dysfunction, etc.

Postural syndrome

The postural syndrome is characterised by intermittent pain brought on only by prolonged static loading of normal tissues. Time is an essential causative component, with pain only occurring following *prolonged loading*. However, the loading period required to induce symptoms may decrease with repeated exposure over time. Patients with the postural syndrome experience *no pain with movement or activity*. Neither do they suffer restriction of movement. No pathological changes occur in this syndrome. Once the aggravating posture is changed, the symptoms cease. The most common posture to provoke pain in this syndrome is slumped sitting.

Pain from the postural syndrome in the spine is caused by mechanical deformation of normal soft tissues arising from prolonged end-range loading affecting the peri-articular structures.

Clinically, patients with pain of postural syndrome rarely present for treatment, as they learn how to abolish symptoms by changing their position. Occasionally concerned parents accompany their teenage children to the clinic with this problem. Often they are individuals who lead a reasonably sedentary lifestyle and their posture is very poor. Although the syndrome is only occasionally seen in the clinic, the role of postural stresses on the genesis and persistence of musculoskeletal conditions is very important. Postural syndrome is not a discrete entity, but part of a continuum. These patients, if they do not alter their postural habits, can progress on to the more clinically common syndrome of derangement. A postural component is invariably present in derangement, which must be addressed to ensure resolution and prevent recurrence.

In the spine, postural pain arises mostly from *joint capsules or adjacent supportive ligaments* and is the result of *prolonged end-range positioning*. Moving from the end-range is sufficient to relieve pain immediately. Only appropriate education in postural correction will remedy pain in this syndrome.

Conclusions

In this chapter an introduction to the three mechanical syndromes and their conceptual models has been made. They describe three separate entities, which present in quite distinct ways and respond very differently to the mechanical evaluation outlined later. Details gained during the history-taking and symptomatic responses to repeated movements and sustained postures would be completely different. This means the three mechanical syndromes are clearly differentiated from each other, allowing the distinct management strategy necessary for each syndrome to be implemented.

Each syndrome must be treated as a separate entity in completely different ways. In the postural syndrome, postural correction must be performed to relieve the development of painful prolonged mechanical loading in normal tissue. In the dysfunction syndrome, structurally impaired tissue must be remodelled by repeatedly stressing the abnormal tissue. In the derangement syndrome, reductive forces must be applied to relocate displaced tissue, and loading strategies are applied that reduce, abolish or centralise symptoms. Appropriate mechanical therapy cannot be applied without correct recognition of these different entities. For instance, treatment of dysfunction requires the regular reproduction of the patient's pain, whereas treatment of derangement is by regular movements that reduce the displacement and cause the reduction, abolition or centralisation of pain.

It must be emphasised that the most common reason for patients to seek assistance is as the result of derangement – this is the entity that is most commonly seen in the clinic. Treatment of derangement is more complex and varied and will be discussed at length; however, the key management decision is to determine the direction of loading that is necessary to reduce the displacement. The means of reduction is identified by a loading strategy that decreases, abolishes or centralises symptoms. The most common derangements are posterior, and thus extension is the most common reductive force used. Lateral and some postero-lateral derangements require lateral forces or lateral forces combined with sagittal ones, and anterior derangements need flexion forces. The means by which these sub-groups can be identified and then treated are discussed in the chapters on management of derangement.

If at first assessment two syndromes are suspected, namely derangement and dysfunction, it is always the derangement that is treated first. Frequently what appeared to be a dysfunction disappears once the derangement is reduced. Once the derangement is reduced, a secondary dysfunction may be present; this should be addressed once the reduction of the derangement is stable.

These non-specific mechanical syndromes include the majority of patients with spinal pain. Failure to clearly identify a mechanical response or an atypical response may require further classification in a limited number of patients. In these instances, various non-mechanical or specific categories of back pain may need to be considered. These are described elsewhere in the book. *Other categories should never be considered without first conducting a thorough mechanical evaluation over several days.* Recognition of these other categories is based on factors in the history-taking, failure to respond in a typical manner to a mechanical loading evaluation pursued over several days and certain responses to mechanical testing.

Figure 8.1   Mechanical and non-mechanical diagnosis – relative roles

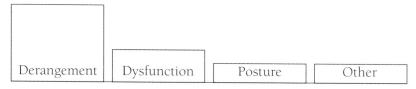

Figure 8.2   Classification algorithm

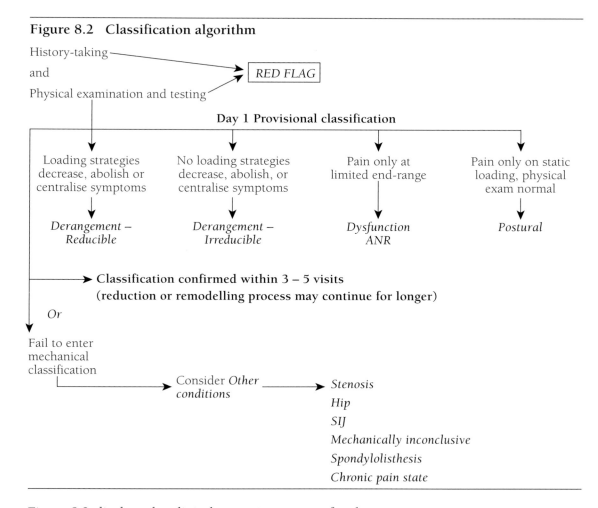

Figure 8.2 displays the clinical reasoning process for determining the mechanical or non-mechanical diagnosis. Suspicion of red flag pathology should mostly be determined by history-taking. Everyone else, about 99%, should been given a thorough physical examination as described later. From this most patients can be classified by a mechanical diagnosis, although initially in some this will be provisional. By five visits the mechanical diagnosis will be confirmed, or, due to an atypical response, one of the 'other' categories may be considered. To be entered for consideration, the patient displays no symptom response that suggests a mechanical diagnosis, as well as displaying signs and symptoms appropriate for that 'other' diagnosis. *The algorithm must be used in conjunction with the criteria and operational definitions in the Appendix – this is essential reading.*

9: Derangement Syndrome – the Conceptual Model

Introduction

The conceptual model that has been used to explain derangement syndrome relates the presentation to internal intervertebral disc displacements (McKenzie 1981, 1990). As derangements are a continuum, these may present in various ways. At its embryonic stage, with minor internal disc displacement, individuals may suffer from brief bouts of back pain and trivial limitations of function that last only a few days and resolve spontaneously. At its most extreme, the internally displaced tissue overcomes the restraining outer wall of the annulus fibrosus and extrudes into the spinal or intervertebral canal, causing predominantly radicular signs and symptoms. The continuum of back pain may start with posture syndrome and later proceed to minor and then major derangement. Back pain may proceed to back and leg pain and then on to sciatica. With the passage of time, dysfunction and nerve root adherence may occur. Irreducible derangement and entrapment are at the extreme end of the continuum, and spinal stenosis may be the culmination of a long history of back pain.

In this chapter a description of the clinical model is presented with the associated signs and symptoms. Evidence that supports this conceptual model is then presented, some of which is considered in more detail in the chapter on intervertebral discs. An understanding of the model allows, in most cases, a reliable prediction to be made regarding the preferred direction of applied forces and the likely response. The conceptual model has diagnostic and pathological implications; however, mechanical diagnosis and therapy are not totally dependent on the model as exceptions to the norm do occur. Ultimately it is a system that utilises repeated movements and loading strategies to treat signs and symptoms.

Sections in this chapter are as follows:

- conceptual model
- loading strategies
- dynamic internal disc model

- lateral shift

- place of the conceptual model.

Conceptual model

Innervation of the disc is absent in the inner part of the annulus fibrosus, and thus considerable occult changes can occur without symptomatology. Over many years of everyday postural stresses, strains and minor trauma, the integrity of the disc is impaired. The annulus fibrosus develops fissures, first circumferentially, then radially, and the homogenous nature of the nucleus pulposus is compromised. At some stage during this normal degenerative process, internal disc disruption and displacement can occur and abnormal morphology can become symptomatic.

Prior to actual disc displacement, pain from prolonged or poor posture may arise from excessive loading of any soft tissues. Early on, brief episodes of back pain may be caused by minor displacements of disc tissue that exert pressure on the outer innervated wall of the annulus fibrosus. Typically these arise following activities involving sustained or repeated flexion; sometimes quite trivial forces can trigger an episode, and this should be viewed against the background of lifestyles in which the ubiquitous posture is flexion. The majority of such episodes arise from minor well-contained posterior or postero-lateral displacements. These may cause back pain, which can be felt centrally or to the right or left of the spine, depending on the site of the pressure within the annulus. Some limitation of function may occur and pain may be experienced during movement, but just as the derangement is minor, so too is the symptomatology. At an early stage displacements are rapidly reversible, and more often than not individuals spontaneously become symptom-free and fully functional.

With the passage of time more persistent episodes may be experienced. There may be a progressive increase in internal disc disruption and displacement posteriorly, and attenuation or rupture of the lamellae of the annulus fibrosus. Symptoms thus become more severe and may radiate into the leg, and functional impairment is more marked – movements and activities are restricted, and after a period of sustained flexion the patient struggles to reverse the spinal curve against an obstructive displacement that prevents extension. Episodes now take longer and more effort to resolve. Failure to fully reduce the displacement leads to residual symptoms and a restriction in the range of motion. As the most common derangements are posterior or postero-lateral; typically there is a failure to regain full extension, and individuals in future refrain from prone lying as this position is painful.

Internal derangements alone may produce symptoms that radiate into the leg; however, peripheral symptoms may also be caused by irritation of the nerve root/dura complex. As long as the outer annular wall is intact and pressure from the displacement is intermittent, the derangement and the symptoms of sciatica are reversible. The phenomena of peripheralisation and centralisation relate to increasing and decreasing stress on the source of pain generation. This may be the outer innervated annular wall or may include the irritated nerve root.

Larger displacements can cause such a disturbance in the normal resting position of the affected motion segment that it forces the body into asymmetrical alignment. The displacement obstructs movement in the opposite direction and fixes the patient in a temporary deformity of kyphosis, in the case of a posterior displacement; lateral shift, in the case of a postero-lateral displacement; and lordosis, in the case of an anterior displacement. The inability of patients to reverse the spinal curve at this stage provides a clue as to the underlying mechanical deformation that is the common aetiological factor in these apparently different disorders.

Ultimately, the outer restraining wall of the annulus fibrosus may be ruptured completely or so attenuated as to become incompetent. At this point displaced or sequestered disc material has interrupted the outer contour of the annulus and posterior longitudinal ligament or invaded the spinal canal. There is constant pressure on the nerve root and/or dura mater and signs and symptoms are consistent with a radiculopathy. A non-specific reversible mechanical backache has progressed into an irreversible and identifiable pathology, thus indicating the likely pathology that exists in many patients with so-called 'non-specific' back pain. With time there will be absorption, fibrosis or adhesions and symptoms will subside or change in nature, but at this stage only surgical intervention will produce a rapid resolution of the pain.

Deformities

Kyphosis   The patient can be locked in a position of *lumbar kyphosis and is unable to extend*. Conceptually, the patient has developed an obstruction to extension caused by excessive posterior internal displacement. The *displacement obstructs curve reversal and locks the patient in a flexed posture they cannot easily correct.*

Lateral shift   The patient can be locked in a position of *lateral shift*. For example, their trunk and shoulders are shifted to the right, a right lateral shift. They are unable to straighten or laterally glide to the left, or, if they can do so, they cannot maintain the correction. Conceptually, the patient has developed an obstruction to left lateral glide caused by excessive postero-lateral internal displacement to the left. *The displacement obstructs curve reversal and locks the patient in a lateral shift deformity that they are unable to correct themselves.*

Lordosis   The patient can be locked in a position of *extension and is unable to flex*. Conceptually, the patient has developed an obstruction to flexion caused by excessive anterior internal displacement. *The displacement obstructs curve reversal and locks the patient in extension they cannot self-correct.*

In all three of these situations, the excessive internal displacement in one direction *locks* the segment in that position and prevents *voluntary* curve reversal or movement in the opposite direction. This is akin to the locked knee joint arising from internal derangement within that joint. These deformities are easily recognised and are the result of *significant* displacements. The greater the displacement, the greater is the deformity. Lesser displacements cause obstruction to movement and problems of curve reversal, but not deformity.

Loading strategies

In earlier stages of derangement, different postural loads will have a marked effect upon symptoms and movement. Unfavourable loading increases the displacement and worsens or peripheralises pain and makes movement more difficult. In contrast, favourable loading decreases the displacement and lessens symptoms and improves movement. Typically patients report a worsening of pain when sitting and an easing of pain when they walk about. Other patterns of pain behaviour occur. Sometimes movements that open the joint space may temporarily reduce the pain, but promote greater displacement and more pain when the person returns to a normal posture. Thus, certain positions can be found that alleviate the pain while the position is maintained, but that aggravate or perpetuate the pain afterwards. For instance, in major postero-lateral derangements, patients find temporary relief in positions of flexion, but afterwards struggle to regain extension and are no better.

During the assessment of patients with spinal disorders, clinicians should be aware of these tendencies for certain favoured and unfavoured postures and movements. Knowledge of these should be used in management, with temporary avoidance of unfavoured loading strategies, and regular use of favoured loading strategies. However, the ability to affect these disorders is related to the state of the annulus fibrosus. In the early stages of derangement, the displacement is well contained by intact lamellae and properly identified repeated movements or sustained postures are easily able to reduce the displacement. At the end stage of derangement, the annular wall has either ruptured (extrusion or sequestration) or become incompetent and is no longer able to restrain displacements (protrusion). As long as the hydrostatic mechanism of the disc is intact with the integrity of the outer wall of the annulus maintained, it is still possible to exert an effect upon the internal displacement using mechanical forces. Once this has been compromised, however, the derangement is not reversible, and no lasting symptomatic changes can be achieved.

The conceptual model as outlined by McKenzie (1981, 1990) makes clear that derangements form a continuum with progressively larger derangements causing more mechanical deformation and consequently more signs and symptoms. For this reason a sub-classification of derangements one to six was outlined that described progressions of the same disturbance within the intervertebral disc. These presented clinically as increasing peripheral pain with or without deformity. These derangements affected the posterior or postero-lateral aspect of the disc, and thus were also capable of causing deformation of the nerve root, thereby producing radicular signs and symptoms. A separate sub-classification (derangement 7) described anterior displacements.

The conceptual model allows determination of therapeutic pathways. It not only describes a pathology and rationale for the origin of many non-specific spinal pains, but also indicates the treatment direction required. Posterior derangements need extension forces in their reduction, anterior derangements need flexion forces and postero-lateral derangements need lateral or extension/lateral forces. Acceptance of the conceptual model allows us to determine, with good reliability, the direction of the required therapeutic motion.

Dynamic internal disc model

Various studies validate the conceptual model. There is now ample evidence concerning the innervation of the disc, and therefore its ability to be a pain-generating source in its own right (Bogduk 1994b, 1997). Pain provocation studies have commonly demonstrated exact reproduction of patients' symptoms with discography (Vanharanta *et al.* 1987; Moneta *et al.* 1994; Aprill and Bogduk 1992; Smith *et al.* 1998; Ricketson *et al.* 1996; Milette *et al.* 1999; Ohnmeiss *et al.* 1997). The disc is the most common cause of mechanical back pain (Schwarzer *et al.* 1995d; Milette *et al.* 1995; Ohnmeiss *et al.* 1997) and the most common cause of back pain and sciatica (Kuslich *et al.* 1991; AHCPR 1994).

Symptomatic presentation

Pain provocation studies at surgery have shown that the site of pressure on the annular wall is reflected in the site of perceived pain (Kuslich *et al.* 1991; Cloward 1959; Murphey 1968). Stimulation centrally produces symmetrical pain, and stimulation laterally produces unilateral pain. This would account for pain that changes site.

Some studies have found that leg pain could only be reproduced by stimulation of an already sensitised nerve root (Kuslich *et al.* 1991; Fernstrom 1960), but discography studies have commonly been able to reproduce leg symptoms in disorders without nerve root involvement (Park *et al.* 1979; McFadden 1988; Milette *et al.* 1995; Donelson *et al.* 1997; Ohnmeiss *et al.* 1997; Colhoun *et al.* 1988; Schellhas *et al.* 1996). Discogenic pain alone can cause radiating symptoms.

The most significant factor in painful discs appears to be radial annular disruptions. Those discs with little or no fissuring of the annulus are rarely painful, but when fissures extend to the outer edge of the disc they frequently are (Vanharanta *et al.* 1987, 1988). Only the presence of outer annular ruptures predicts a painful disc; neither inner annular tears nor general disc degeneration are associated with painful discs

(Moneta *et al.* 1994). In these instances, the extent of pain referral may reflect the degree of mechanical pressure to which the ruptured and weakened annular fibres are subjected.

The degree of radiation of somatic symptoms can be a reflection of the intensity of the stimulation of the pain-generating mechanism. Several experimental studies have shown this to be the case (Kellgren 1939, 1977; Feinstein *et al.* 1954; Mooney and Robertson 1976; Moriwaki and Yuge 1999). More mechanical pressure is associated with more distal referral of symptoms.

Mechanical stimulation of intervertebral discs in patients with radicular syndromes produces their back pain, while their leg pain could only be produced by stimulation of a sensitised nerve root (Kuslich *et al.* 1991; Fernstrom 1960; Smyth and Wright 1958). The distal extent of the radicular pain, its severity and frequency all appear to be a function of the amount of pressure exerted on the nerve root (Smyth and Wright 1958; Thelander *et al.* 1994). Thus increased discal pressure on the nerve results in more distal pain and a reduction of pressure causes the pain to move proximally.

Pople and Griffith (1994) found that the pain distribution pre-operatively was highly predictive of findings at surgery in 100 patients (Table 9.1). When the leg pain was predominant this usually indicated a disc extrusion, whereas if the back pain was worse than the leg pain this was more likely to indicate a protrusion. When pressure was still being exerted on the disc back pain was dominant, and when pressure was mostly on the nerve root leg pain dominated. Furthermore, when an extrusion was present, back pain tended to decrease or go completely.

Table 9.1   Pre-operative pain distribution and operative findings

Pain	Extrusion	Protrusion	Total
Leg pain only	96%	4%	27
90 – 99% leg pain	58%	42%	12
50 – 90% leg pain	37%	63%	49
Back > leg pain	17%	83%	12
Total	53	47	100

Source: Pople and Griffith 1994

The study by Donelson *et al.* (1997) correlated findings from a mechanical assessment and discography. Whereas 70% of those whose pain centralised or peripheralised had a positive discography, only 12% of those whose symptoms did not change had disc-related pain. Among those who centralised their pain, 91% had a competent annular wall according to discography, compared to 54% among those whose pain peripheralised.

These studies demonstrate that the site of pain from internal disc lesions is reflected in the symmetry or unilateral nature of the pain perceived, and that these are capable of causing radiating symptoms. More extensive radiation of symptoms can be caused by more mechanical pressure. If the nerve root is involved then pain is referred down the leg, and neurological signs and symptoms may also occur. The accumulative evidence to date attests to the importance of discogenic pain in the back pain population, and also provides the theoretical background for an understanding of the phenomenon of peripheralisation and centralisation. Increased displacement or pressure on the outer annulus or nerve root produces more peripheral symptoms, while reduced pressure relieves these symptoms.

Figure 9.1   Centralisation of pain – the progressive abolition of distal pain

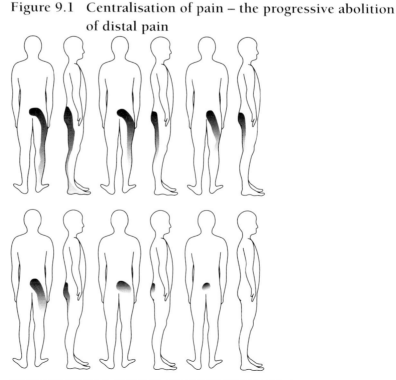

Pathological model

Numerous studies have shown the internal disc to be mobile. This effect has been demonstrated in cadaveric experiments (Shah *et al.* 1978; Krag *et al.* 1987; Shepperd *et al.* 1990; Shepperd 1995) and in living subjects (Schnebel *et al.* 1988; Beattie *et al.* 1994; Fennell *et al.* 1996; Brault *et al.* 1997; Edmondston *et al.* 2000). These have shown a posterior displacement of the nucleus pulposus with flexion and an anterior displacement accompanying extension of the lumbar spine. These studies support McKenzie's (1981) proposal that anterior to posterior displacement resulted in an obstruction to extension in a majority of patients with low back pain.

Kramer (1990) hypothesised that a combination of factors trigger pathological displacement of disc tissue:

- high loading pressure on the disc

- high expansion pressure of the disc

- structural disruption and demarcation of disc tissue, such that internal loose fragments of disc tissue can become displaced down existing fissures as a result of asymmetrical loading

- pushing and shearing forces encountered in ordinary activity.

Kramer (1990) suggests that external mechanical forces act as a trigger on tissue that may be predisposed to symptoms because of the other factors. Therefore, minor additional postural stresses can lead to deformation, tearing of annulus fibres or displacement of disc tissue. This displacement may be internal or may exceed physiological dimensions and lead to protrusions and extrusions.

There is thus a continuum between asymptomatic disc degeneration and symptomatic structural changes to the annulus. The process develops in a sequential manner, with the distortion, then failure of the annulus leading to the formation of radial fissures, which are a prerequisite of displacement. In its turn the displacement can be checked by the outer annular wall or this can be ruptured also and a complete herniation results. Once the annular wall has been completely breached and the hydrostatic mechanism of the disc is impaired, it is no longer possible to influence the displaced tissue (Kramer 1990).

Radial fissures are a common finding in cadaveric studies (Hirsch and Schajowicz 1953; Yu *et al.* 1988a; Osti *et al.* 1992). Various experimental and clinical studies describe the sequential way in which radial fissures develop, which may culminate with disc herniation (Adams and Hutton 1985a; Adams *et al.* 1986; Bernard 1990; Buirski 1992). For instance, Adams *et al.* (1986) describe the stages of disc degeneration as shown on discograms in cadavers; with fissures and clefts in the nucleus and inner annulus, leading to outer annular tears and complete radial fissures. In vivo discography studies (Bernard 1990; Buirski 1992) show the stages of disc disruption, with early annular fissuring and later radial tears sometimes associated with discal protrusion.

In vitro experiments have demonstrated that fatigue flexion loading of discs can lead to distortion and rupture of the annulus, which may be followed by extrusion of disc material (Adams and Hutton 1983, 1985a; Gordan *et al.* 1991; Wilder *et al.* 1988). Computer-generated disc models predict annular fissuring will occur with flexion loads (Natarajan and Andersson 1994; Shiraz-Adl 1989). These models also predict that failure is most likely to occur in the posterolateral section of the annulus fibrosus (Hickey and Hukins 1980; Shiraz-Adl 1989).

Other experimental and clinical studies (Brinckmann and Porter 1994; Moore *et al.* 1996; Cloward 1952) support this *dynamic internal disc model* because in the presence of fissures and disc fragments, the effects of normal loading can lead to the non-physiological displacement of discal material, protrusions and extrusions. The development of radial fissures would seem to be the key factor in the pathology of disc problems. These entities can be painful in themselves, but in some patients these fissures may act as conduits for intradiscal material to be displaced, to protrude or to be extruded beyond the contours of the annulus. The study by Milette *et al.* (1999) shows that in patients with discogenic pain, radial fissures may be more significant than protrusions. This study also found that bulging and protruded discs were significantly associated with grade 2 or grade 3 fissures (see Table 4.1). This also would indicate a continuum between these entities, with abnormal disc contour and possible nerve root involvement being impossible without pre-existing disruption of the annulus.

Although some posterior herniations can be asymptomatic, many do cause somatic and radicular pain. It is in the posterior aspect of the disc that the majority of pain-generating pathology has been identified. This relates both to radial fissures and actual herniations. It is primarily postero-central or postero-lateral herniations that are the cause of nerve root symptomatology. These are likely to be worsened with flexion loading, which experimentally has been shown to cause disruption and displacement (Adams and Hutton 1983, 1985a; Gordan et al. 1991; Wilder et al. 1988).

Although the end result may be actual disc herniation with nerve root involvement, this only represents the extreme end of the continuum and a minority of patients. The majority of patients present at an earlier stage in this continuum with the outer annular wall still intact, when the displaced tissue can be influenced by movement and positioning and when the symptom-generating mechanism is reversible. At this stage the mechanism of symptom generation is primarily from the disc, although there may be intermittent irritation of a nerve root.

Lateral shift

What will be referred to in this text as a lateral shift has also been described as a (gravity-induced) trunk list or (acute) lumbar, lumbosacral or sciatic scoliosis. The Scoliosis Research Society recognises the lumbosacral list as a non-structural shift caused by nerve root irritation from a disc herniation or tumour (Lorio et al. 1995). Longstanding scoliosis may be the result of a primary structural deformity in the vertebrae of the lumbar spine, while a secondary curve can develop to compensate for a morphological abnormality, such as a leg length inequality or contracture around the hip joint. In contrast to such entities, the lateral shift is an acute and temporary occurrence that accompanies the onset of an episode of back and leg pain. However, it should be noted that very rare causes of non-mechanical back pain, such as osteoid-osteoma and discitis, are also associated with rapid onset scoliosis (Keim and Reina 1975; Greene 2001).

Typically the patient has an asymmetrical alignment of the spine. With the onset of this episode of back, and usually referred leg pain, they develop a shift to one side. If they have had previous episodes of back pain, a history of previous s`afts is not uncommon. The shift is temporary and resolves as the episode of back pain resolves. The shift is gravity-induced and often worsens the more the patient stands or walks. When they lie down the shift is abolished.

The prevalence of lateral shifts within the back pain population is unclear and there is considerable variability in the reported proportion that present with this sign (Table 9.2). As clear-cut definitions are usually not included in these reports, the variability may simply reflect different operational definitions.

Table 9.2   Prevalence of lateral shift

Reference	Patient population	Total sample	N (%) with shift	% shift who had surgery
Porter and Miller 1986	Back pain clinic in hospital	1,776	100 (6%)	20%
O'Connell 1951	Surgical cases; DH	500	244 (49%)	100%
Falconer et al. 1948	Surgical cases; DH	100	50 (50%)	100%
Khuffash and Porter 1989	Back pain clinic in hospital; DH	113	32 (28%)	41%
Matsui et al. 1998	Surgical cases; DH	446	40 (9%)	100%

DH = symptomatic disc herniation for which patient was treated surgically

Lateral shifts are strongly associated with symptomatic disc herniations. In Porter and Miller's (1986) sample of 100, 49% fulfilled three or more of the criteria for a symptomatic disc herniation. Shifts also appear to be particularly associated with disc herniations at the extreme end of the pathological continuum and to augur a poor prognosis requiring surgical intervention (O'Connell 1943, 1951; Falconer et al. 1948; Porter and Miller 1986; Khuffash and Porter 1989). Compared to patients without a shift and without cross leg pain, patients with a shift were three times more likely to come to surgery, and those with a shift and cross leg pain six times more likely (Khuffash and Porter 1989). The pressure on the nerve root from the disc herniation in patients undergoing surgery has been found to be significantly higher in those with a shift compared to those without (Takahashi et al. 1999).

The evidence makes clear that some of the previous assumptions that had been made about lateral shifts are incorrect. Although the shift most commonly occurs in those with leg or radicular pain, it has also been reported to occur in those with back pain only (Falconer et al. 1948; Porter and Miller 1986; Gillan et al. 1998). Gillan et al.

(1998) reported 55% of forty patients to have back pain only. Porter and Miller (1986) reported back pain in 16%, thigh pain in 13% and nerve root pain in 71% of 100 patients.

Multiple studies have found no consistency between the direction of the shift and the topographical relationship of the disc herniation to the nerve root found during surgery (Falconer *et al.* 1948; Porter and Miller 1986; Lorio *et al.* 1995; Laslett *et al.* 1992; Suk *et al.* 2001; Matsui *et al.* 1998). Traditional concepts relating the shift to a certain topographical relationship between the herniation and the nerve root are no longer tenable.

Different terminology has been used to describe the direction of the shift (Table 9.3). Earlier studies relate the convexity or concavity to the side of the pain, while more recent studies mostly use the terms 'contra' and 'ipsilateral'. Several reports mention the existence of alternating shifts – that is, patients whose shift might change sides.

Table 9.3   Sidedness of lateral shifts

Reference	Convex to side of pain	Concave to side of pain	Contra-lateral shift	Ipsila-teral shift	Alter-nating shift
O'Connell 1951	73%	17%			10%
Falconer *et al.* 1948[1]	53%	36%			11%
McKenzie 1972[2]			91%	9%	Some present
Porter and Miller 1986[3]			54%	46%	
Suk *et al.* 2001			67%	33%	
Matsui *et al.* 1998	80%	20%			
Tenhula *et al.* 1990[4]			68%	32%	

1 = 47/50 with leg pain
2 = 526 patients
3 = 67/100 with unilateral leg pain
4 = 22/24 with unilateral symptoms

Only a few authors have discussed conservative management of the lateral shift. McKenzie (1972) reported on 526 patients treated with lateral shift correction followed by restoration of extension. A further sixteen patients had increased pain on test movements and were rejected as unsuitable for conservative treatment, and 470 (89%) patients were symptom-free at the end of one week with no residual deformity, with the majority greatly improved within forty-eight hours. Of the remaining twenty-four (5%), eighteen were symptom-free, but with residual deformity at the end of one week. The other six patients took several weeks to resolve or still had minor symptoms or residual deformity. Of the thirty-two (6%) who failed to respond to treatment, 84% had had symptoms for more than twelve weeks and 66% had root compression with neurological deficit.

Gillan *et al.* (1998) conducted a randomised controlled trial to compare lateral shift correction by a McKenzie-trained therapist with massage and standard back care advice. Disability scores improved in both groups at twenty-eight and ninety days' follow-up, with no significant difference between the groups. After twenty-eight days the shift had resolved in 64% of the McKenzie group and 50% of the control group. At ninety days shift resolution was significantly different, at 91% and 50% respectively. Unfortunately there was considerable loss to follow-up, with only twenty-five of forty patients being available at ninety days. Patients included in this trial had had symptoms for less than twelve weeks; outcomes in the control group demonstrate that the natural history for many patients with a lateral shift is towards resolution.

Place of the conceptual model

This conceptual model (McKenzie 1981, 1990), when applied to the clinical situation, becomes an effective and reliable diagnostic and therapeutic tool (Donelson *et al.* 1997; Kopp *et al.* 1986; Alexander *et al.* 1991; Nwuga and Nwuga 1985). Using it during a mechanical evaluation enables the prediction of discogenic pain and the state of the annular wall (Donelson *et al.* 1997).

Patients' response to repeated movements enables the prediction of suitability for conservative care (Kopp *et al.* 1986; Alexander *et al.* 1992). Patients presenting with signs and symptoms of disc herniations with nerve root involvement were given extension exercises as long as this did not increase radicular pain. Thirty-five (52%) of them responded to conservative therapy, of which thirty-four (97%) achieved full extension, mostly in the first few days of extension exercises. Thirty-two failed to improve with conservative treatment or rest, and went to surgery. Of these, twenty-four (75%) had sequestrations or evidence of nerve root displacement, but only two (6%) achieved full extension pre-operatively (Kopp *et al.* 1986). Failure to achieve extension in this study had clear predictive implications, and a larger study replicated the same findings (Alexander *et al.* 1992). Neurological signs and symptoms, straight leg raising and abnormal imaging studies in those with disc herniation were unable to differentiate between those who responded to a McKenzie regime and those who needed surgery. In contrast, the ability to achieve extension in the first five days was highly predictive of treatment group (P = 0.0001).

The conceptual model provides a hypothetical pathology to explain various presentations that are encountered in the clinic such as centralisation and peripheralisation, pain that changes sides, pain that fluctuates with different loading strategies, deformity, obstruction to movement, curve reversal and so on. There is an intimate connection between the symptomatic presentation, the mechanical presentation and the degree of derangement. Greater displacements produce more extreme presentations of pain and altered mechanics, and as the derangement is reduced symptoms and movement, aberrations will return to normal.

Repeated movements or postures that increase the displacement also increase the obstruction, which in turn increases the pain. Repeated movements that progressively reduce the pain also progressively reduce the obstruction and derangement and allow the restoration of normal pain-free movement. Disc displacements occur predominantly in a posterior or postero-lateral direction; according to the conceptual model, this type of derangement requires the extension principle in its reduction, or a combination of extension and lateral forces. An anterior displacement requires the flexion principle, and lateral displacements require the lateral principle of treatment.

The dynamic internal disc model allows the clinician to determine the direction of therapeutic motion that needs to be employed to reduce the displacement, as well as the direction of movement that can worsen the displacement and therefore needs to be temporarily avoided. Clinical findings suggest that a large proportion of displacements are primarily affected by sagittal plane procedures and will be reduced by extension forces and aggravated by flexion forces (McKenzie 1981). A smaller proportion of displacements occur in the frontal plane and require lateral or torsional forces in their reduction. A small proportion of displacements are anterior and will need flexion forces in their reduction (McKenzie 1981). Figure 9.2 relates direction of displacement to specific mechanical procedures.

Figure 9.2   Conceptual model and procedures; relating procedures to direction of derangement

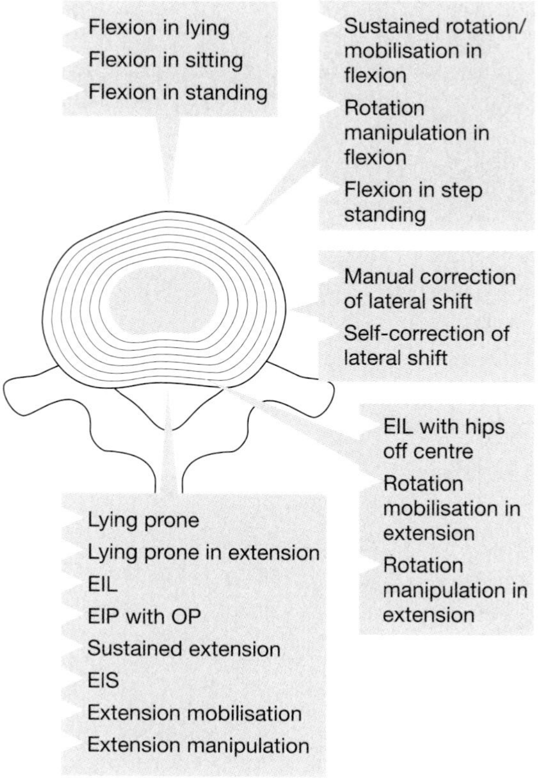

Flexion in lying
Flexion in sitting
Flexion in standing

Sustained rotation/mobilisation in flexion

Rotation manipulation in flexion

Flexion in step standing

Manual correction of lateral shift

Self-correction of lateral shift

EIL with hips off centre

Rotation mobilisation in extension

Rotation manipulation in extension

Lying prone
Lying prone in extension
EIL
EIP with OP
Sustained extension
EIS
Extension mobilisation
Extension manipulation

This model not only provides a useful indicator of appropriate management, it is also useful as a teaching tool for patients. Most patients are more satisfied attending clinicians who provide logical and utilisable models of pathology. It is important for the patient to know that the disc is a source of pain generation and is a mobile structure influenced by everyday postures and movements. This enables them to achieve and improve compliance with their posture and exercise. Understanding the model teaches self-reduction and preventive techniques.

A better explanation may eventually be found for some of the features of back pain, but until that time this is a reasonable and reliable model upon which to base mechanical therapy. Since the model was first suggested (McKenzie 1981), numerous studies have been conducted that have increased our knowledge concerning disc disease, many of which endorse an internal dynamic disc model of pathology as noted above.

Although the definition of derangement relates to internal articular displacement, it could also be defined by its characteristic symptomatic and mechanical presentations. This mechanical syndrome is present when, for example, there is sudden onset of pain, peripheralisation, centralisation, spontaneous resolution of pain, improvement and worsening with loading strategies, deformity, sudden loss of range of movement and so on. It is most clearly defined by its response to the appropriate loading strategies, which is a rapid and lasting change in pain intensity and location. This only occurs in derangement syndrome – a syndrome being a collection of commonly observed signs and symptoms. Management of derangement is based upon symptomatic and mechanical responses to loading strategies.

Conclusions

This chapter describes the pathophysiological model that may be the explanation for derangement. It presents some of the clinical and experimental studies that support this explanation. The conceptual model suggests that derangement is related to internal disc dynamics and is initially a form of discogenic pain that may later, in a minority, involve the nerve root. The model embraces a continuum, which would account for the varied presentation of derangement, and offers an explanatory model for such clinical phenomenon as acute spinal deformities, blockage to movement, centralisation and peripheralisation. At the end of the pathological continuum is the irreducible derangement in which the hydrostatic mechanism of the disc is no longer intact and internal disc mechanics can no longer be influenced. When the outer annular wall is intact, posture and movement can influence disc displacement, and thus the conceptual model allows for the logical formulation of therapeutic loading. The model is a possible explanation for clinical events, but ultimately the treatment of derangement is dependent upon symptomatic and mechanical responses.

Introduction

Centralisation describes the progressive reduction and abolition of distal pain in response to therapeutic loading strategies. It is one of the key symptomatic responses that denotes derangement, the others being reduction or abolition of pain. Centralisation occurs during the reduction of a derangement. This chapter presents a detailed description of this phenomenon, as well as outlining its characteristics.

Sections in the chapter are as follows:

- definition
- description of the centralisation phenomenon
- discovery and development of centralisation
- characteristics of centralisation
- literature on centralisation
- reliability of assessment of symptomatic response.

Definition

- in response to therapeutic loading strategies, pain is progressively abolished in a distal-to-proximal direction with each progressive abolition being retained over time until all symptoms are abolished
- if back pain only is present, this moves from a widespread to a more central location and then is abolished.

Description of the centralisation phenomenon

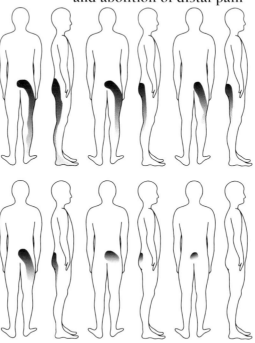

Figure 10.1 Centralisation of pain – the progressive reduction and abolition of distal pain

Centralisation describes the phenomenon by which distal limb pain emanating from the spine, although not necessarily felt there, is immediately or eventually abolished in response to the deliberate application of loading strategies. Such loading causes reduction, then abolition of peripheral pain that appears to progressively retreat in a proximal direction. As this occurs there may be a simultaneous development or increase in proximal pain.

The perceived movement of pain either distally or proximally can occur during the natural history of an episode of pain and during the different activities of daily function. The identification of this pain behaviour during the history-taking provides an indication of the stage of the disorder and helps to identify appropriate management strategies. Centralisation specifically describes the abolition of distal pain that occurs *in response to clinically prescribed repeated end-range movement, static end-range loading or maintenance of corrective postural habits.*

The retreat of distal pain can occur immediately during the first assessment on the first day, and centralisation and final reduction can be a rapid process. Alternatively, it may be apparent from an initial assessment that a particular loading strategy is having a centralising effect, which may, if pursued over a longer time period, result in the abolition of distal symptoms and a more gradual process of centralisation.

The term 'centralisation' also applies if pain felt only in the back localises to the centre of the spine. Continuing application of the appropriate loading results in decrease and finally, abolition of pain.

The phenomenon only occurs in derangement syndrome (McKenzie 1981, 1990). Reduction describes the process by which the derangement is progressively lessened. During this process symptomatic and mechanical presentations are gradually improved, thus centralisation occurs and movement is restored. The process of reduction and centralisation are intimately related and occur together. When the derangement is fully reduced, pain is abolished and full-range, pain-free movement is regained. Maintenance of reduction is highly variable. Some reductions are stable in a short period of time and with a limited application of loading strategies, while others need a strict application of loading strategies over a more protracted period to bring about and maintain reduction. Some reductions are so unstable that simply a change in loading causes re-derangement. On occasion the derangement may be reduced, but pain on end-range movement, which may be limited, persists because of dysfunctional tissue.

Centralising means that in response to the application of loading strategies, distal symptoms are decreasing or being abolished. Symptoms are in the *process* of becoming centralised, but this will only be confirmed once the distal symptoms are abolished. This process can be rapid or may occur gradually over time with repeated exposure to the appropriate loading. The centralising phenomenon indicates that reduction of the derangement is in progress. The reductive process is continuing when pain is reported to be progressively centralising, decreasing or has ceased distally, or if pain located in the back is centralising, decreasing or ceasing.

Reduction is complete only when the patient reports no back or referred pain when undertaking normal daily activities and pain-free movement is fully restored. During the process of reduction the patient may undertake certain activities that impede or reverse the process and cause distal symptoms to reappear. With cessation of the aggravating positions and performance of the appropriate end-range movements, symptoms should once again start centralising.

Centralised means that as a result of the application of the appropriate loading strategies, the patient reports that all of the distal radiating or referred symptoms are abolished and have not recurred during normal activity. They may be left with back pain. The reductive process has been stabilised, and further end-range movements will decrease and then abolish the remaining spinal symptoms.

Pain that is centralising during the application of loading strategies may be a stable or an unstable phenomenon. If, following repeated end-range movements performed in lying, pain has centralised and remains better on resuming the upright position and being normally active, the centralisation process is stable (but not necessarily complete). *Stable symptomatic improvement resulting from end-range loading indicates the stable nature of the reduction of the derangement and generally offers a good prognosis.*

Stability of reduction process is evidenced when any symptomatic improvement achieved *from end-range loading applied in lying* is maintained on and after the resumption of weight-bearing and normal activity. If symptomatic improvement is stable, further reduction will occur with a continuation of the same management.

Although symptoms may return if aggravating postures are maintained, any increase in intensity or peripheralisation of pain will cease and be reversed by more rigorous application of the appropriate loading strategies. Centralisation of symptoms occurring during loading applied *in standing* is usually stable.

Temporary cessation or centralisation of pain in response to end-range loading performed in the lying position is an *indication* that reduction *may* be occurring. Should pain *immediately* reappear on weight-bearing, the reduction is unstable. An unstable centralising process indicates the need for more persistent and strict application of loading strategies and complete avoidance of aggravating postures.

Unstable reduction may indicate that a good prognosis can be achieved over a protracted period if rigorous application of management is applied; however, frequently it indicates a derangement that is not amenable to lasting reduction, and prognosis in these cases is poor. It can generally be determined over a test period of a few days whether or not stability of reduction and a lasting centralising effect are being achieved.

Spontaneous abolition of pain achieved by adopting the lying position is not an indication that the derangement has been reduced. Pain in this case has ceased because of removal of compressive loading and will return with the resumption of weight-bearing. In this situation it is inappropriate to consider that centralisation has been achieved or that reduction has occurred.

Peripheralisation describes the phenomenon when pain emanating from the spine, although not necessarily felt in it, spreads distally into or further down the limb. This is the reverse of centralisation. Loading strategies may produce temporary or lasting distal pain. In response to repeated movements or a sustained posture, if pain is produced and remains in the limb, spreads distally or increases distally, that loading strategy should be avoided. In some situations an instant but short-lived production of distal pain may occur with a particular loading strategy. This is not peripheralisation.

Centralisation

- only occurs in derangement syndrome

- occurs with the reduction of the derangement

- involves lasting abolition of peripheral or radiating pain

- may occur rapidly or gradually

- is accompanied by improvements in mechanical presentation

- occurs in response to loading strategies (repeated movements or postural correction).

Peripheralisation

- only occurs in derangement syndrome

- distal symptoms are produced and remain or distal symptoms are made more severe

- occurs in response to loading strategies (repeated movements or postures).

Discovery and development of centralisation

McKenzie's first experience with what he was to call the 'Centralisation Phenomenon' occurred in 1956. A patient, 'Mr Smith', who had pain extending from his back to his knee, had undergone treatment for three weeks without any improvement. He could bend forward, but his extension was painful and limited. He was told to undress and lie face down on the treatment table, the end of which had been raised for a previous patient. Without adjusting the table, he lay in a hyperextended position unknown to staff in the clinic. On being found five minutes later, he reported that he was the best he had been all week – the pain had disappeared from his leg, the pain in his back had shifted from the right to the centre, and his restricted range of extension had markedly improved. When he stood up he remained better, with no recurrence of his leg pain. The position was adopted again the following day and resulted in the complete resolution of his remaining central back pain.

During the following two or three years, every patient with back or referred leg pain was placed in either the extended position or was asked to repeat extension movements ten or fifteen times while lying in the prone position. There emerged a consistency of response to these exercises that could not have been coincidental.

Patients with certain referred pain patterns would become symptom-free within two or three days. Whenever this rapid resolution occurred, recovery was preceded by a change in the location of the pain from a referred to a near central midline position. Referred symptoms were seen to rapidly disappear at the same time as localised central back pain appeared or increased. Once symptoms centralised, referred symptoms would not reappear as long as patients avoided flexed postures. Continuation of the centralising manoeuvre caused rapid resolution of the central back pain. Consistently, concomitant restriction of extension mobility improved and patients *remained better as a result* of performing the exercises.

Some individuals with unilateral pain would not experience improvement as a result of sagittal plane extension movements, but did after applying lateral flexion in a loaded position – after which centralisation occurred. In others, if lateral flexion was too vigorously applied, the pain would disappear from one side, but appear on the other. It became clear that by performing certain movements one could influence the site of pain radiation. This suggested that when pain changed location, something with the segment had also changed location and when pain centralised, reduction of displacement was occurring. If centralisation of pain occurred, the prognosis was invariably excellent and a rapid response would usually follow.

Patients whose pain extended below the knee and never abated reacted in an unpredictable manner, many being significantly aggravated rather than improved by these manoeuvres. Referred pain and neurological symptoms were sometimes exacerbated or produced by repeated movements, both in the sagittal and frontal planes. If extension was maintained for an excessive period of time or if the exercise was forced to an excessive degree, some of these patients, in the experimental years, remained worse as a result of the procedures. Many of these patients did not respond to mechanical therapy.

Characteristics of centralisation

With the realisation that movements that cause pain to centralise are therapeutic and cause a good outcome, the *prognostic significance* of centralisation became apparent. Movements that caused centralisation also indicate the direction in which any mobilising or manipulation procedures should be applied when an *increase of force* is necessary because of incomplete or partial responses to self-treatment exercises. Likewise, it became clear that movements that caused symptoms to peripheralise were undesirable and therefore contraindicated.

The phenomenon of centralisation most commonly occurs in patients who also demonstrate *significant obstruction* to full range of extension. When these patients are subjected to repeated end-range unloaded extension movements, centralisation of pain develops in conjunction with and directly proportional to the rapid recovery of extension that follows.

Although many patients with back pain experience centralisation with the performance of *extension exercises* carried out from the prone lying position, there are others, identified during mechanical evaluation, who must perform extension from a prone hips off-centre position. Some patients respond to lateral movements, and a further group must repeat flexion movements in order to cause centralisation of pain.

The prognostic value of centralisation derives partly from the fact that the change in pain location that it describes is of a *lasting nature*. Furthermore, while one direction – often but not always extension – produces this desirable change in pain location, very often the opposite movement – often flexion – causes the peripheral pain to return and the condition to worsen. Patients frequently exhibit this *directional preference* in which one direction improves and the opposite worsens the symptoms.

Literature on centralisation

More detail about many of the studies mentioned in this section are provided in Chapter 11, which includes a literature review of centralisation and relevant reliability studies. Centralisation has been commonly identified during repeated movement tests (Donelson *et al.* 1990, 1991, 1997; Williams *et al.* 1991; Long 1995; Sufka *et al.* 1998; Erhard *et al.* 1994; Karas *et al.* 1997; Delitto *et al.* 1993; Kilby *et al.* 1990; Kopp *et al.* 1986; Werneke *et al.* 1999; Werneke and Hart 2000, 2001). This has occurred in between half and three-quarters of the patient groups evaluated. Studies that have examined centralisation have done much to confirm the characteristics of the phenomenon as outlined above.

Centralisation has been associated with good outcomes in both acute and chronic back pain populations (Donelson *et al.* 1990; Sufka *et al.* 1998; Long 1995; Rath and Rath 1996). Centralisation has been associated with improved functional disability scores and better return-to-work rates compared to individuals whose symptoms did not centralise (Werneke *et al.* 1999; Sufka *et al.* 1998; Karas *et al.* 1997). Donelson *et al.* (1990) found it to be an excellent predictor of outcome in 87 patients with acute and chronic referred pain; in 87% centralisation occurred with sagittal or frontal plane repeated movements. There was a correlation between the occurrence of centralisation and better outcomes.

Table 10.1 Prognostic significance of centralisation

Outcome	No. of patients with each outcome (%)	Occurrence of centralisation in each outcome group (N)
Excellent	59 (68%)	100% (59)
Good	13 (15%)	77% (10)
Fair	7 (8%)	57% (4)
Poor	8 (9%)	37% (3)
Total	87 (100%)	87% (76)

Source: Donelson *et al.* 1990

Centralisation occurred in over 80% of all patients, regardless of how long the symptoms had been present. However, centralisation was more definitely associated with a good or excellent outcome in those with acute symptoms (88%) compared to those with symptoms that had been present for over one month (67%) (Donelson *et al.* 1990). Centralisation readily occurs in those with more recent onset of symptoms, but it can also be gained in many patients with chronic back and referred pain (Donelson *et al.* 1990; Sufka *et al.* 1998). In one study in which centralisation occurred in twenty-five out of thirty-six patients (69%), the rates on centralisation decreased with the longevity of symptoms (Sufka *et al.* 1998).

Table 10.2 Occurrence of centralisation in acute, sub-acute and chronic back pain

Duration of back pain	Occurrence of centralisation %
< 7 days	83%
7 days to 7 months	73%
> 7 months	60%
Total	69%

Source: Sufka *et al.* 1998

In studies of chronic populations, about 50 – 60% of patients describe centralisation of their pain (Long 1995; Donelson *et al.* 1997; Sufka *et al.* 1998), again associated with a better outcome (Long 1995). It is thus independent of the duration of symptoms, but tends to be observed somewhat less frequently in those with chronic back pain.

Just as centralisation tends to be strongly associated with greater improvements in pain severity and perceived functional limitations, failure of centralisation to occur is strongly associated with poor overall response (Donelson *et al.* 1990; Karas *et al.* 1997; Werneke *et al.* 1999; Werneke and Hart 2000). *"Failure to centralize or abolish pain rapidly indicates a lack of response to mechanical treatment and presages a poor result"* (Karas *et al.* 1997). Werneke *et al.* (1999) found that some patients experienced centralisation rapidly (average four visits), while in some it occurred more gradually or partially (average eight visits) and was not directly related to observed therapeutic loading in the clinic. If patients had failed to show a decrease in pain intensity by the seventh visit, no significant improvements in pain or function were found.

Failure to achieve centralisation as a prognostic factor was compared to other historical, work-related and psychosocial variables in predicting outcomes at one year (Werneke and Hart 2001). This included Waddell's non-organic physical signs, depression, somatisation and fear–avoidance beliefs. In a multivariate analysis that included all the significant independent variables, only leg pain at intake and non-centralisation significantly predicted outcomes at one year. This study is of great importance; for the first time it identifies a clinical variable that is more predictive of outcome than a psychosocial one.

When using sagittal or frontal plane repeated movements, 87% of patients experienced centralisation (Donelson *et al.* 1990). In a single testing protocol when only sagittal plane movements were used, centralisation occurred in 40% of patients with extension and 7% with flexion (Donelson *et al.* 1991). Movements in the opposite direction can worsen pain, and thus patients' conditions are deemed to have a preferential direction of movement. Centralisation can occur rapidly and be lasting in nature. It occurs with end-range repeated movements, and can demonstrate paradoxical responses in that a single movement may increase symptoms, but repeated movements leave the patient better overall. Sometimes it is associated with a concomitant increase in spinal pain (Donelson *et al.* 1990, 1991).

Centralisation can occur with posture correction only. Those adopting a lordotic sitting posture over a twenty-four- to forty-eight-hour period experienced a 56% reduction in leg pain and 21% decrease in back pain. Those who adopted a flexed posture over the same period experienced an increase in back pain and no change in leg symptoms (Williams *et al.* 1991).

Although centralisation by its very nature seems more likely to be described when peripheral symptoms are present, in fact there is some indication that it is more likely to occur with back, buttock and thigh pain rather than leg pain (Werneke *et al.* 1999; Sufka *et al.* 1998).

Table 10.3 Occurrence of centralisation according to site of referred pain

Referral of symptoms	Occurrence of centralisation %
Back	80%
Thigh	73%
Calf	43%
Total	69%

Source: Sufka *et al.* 1998

Different studies have used slightly different operational terms to define centralisation. Most have termed it *abolition* of distal pain during repeated end-range movements, with classification usually made during the initial assessment (Long 1995; Donelson *et al.* 1990, 1997); some studies have included *reduction* of distal pain also (Karas *et al.* 1997; Erhard *et al.* 1994; Delitto *et al.* 1993). In these studies, the rate of centralisation varied from 47% to 87%. Sufka *et al.* (1998) defined centralisation as reduction to central pain only within fourteen days, which occurred in 69% of their sample. The consensus from these studies suggests that the important qualitative distinction is that changes in pain status are rapid and occur over a period of days to a week or two, and are lasting in nature.

Werneke *et al.* (1999) employed a much stricter definition of centralisation in which symptoms had to retreat during the initial assessment, remain better, and at each subsequent session display further progressive abolition of symptoms. They found that 31% fitted these criteria, while a further 46% centralised fully or partially in between treatment sessions or during some sessions only. Although the full centralisation group required significantly fewer treatment sessions (four sessions compared to eight in the partial centralisation group), both groups had significant improvements in pain and function compared to the non-centralisation group. There were no significant differences in outcomes between the partial and fully centralising groups except the number of treatment sessions. If symptoms had not centralised by the seventh treatment session, any improvement was unlikely.

In summary, centralisation can thus occur or start to occur on the first day; however, in other patients it occurs over a period of a few weeks. It can occur both during treatment sessions and gradually in the time between sessions. However, the key distinction is between those who fail to centralise at all and those who may experience centralisation rapidly or more slowly. Outcomes are likely to be good in those experiencing centralisation – abolition of distal symptoms that remain better afterwards. After a thorough trial of up to seven therapy sessions, failure to alter symptoms is associated with a poor outcome.

Table 10.4 Characteristics of centralisation

- refers to the immediate or eventual abolition of distal pain in response to therapeutic loading strategies
- may be accompanied by increase in spinal pain
- usually a rapid change in pain over a few treatment sessions
- always a lasting change in pain
- occurs in acute and chronic patients
- often occurs in patients with obstruction to movement
- occurs most commonly with extension
- occurs with end-range repeated movements or postural correction
- occurs less commonly with lateral movements or flexion
- indicates directional preference
- indicates good prognosis
- failure to achieve indicates poor prognosis.

Reliability of assessment of symptomatic response

As the phenomenon of centralisation is entirely based upon the patient's report of pain location and behaviour, it is important to know that this subjective response can be reliably assessed. The Kappa value is a numerical expression of agreement between testers that seeks to exclude the role of chance (see Glossary).

The ability of different clinicians to concur on the existence of centralisation occurring in an individual has been found to be good to excellent, with rates of agreement of about 90% and Kappa scores of 0.92 – 1.0 (Sufka *et al.* 1998; Werneke *et al.* 1999). In one study involving eighty physical clinicians and physical therapy students who were evaluated on their ability to assess pain changes during movement from a video, agreement was 88% and Kappa value 0.79 (Fritz *et al.* 2000a).

Several studies have examined how much agreement there is between clinicians when interpreting pain responses in general to the performance of movements. These studies have shown that judgements about the site of pain and the behaviour of pain on movement can be reliably assessed (Spratt *et al.* 1990; Donahue *et al.* 1996; Kilby *et al.* 1990; McCombe *et al.* 1989; Strender *et al.* 1997). Tests involving pain responses are invariably more reliably assessed than tests involving visual or palpatory queues (Donahue *et al.* 1996; Kilby *et al.* 1990; Strender *et al.* 1997; Potter and Rothstein 1985).

"In lieu of the common limitation of imaging and other diagnostic studies in identifying the underlying disorder, pain and, in particular, its location would seem to be useful as a reflection of the nature of that underlying disorder" (Donelson *et al.* 1991).

Conclusions

This chapter has considered the phenomenon of centralisation, which refers to the lasting abolition of distal, referred symptoms in response to therapeutic loading. Various studies have demonstrated its frequent occurrence in the back pain population and its use as a favourable prognostic indicator. This clinically induced change in pain location has been reported in both acute and chronic patients with back, and back and leg, symptoms. This occurs with repeated end-range movements, particularly but not only with extension, and postural correction. As it can be consistently assessed, it is a reliable occurrence upon which to base treatment. The failure to alter the site of distal symptoms is conversely associated with poor outcomes. A description of this phenomenon and its characteristics have been presented in this chapter, while the following chapter provides a more detailed analysis of the articles mentioned here.

11: Literature Review

Introduction

Since the publication of the first edition of this book (McKenzie 1981), there has been a considerable amount of research into different aspects of the approach. Different types of study design that relate to mechanical diagnosis and therapy are considered in this chapter. Within the hierarchy of evidence, systematic reviews and randomised controlled trials (RCTs) are considered the strongest study design when evaluating interventions (Gray 1997). The relevant research is described as well as some of its limitations.

Other study designs must be considered when investigating other issues, such as the reliability of assessment process or the value of prognostic factors. It is also important to consider the evidence that relates to other aspects of the McKenzie approach. Key elements are the use of symptomatic response to guide treatment, the phenomenon of centralisation and the concept of directional preference. Some of these other issues are also considered and the available published literature presented.

The chapter considers the evidence under the following headings:

- systematic reviews and guidelines
- controlled trials and randomised controlled trials
- other efficacy trials
- studies into directional preference
- reliability studies
- reliability of palpation studies
- studies into the prognostic and diagnostic utility of centralisation.

Systematic reviews and guidelines

Various systematic reviews have evaluated the efficacy of exercise in general for back pain, some of which have included an analysis of McKenzie trials, and also some reviews have specifically focused on the McKenzie approach. For systematic reviews an electronic database and hand search is conducted, and only RCTs are included in the analysis. There are predefined inclusion criteria, quality control standards and outcome measures. The methodological quality of the studies is considered, and often a method score for the different trials is given in an attempt to rate their quality. These show the modest methodological quality of most research, with scores from three reviews averaging 50% or less (Koes *et al.* 1991; Faas 1996; Rebbeck 1997). Common weaknesses in the literature include small sample sizes, lack of a placebo control group, inadequate follow-up, patient attrition, failure to measure compliance, use of other interventions and insufficient description of interventions (Koes *et al.* 1991; Faas 1996). However, an improvement over time has been noted, with a recent review noting high quality in 41% of studies compared to 17% in 1991 (van Tulder *et al.* 2000a).

Although the methodological scoring system is meant to objectify analysis of the different trials, qualitative judgements have to be made in defining aspects of the methods. Comparison between different reviews reveals a lack of agreement over the quality of certain trials. Rebbeck (1997) adopted a slightly modified version of the scoring system proposed by Koes *et al.* (1991), yet their scores for the same trials reveal considerable disparity.

Table 11.1 Comparison of method scores for the same trials

Reference	Score: Rebbeck 1997	Score: Koes et al. 1991
Nwuga and Nwuga (1985)	46%	28%
Stankovic and Johnell (1990)	61%	42%

Koes *et al.* (1991) reviewed sixteen RCTs into exercise for back pain, from which they decided that no conclusion could be drawn about whether exercise therapy is better than other conservative treatments for back pain or whether a specific type of exercise is more effective. Belanger *et al.* (1991) found three 'scientifically admissible' trials into the McKenzie approach, all of which favoured the approach for acute back pain, but these were criticised for lack of randomisation, blinding and use of a control group. Faas (1996) reviewed eleven RCTs from the literature between 1991 and 1995 to update the earlier review by Koes *et al.* (1991). In patients with acute back pain exercise was deemed to be ineffective, but two trials favoured McKenzie therapy compared with the reference therapy. As both had low method scores, the necessity of additional trials to clarify the efficacy of the system were indicated. For sub-acute and chronic back pain there is some evidence for the benefits of exercise therapy, but conclusions about which type of exercise is most suitable could not be made.

Rebbeck (1997) located twelve clinical trials in the literature that used the McKenzie regime. Seven were excluded from the review, five of which found the system superior to the comparison regime. Failure to be included resulted from lack of a pure McKenzie approach or lack of publication in a peer-reviewed journal. Of the five acceptable trials, four demonstrated statistically significant improvements compared to the reference therapy. As the trials in acute patients did not include a control group, given the tendency for many to recover quickly, it cannot be definitively known that the McKenzie regime is superior to the natural history. Evidence for a positive effect is more apparent in chronic patients. In an overview of all twelve trials, the McKenzie regime was shown to be significantly better in reducing back and leg pain than flexion regimes, a mini back school, traction, an NSAID or a non-specific exercise programme. However, it was not better than a combination of extension, flexion and manipulation, or chiropractic manipulation. Overall trials were too few and methodologically of poor quality to make absolute recommendations.

Maher *et al.* (1999) reviewed sixty-two trials in the attempt to answer the question: Prescription of activity for low back pain: what works? Relative to acute and sub-acute back pain, few of the relevant trials demonstrated that exercises were more effective than the control treatment. The only clinical trial that did note an improvement used the McKenzie approach, with exercises being supplemented by posture correction and postural advice (Stankovic and Johnell 1990, 1995), the benefits of which were quite substantial in certain outcomes. The review recommends that patients with acute back pain be advised to avoid bed-rest and return to normal activity using time rather than pain as a guide. This advice may be supplemented by the provision of McKenzie therapy or manipulative therapy. For chronic back pain, there is strong evidence to support the use of general intensive exercises. They also found convincing evidence that exercise has a preventative effect on future back pain.

Van Tulder *et al.* (2000a) identified thirty-nine trials for their systematic review of exercises for back pain in the Cochrane Library. Their conclusions were similar to earlier reviews – for acute back pain exercises appear to be no more effective than other treatments, whereas for chronic back pain exercises appear to be helpful. They also reported specifically on flexion and extension exercises, including the McKenzie approach. Three low-quality studies evaluated flexion exercises for acute back pain, which showed they were ineffective or produced worse outcomes than comparison treatments. Four studies evaluated extension exercises in acute back pain, two of good quality (Cherkin *et al.* 1998; Malmivaara *et al.* 1995), and two of low quality (Stankovic and Johnell 1990, 1995; Underwood and Morgan 1998). Three of them failed to show a significant difference in favour of the extension exercises, and one of these showed they were significantly less effective than comparison treatments. They concluded, somewhat confusingly, that extension exercises are more effective than flexion exercises, but that both are not effective in the treatment of acute back pain. For chronic back pain, no trials were found exploring the role of flexion or extension exercises compared to other treatments, and the three comparisons between the two types of exercise produced conflicting results.

Two guidelines about the general management of back pain, which use a thorough and systematic review of the literature, include mention of exercise therapy according to McKenzie (DIHTA 1999; Philadelphia Panel 2001a). The Danish Institute for Health Technology Assessment (DIHTA 1999) in a chapter on *Treatments that could generally be recommended* included the following summary. They separated the approach into a treatment and a diagnostic method. As a treatment method they concluded that "*McKenzie exercises can be considered as a treatment method for both acute and chronic low-back pan*". A few studies showed a positive clinical effect in both patient groups, with or without radiating symptoms. This meant that this recommendation was weighted as strength C – "*Limited research based documentation such that there is at least one relevant medium quality study, which supports the usefulness of a particular technology*".

As a diagnostic method they concluded that several studies indicate the method has value as both a diagnostic tool and prognostic indicator. They recommended that the approach could be used for both acute and chronic back pain. This recommendation was weighted as strength B – "*Moderate research based documentation such that there is at least one relevant high quality study or several medium quality studies, which support the usefulness of a particular technology*".

The Philadelphia panel evidence-based clinical practice guidelines have been developed using a structured and rigorous methodology (Philadelphia Panel 2001b). A whole edition of *Physical Therapy* records their findings according to back, neck, shoulder and knee conditions (*Physical Therapy 2001*, volume 81, number 10). They compare their findings with other guidelines and also include practitioner comments. For acute back pain, they find no evidence for therapeutic exercise. For sub-acute and chronic back pain, they recommend that there is good evidence to include extension, flexion and strengthening exercises, which include the McKenzie Method (Philadelphia Panel 2001a).

In summary, there is no straightforward consensus concerning McKenzie therapy from these systematic reviews. In some the evidence is seen as quite supportive, while in others the evidence is seen to be absent. Its apparent benefit is undermined by the low quality of the supportive trials and insufficient high-quality trials. The evidence concerning exercise in general is more positive in chronic rather than acute back pain. Part of the problem with evaluating the McKenzie Method is the fact that it does not fit neatly into one type of treatment. It uses exercise and postural instruction, but also can employ mobilisation and manipulation. While in some reviews a lot of effort is expended on determining the methodological quality of a trial, often the quality and type of intervention is not considered. Ultimately systematic reviews are only as useful as the trials on which they are based, so it would be helpful next to consider the individual trials included by the reviews, as well as other studies not included.

Controlled trials and randomised controlled trials

Some earlier reports of exercise therapy for back pain that utilised extension involved active backwards bending (Kendall and Jenkins 1968; Davies *et al.* 1979; Zylbergold and Piper 1981). As this is different from extension in lying, the procedure advocated by McKenzie (1981), these studies are not included in the literature review. Included is research that includes the extension exercises proposed by McKenzie (1981), as well as studies that sought to replicate the McKenzie approach in a more thorough manner. Some of the main outcomes are summarised in Table 11.2. To give some idea of the strength of the different studies, where available, the method score for that trial is given, as well as the source of that score. All of these studies are randomised controlled trials (RCTs), excepting two stated instances.

Buswell (1982) compared a programme of extension exercises and postural advice, incorporating some of McKenzie's ideas, with one of flexion exercises and advice in fifty patients with an acute exacerbation of back pain. Both groups improved significantly with no important difference between them. Method score – 30% (Koes *et al.* 1991).

Ponte *et al.* (1984) assigned, not randomised, twenty-two acute patients to Williams' flexion exercises and postural instruction or a McKenzie exercise and posture protocol in which extension, lateral or flexion exercises were selected. Improvements in pain, sitting tolerance, forward flexion and straight leg raise were significantly better in the McKenzie group, of whom 67% were pain-free at the post-treatment evaluation compared to 10% in the Williams group. Patients in the McKenzie group received an average of 7.7 treatment sessions compared to 10.4 in the other group; this difference was also significant. Method score – 43% (Rebbeck 1997).

Nwuga and Nwuga (1985) used a sample of sixty-two women with disc protrusions and root compression of recent onset, which had been confirmed by investigations. These were assigned, not randomised, to McKenzie extension exercises and posture instruction, or Williams' flexion exercises. Re-evaluation of patients occurred at six weeks and was conducted by a blinded assessor. There were significant improvements in pain, sitting endurance and straight leg raising in the McKenzie group, but not in the Williams group, and mean treatment time was significantly less in the McKenzie group. Method score – 28% (Koes *et al.* 1991), 46% (Rebbeck 1997).

Stankovic and Johnell (1990) randomised 100 patients with acute back and leg pain to a McKenzie protocol involving extension exercises, preceded by lateral correction if necessary, and then flexion exercises, or a 'mini back school'. This involved education, advice on resting positions and keeping as active as possible, but refraining from exercises. Follow-ups were performed at three weeks and one year; there were significant differences between the groups at various points. All patients in the McKenzie group had returned to work within six weeks, as opposed to eleven weeks in the other group. There was significantly less pain in the McKenzie group at three and fifty-two weeks, there were fewer recurrences and fewer had to seek medical help. Method score – 42% (Koes *et al*. 1991), 61% (Rebbeck 1997).

Eighty-nine patients from this trial were followed up five years later (Stankovic and Johnell 1995). Differences were much less than previously, but were still significant as far as recurrences of back pain and sick leave were concerned. There were no differences between the groups in seeking health care or in ability to self-help. Pain was present in 64% of the McKenzie group and 88% of the other group. Method score – 41% (Faas 1996).

Unlike all the trials mentioned so far, Elnaggar *et al*. (1991) chose to explore the effects of flexion and extension exercises in patients with chronic back pain. Postural instructions were not given, exercises were performed only for one session a day for two weeks and a pure McKenzie regime was not adopted. Both groups had a significant reduction in pain post-treatment, but no significant difference between the groups. Method score – 36% (Koes *et al*. 1991).

Spratt *et al*. (1993) explored the use of extension and flexion exercises and postures, incorporating braces and a no-treatment control group in fifty-six patients with chronic back pain and specific radiographic findings. These were spondylolisthesis, retrodisplacement or normal sagittal translation. Patients were reviewed after a month, at which point the extension group pain score was significantly better than the other two groups, and was the only one that showed a significant improvement across time. The pattern of treatment response was similar across all translation sub-groups. Method score – 45% (Faas 1996).

Delitto *et al*. (1993) and Erhard *et al*. (1994) investigated exercises in small groups of patients who were classified as extension responders by showing reduction or centralisation of symptoms with extension and worsening of symptoms with flexion. Once so-classified, twenty-four patients were then randomised to either a manipulation procedure followed by extension exercises or a flexion exercise regime. There was a significantly greater improvement in Oswestry disability score in favour of the manipulation/extension group (Delitto *et al*. 1993). Method score – 30% (Faas 1996). In the second trial (Erhard *et al*. 1994), twenty-four patients were randomised to an extension group or a group who received a manipulation and then performed a spinal flexion/extension exercise.

At a week, only two of the first group met the discharge criteria, while nine of the second group did so. Follow-up at one month was only 50%, but also favoured the manipulation group. Method score – 52% (Rebbeck 1997).

Dettori *et al.* (1995) recruited 149 soldiers with acute back and leg pain. These were randomised to extension, flexion and control groups, but then at the end of week two, half of each of the active exercise groups also performed the other exercise. Exercises were done three times daily and patients were instructed in the appropriate postural advice according to their group. The control group lay prone with an ice pack over the lumbar spine. All groups improved rapidly over the eight weeks of the trial with no statistically significant differences in pain or function over this period. There was a tendency for both exercise groups to show a better return of function in the first week, at which time there was very little change in the control group; when the two exercise groups were combined and compared with the control group, this was significant at this point. In the six- to twelve-month follow-up, recurrences of back pain were similar in all groups, at over 60%. However, control group patients were more likely to require medical care than those who had exercised, and those who had been in the extension group, particularly, were less likely to need medical care and work limitation.

Malmivaara *et al.* (1995) did not refer to the McKenzie approach; however, backward bending and lateral bending exercises were used in one of the treatment arms; other patients were randomised to either a bed-rest or a normal activity control group. It is not indicated if exercises were performed in lying or standing, and they were done only three times a day. One hundred and eighty-six patients with acute back and leg pain were entered in the trial. At three weeks there were significant improvements in favour of the control group over the exercise group in terms of sick days, duration of pain and Oswestry scores. At twelve weeks some of the outcomes still favoured the control group, but these were not stated to be significant. Method score – 63% (Faas 1996).

Underwood and Morgan (1998) randomised seventy-five patients with acute back pain to either a single back class lasting up to one hour with one to five patients in which the 'teaching was as described by McKenzie', or to receive conventional management. At no point during the follow-up year were there any statistical differences between the two groups in terms of pain or Oswestry score. There was a statistically significant difference at one year when 50% of the class group reported 'back pain no problem' in the previous six months compared to 14% of the control group.

Gillan *et al.* (1998) attempted to study the natural history of lateral shift and the effect of McKenzie management. Forty patients were recruited to the trial and randomised to the McKenzie group or a non-specific back massage and standard back advice group. Patients were followed up at twenty-eight and ninety days, but 37% of patients were lost by the last follow-up. Resolution of shift occurred more frequently in the McKenzie group, with a significant difference at ninety days. However, there was no difference in functional outcome at any point.

Cherkin *et al.* (1998) randomised 323 acute back pain patients to one of three groups: a McKenzie regime, chiropractor manipulation or a control group who were given an educational booklet. This was the first study to recognise the importance of using trained clinicians, but rather than using experienced McKenzie clinicians, they were trained prior to the study. The trial, because of exclusion criteria, ultimately recruited only 8.5% of those who attended their primary care physician with back pain. At four weeks the chiropractic group (P= 0.02) and the McKenzie group (P=0.06) had less severe symptoms than the booklet group, but not different Roland-Morris disability scores. At twelve weeks there were no significant differences in symptoms or function between the three groups, and there had been no further improvement in outcomes. In the subsequent two years recurrences were similar in all groups, as was care-seeking. Costs were substantially lower in the booklet group, but satisfaction with care was significantly worse than in the two other interventions.

In summary, several trials are supportive of the McKenzie approach (Nwuga and Nwuga 1985; Ponte *et al.* 1984; Stankovic and Johnell 1990, 1995; Spratt *et al.* 1993; Delitto *et al.* 1993). Several of these trials are of poor or moderate quality, which can have the tendency to exaggerate treatment effects (Gray 1997). Many of the trials have small numbers, which can mean the trial has insufficient power and therefore is unable to detect important clinical differences, although in fact all did. Two trials appear to show parts of the McKenzie system perform less well against comparison (Erhard *et al.* 1994; Malmivaara *et al.* 1995); however, the interventions bear so little resemblance to the approach if used properly that such a conclusion would be erroneous.

Several trials have ambivalent conclusions; for instance, that neither extension nor flexion exercises are necessarily better (Buswell 1982; Elnaggar *et al.* 1991; Dettori *et al.* 1995), and that a single 'McKenzie class' is no better than usual care in the short-term (Underwood and Morgan 1998). Again, with these trials the approach is not rigorously mechanical diagnosis and therapy; for instance, there is lack of attention to patient selection. The study by Cherkin *et al.* (1998) also has an ambivalent outcome. That mechanical diagnosis and therapy performed as well as chiropractic manipulation is very positive, given the support for manipulation by numerous systematic reviews. Only 10% of patients had pain below the knee, thus it is likely that there was a preponderance of patients with back pain only without referred symptoms. It is precisely this group, acute simple back pain, which is supposed to be the optimal group to receive manipulation (AHCPR 1994). However, neither intervention was more than marginally better than a cheap booklet.

Table 11.2. Main outcomes from published randomised controlled trials using extension exercises or purporting to use McKenzie regime (see text for more detail)

Reference	Group 1	Group 2	Group 3	Outcomes *Statistically significant improvements supporting McKenzie intervention. Not supportive.*
Buswell 1982	Extension	Flexion		Improvements both groups NS difference
Ponte *et al.* 1984	McKenzie protocol	Flexion		*Pain (10):* *1: -4.9* *2: -3.2 (P =0.001)*
Nwuga and Nwuga 1985	McKenzie protocol	Flexion		*Pain (10):* *1: -5.3* *2: -2.7 (P<0.01)*
Stankovic and Johnell 1990	McKenzie protocol	Education Normal activity		*Sick leave (days):* *1: 11.9* *2: 21.6 (P<0.001)* *Recurrences:* *1: 22* *2: 37 (P<0.001)*
Elnaggar *et al.* 1991	Extension	Flexion		Improvements both groups. NS difference

Continued next page

Reference	Group 1	Group 2	Group 3	Outcomes
Spratt et al. 1993	Extension	Flexion	Control	*Pain: Only 1 improved post treatment (<0.004)*
Delitto et al. 1993	Manipu-lation Extension	Flexion		*Oswestry:* 1: -23% 2: -10%
Erhard et al. 1994	Extension	Manipu-lation Flex / Ext		Discharge criteria: 1: 2/12 2: 9/12 (P<0.05)
Stankovic and Johnell 1995	See 1990 study			*Sick leave:* 1: 51% 2: 74% (P<0.03) *Recurrences:* 1: 64% 2: 88% (P<0.01)
Dettori et al. 1995	Extension (+flexion)	Flexion (+exten-sion)	Control	Improvements all groups NS difference
Malmivaara et al. 1995	Extension + side-bending	Usual activity	Bed-rest	Sick days: 1: 5.7, 2: 4.1, 3: 7.5 Oswestry: 1: -15, 2: -22, 3: -19
Underwood and Morgan 1998	'McKenzie class'	Usual manage-ment		Improvements both groups. NS difference *Chronic back pain:* 1: 50% 2: 14% (P<0.007)
Gillan et al. 1998	McKenzie lateral shift protocol	Massage and advice		*Resolution of shift > 5mm:* 1: 91% 2: 50% (P = 0.04) Oswestry NS
Cherkin et al. 1998	McKenzie regime	Chiro-practor manipu-lation	Booklet control	Improvements all groups

NS = any differences are non-significant

It should be emphasised that nearly every trial makes no selection of patient appropriateness for a given exercise regime. Exercise programmes are invariably standardised, are prescribed routinely or implemented in groups, and by clinicians of unknown skill or experience in the McKenzie approach. No attempt is made to assess for suitability, which is a key component of the approach. The only trials that attempt patient selection are those by Delitto et al. (1993) and Erhard et al. (1994). These suffer from very small numbers, considerable loss to follow-up and confusion as to exactly which component of the interventions was responsible for the effects observed.

The importance of individual assessment of suitability for exercise regimes is highlighted by the study by Donelson *et al.* (1991) – method score 57% (Rebbeck 1997). This showed that back pain frequently responds differently to different movements – nearly one-half of this group had a clear directional preference, most for extension, but a few for flexion. Not only did one direction clearly centralise symptoms, but also the opposite movement typically intensified and/or peripheralised it. This study was only short-term, but illustrated the importance of directional preference as a key to the management of mechanical back pain. Other studies have shown the good prognostic significance of identifying centralisation early on (Donelson *et al.* 1990; Sufka *et al.* 1998; Long 1995; Werneke *et al.* 1999; Karas *et al.* 1997). More patients may have demonstrated centralisation or a decrease in symptoms if testing had been pursued over a longer time period, and if other movements, besides sagittal ones, had been employed. For instance, in a study of eighty patients in which frontal and sagittal plane movements were used, 87% of them demonstrated centralisation (Donelson *et al.* 1990). If this directional preference is not taken into account and exercises are dispensed to all comers, then some in that group might respond, but some may be made worse and overall such a trial would show no value in a particular exercise.

Most of these trials have been conducted in patients with acute back pain. In this group there is a marked tendency for spontaneous recovery with whatever intervention is used, or if none is used. This is well-illustrated in the study by Cherkin *et al.* (1998). Disability is seen to fall rapidly from a starting point of twelve out of a twenty-four-point scale to seven at week one, and about four at week four *in all groups*. After this at weeks twelve, fifty-two and 104 the scores remain virtually unchanged, except for some minor further improvements in the physical therapy group. There is, in other words, a minor level of functional disability after recovery from the acute episode that remains largely unchanged two years later.

Various other shortcomings, which are common characteristics of these trials, limit their generalisability for mechanical diagnosis and therapy. A distinction is often not made between those with back pain only and those with referral of symptoms or with sciatica. Frequently interventions are inadequately described, performed with inadequate regularity and with adherence to exercise programmes not monitored. None of the trials excluded patients in whom no movement or position could be found to abolish, reduce or centralise symptoms. Such patients should be excluded from treatment groups (McKenzie 1981). Randomisation should be made after a mechanical evaluation – if a patient is intolerant of penicillin, they don't get it! The level of skills and experience of the participating clinicians is rarely considered, but this affects clinical efficiency as seen in the section on reliability studies. Lack of understanding of the McKenzie approach has a deleterious effect on its application. Trials that need to be performed include the effects of mechanical diagnosis and therapy, using suitably trained clinicians, involving patients with chronic and recurrent back pain and also to distinguish its effects in patients with back pain and in those with referred symptoms.

Other efficacy trials

Besides the evidence reviewed above, there are also a number of studies that have either not been published in peer-reviewed journals, and therefore have not gone through the critical appraisal process that is necessary prior to publication, or else lack a control group. Despite weaknesses, it is still worth considering this other literature, which on the whole is supportive of the approach. Principle findings are summarised in Table 11.3.

Kopp *et al.* (1986) included sixty-seven patients with acute disc prolapse, displaying radicular pain and at least one sign of nerve root irritation, and evaluated their response to an extension exercise protocol. If extension exercises worsened radicular pain, further attempts were abandoned. If extension was limited and produced back pain without worsening the leg pain, gradual extension procedures after the method of McKenzie (1981) were implemented. Thirty-five of these patients responded to the extension programme, and 97% of them achieved full-range extension within a matter of days. Thirty-two patients failed to respond and came to surgery, and of these only two (6%) were able to achieve extension. At surgery 75% had either a sequestered or protruding disc with nerve root displacement or deformity. There was no difference between the two groups in referred pain, positive straight leg raise or neurological signs and symptoms. The authors coined the phrase the 'extension sign' – being the inability to achieve extension – as an early predictor of the need for surgical intervention. At long-term follow-up, average six years, the extension sign was able to predict a favourable response to non-operative treatment in 91% of cases (Alexander *et al.* 1991).

Alexander *et al.* (1992), in a further report dealing with a total of 154 patients with disc herniation, reported on seventy-three patients who were selected for conservative management based on their ability to achieve full-range extension in lying. The decision to proceed with a McKenzie approach was made by the fifth day, by which time most had achieved extension if they were going to. These patients were then discharged and instructed to continue with extension exercises. Those in whom the extension sign remained positive were managed surgically. Thirty-three (45%) of the conservatively managed patients were traced about five years later. Symptoms were resolved or slight in 82%, functional limitations nil or minor in 85%, and 94% were satisfied with their treatment.

In those who initially had a positive extension sign that became negative, complete resolution was reported in 47%, compared to 21% in those who had a negative extension sign at admission and at five days. Patients (nineteen of thirty-three) whose extension sign changed from positive to negative (achieving extension) within five days had consistently better outcomes, and this mechanical presentation was a strong predictor of successful conservative management. This ability to regain extension in the acute stage was highly significant in predicting the treatment group, conservative or surgical. Other factors, such as neurological signs and symptoms, straight leg raising or abnormal imaging studies, were unable to differentiate between the two groups.

Numerous studies have only been published as abstracts (Vanharanta *et al.* 1986; Adams 1993; Kay and Helewa 1994; Goldby 1995; Fowler and Oyekoya 1995; Udermann *et al.* 2000, 2001; Schenk 2000; Borrows and Herbison 1995a) or as a dissertation or separate publication (Roberts 1991; Borrows and Herbison 1995b); detailed evaluation of these is not always available.

Vanharanta *et al.* (1986) allocated 138 patients to back school, McKenzie exercises or a home traction device according to date of birth. In the McKenzie group 97% had improved after one week, while less than 50% improved in the other two groups. After two weeks 36% of the back school group and 37% of the traction group had to change treatment because of lack of improvement; no changes were necessary in the McKenzie group. The McKenzie and traction groups recovered more quickly, with a statistically significant difference at one month, but no group differences at six months.

Roberts (1991) compared McKenzie therapy to treatment with a non-steroidal anti-inflammatory drug (NSAID) in patients with acute back pain, all of whom were encouraged to mobilise actively. At seven weeks the McKenzie group was less disabled, a difference that was significant in the sub-group of patients who were classified according to the mechanical syndromes at the first assessment. However, sick leave was greater in the McKenzie group.

Adams (1993, Adams *et al.* 1995) gave twenty-three chronic back pain patients a standardised six-week treatment programme of McKenzie extension procedures. Post-treatment values showed a significant reduction in pain scale rating. While prior to treatment patients showed a higher psychological involvement, reduced range of movement and increased EMG activity compared to matched non-pain controls, after treatment these differences were no longer significant.

Fowler and Oyekoya (1995) did a retrospective note review of twenty-seven subjects, twenty (74%) of whom had excellent recovery using McKenzie treatment within a shorter time period than other therapies previously or concurrently applied.

Kay and Helewa (1994) randomly assigned twelve patients with acute back pain to a McKenzie or Maitland protocol. At three weeks the McKenzie group showed an eighteen-point reduction on the pain scale, while the Maitland group reported a sixteen-point increase (P=0.029). There were no significant differences in range of movement or disability. Longer-term follow-up was not reported.

Goldby (1995) conducted a double blind randomised controlled trial on fifty patients with chronic back pain, of whom complete data existed on thirty-six. One group was treated along the McKenzie principles and one group received a non-specific exercise programme. There were improvements in both groups that were significant. Comparisons between the two groups found significant differences in favour of the McKenzie regime and significant changes in health locus of control that were not found in the non-specific exercise group.

Borrows and Herbison (1995b) reported on the Accident Rehabilitation and Compensation Insurance Corporation (ACC) evaluation of the effectiveness of four treatment programmes for chronic compensated back pain patients in New Zealand. All programmes used different exercise and rehabilitation regimes, three on an outpatient basis, while the McKenzie regime was a fourteen-day residential programme. Nearly 800 patients with an average of twenty months on compensation were allocated, not randomised, to the different programmes. The main outcome was 'Fitness to Work'; at one month this had improved by 35% in the McKenzie programme compared to 20% in the next best intervention, and by less than 4% in the other two. Secondary outcomes showed a similar picture, with the best two interventions producing substantially greater improvements in functional disability scores (about eight points on a twenty-four-point scale) and depression (five- to six-point improvement) than the other programmes (about three points and less than two points respectively). Long-term outcomes were missing in this study, and all programmes achieved a 20% return to work rate at three months. Nonetheless, two of the programmes, including the McKenzie one, showed significant and clinically meaningful greater improvements. The authors made various attempts in their analysis of the results to ensure against bias or confounding as a randomisation process was not used, and felt confident that the improvements were the true effect of treatment. While the McKenzie residential programme lasted nine days, the other programmes had an average duration of 103 to 127 days. This programme is described in more detail in the section on treatment of chronic pain.

Udermann *et al.* (2000) reported on the value of a purely educational approach, using *Treat Your Own Back* (McKenzie 1997) in sixty-two volunteers with chronic back pain, of whom 81% were available for follow-up nine months after reading the book. At this point 87% were still exercising regularly, 91% still used good posture, 82% noted less back pain and 60% were pain-free. Mean pain severity had dropped from 1.3 on a four-point scale to 0.44, and mean number of episodes from 4.1 to 1.0 per annum. Over 70% had found extension exercises to be most beneficial. Although there was no control group in this study, with a mean length of duration of back pain of over ten years prior to the intervention, this chronic sample served as its own control. At eighteen months fifty-four (87%) were contacted again (Udermann *et al.* 2001). Over 92% still claimed to be exercising regularly and focusing on posture. Pain severity had decreased to 0.33 and episodes per annum to 0.15.

From thirty-four patients recruited with lumbar radiculopathy, Schenk (2000) classified twenty-five as derangements, who were then randomly assigned to McKenzie exercises or joint mobilisation. The McKenzie group demonstrated significantly greater improvements in pain and function after three sessions.

Table 11.3 Other literature – abstracts, uncontrolled trials, etc.
(see text for more detail)

Reference	Group 1	Group 2	Results *Statistically significant improvements supporting McKenzie intervention.*
Kopp *et al.* 1986	Negative extension sign: McKenzie	Positive extension sign: Surgery	*Achieved full extension:* *1: 97%* *2: 6% (P<0.005)*
Alexander *et al.* 1992	Negative extension sign: McKenzie	Positive extension sign: Surgery	*Mechanical response predicted treatment group (P = 0.0001)*
Vanharanta *et al.* 1986	McKenzie (extension)	2. Back school 3. Back Traction	*Significant difference in pain at one month*
Roberts 1991	McKenzie	NSAID	*Significant difference in disability at seven weeks in those classified by mechanical syndrome*
Adams 1993	Extension		*Pain reduction (P<0.001)* *Increased ROM (P<0.05)*
Kay and Helewa 1994	McKenzie	Maitland	*Pain:* *1: -18* *2: +16 (P=0.029)*
Goldby 1995	McKenzie	Non-prescriptive exercise	*Significant differences in pain, Oswestry, HLC*
Fowler and Oyekoya 1995	McKenzie	Other therapies	*74% responded quicker to McKenzie*
Borrows and Herbison 1995a, 1995b	McKenzie residential rehabilitation programme	2. 3. and 4. Gym-based exercise and rehabilitation programmes	*Impairment:* *1: -7* *2: 0* *3: -1* *4: -4 (P=0.0005)* *Oswestry:* *1: -7%* *2: -3%* *3: -3.5%* *4: -9% (P= 0.0005)*

Continued next page

Reference	Group 1	Group 2	Results
Udermann *et al.* 2000	*Treat Your Own Back*		*Pain: -0.9 (4 point scale) Episodes: -3 (P<0.0001)*
Schenk 2000	McKenzie	Mobilisation	*Significant differences: pain (P<0.014) function (P<0.032)*

Positive extension sign = increase in radicular pain on extension in lying
HLC = health locus of control

Studies into directional preference

Directional preference describes the propensity of mechanical back and referred pain to lessen if movements or positions in one direction are performed and to worsen if movements or postures in the opposite direction are performed. Likewise, opposite postures or movements may centralise or peripheralise patients' symptoms. Studies included in this section have specifically investigated the phenomenon of directional preference. This has been done by randomly exposing patients to repeated movements or postural practises with different loading strategies and examining their symptomatic response. Studies have been conducted on the effects of extension and flexion and into control or limitation of flexion – main findings are summarised in Table 11.4.

Donelson *et al.* (1991) examined the effects of flexion and extension on symptoms in the short-term by randomising 145 patients to two different protocols. In one group flexion movements were performed first and then extension movements, first in standing and then in lying; in the other group the order of movements was reversed. Whichever protocol was performed, flexion generally had the effect of increasing symptoms and extension generally had the effect of decreasing symptoms. Individually, back pain decreased in fourteen subjects (10%) during flexion and in thirty-one subjects (21%) during extension. Individually distal leg pain decreased in eleven subjects (8%) during flexion and in fifty-six subjects (39%) during extension. Interestingly, only one patient reported improvement with both flexion and extension movements. An analysis model that assumed different responses to flexion and extension in central and peripheral pain and centralisation/peripheralisation was tested out, which found significant differences in pain behaviour to the different movements (P<0.0001). Methods score – 57% (Rebbeck 1997).

Williams *et al.* (1991) compared the effects of two sitting postures on back and referred pain over a twenty-four- to forty-eight-hour period. Two hundred and ten patients with acute and chronic symptoms were randomised to a kyphotic or lordotic sitting group. Patients' response to the different sitting postures was assessed while in the clinic, and then over the next day or two they were instructed, when they sat, to assume a particular posture. The lordotic group was provided with a lumbar roll and instructed to maintain their lordosis; the kyphotic group with a portable cushion and instructed to sit with the spine in flexion. Back and referred symptoms were again assessed on return to the clinic.

There was a significant reduction in back and leg pain at all test points in the lordotic group compared to baseline, but no change in the kyphotic group. Whereas at baseline there was no significant difference between the two groups after the intervention, they differed significantly in terms of back (P = 0.009) and leg (P = 0.018) pain. There was a 21% and 56% reduction in intensity of back and leg pain respectively in the lordotic group, while in the kyphotic group back pain increased by 14%, and there was no change in leg pain intensity. Pain peripheralised to below the knee in 6% of the lordotic group and in 24% of the kyphotic group (P = 0.017). Conversely, pain centralised above the knee in 56% of the lordotic group and 10% of the kyphotic group (P = 0.001).

Snook *et al.* (1998) tested the effect of controlling early morning flexion in a group of patients with chronic back pain whose mean duration of symptoms was seventeen years. After recruitment symptoms were monitored for six months, patients were then randomised to the intervention or a control group who performed flexion exercises, which a previous study had found to be ineffective. The intervention group received instructions and help in a strict regimen of abstaining from flexion in the first two hours after rising, and relative restriction on flexion activities thereafter. After six months the control group was instructed in the intervention.

At six months there were significant improvements in pain intensity (P < 0.01), days in pain (P < 0.05) and medication use (P < 0.05) for the intervention group that were not found in the control group. At one year there were further improvements in pain for the intervention group and a number of significant changes in both groups relating to pain and disability compared to baseline.

The drop-out rate from this study was high, especially from the intervention group, with a 30% attrition rate following randomisation. This perhaps attests to the difficulty of making such behavioural changes; the postural rules expected of the patients were extremely strict and demanding. Fifty-three of the sixty patients who completed the trial were followed up at three years (Snook 2000). Sixty-two percent of this group were still finding the intervention useful and restricting their flexion, and 74% reported a further reduction in days in pain.

Table 11.4. Studies into directional preference

Reference	Intervention	Effects of extension	Effects of flexion	Difference between groups
Donelson et al. 1991	Repeated movements in single assessment. Randomised: 1. extension/ flexion 2. flexion/ extension	LBP better: 21% Leg pain better: 39%	LBP better: 10% Leg pain better: 8%	P = 0.0001
Williams et al. 1991	Two-day period Randomised: 1. lordotic sitting 2. kyphotic sitting	LBP better: 21% Leg pain better: 56% Centralisa- tion: 56% Periphera- lisation: 6%	LBP worse: 14% Leg pain: no change Centralisa- tion: 10% Periphera- lisation: 24%	P = 0.009 P = 0.018 P = 0.001 P = 0.017
		Control of morning flexion		*Difference from baseline*
Snook et al. 1998	One year study Randomised: 1. flexion control / flexion control 2. sham / flexion control	Pain intensity reduced Pain days reduced Impairment days reduced Medication days reduced		1 and 2: P < 0.001 1: P < .001 2: P < 0.05 1: P< 0.05 2: P < 0.01 1 and 2: P<0.05

LBP = low back pain

These trials and those mentioned in other sections in this chapter (for instance, Kopp *et al.* 1986; Alexander *et al.* 1992; Donelson *et al.*

1990) illustrate the effect that different loading strategies can have on back pain. All movements are not the same. Commonly in these studies, extension or control of flexion is the direction of preference. Donelson *et al.* (1991) demonstrated that in a single session without the use of force progressions, 40% showed a clear preference for extension, and Williams *et al.* (1991) states that nearly 60% showed a preference for an extended posture when sitting. In the long-term follow-up conducted by Snook (2000), about 60% of those who completed the trial still found limitation of flexion helpful. However, a minority of patients demonstrate other directional preferences, with 7% showing a clear preference for flexion in one trial (Donelson *et al.* 1991). Patients at all stages of the natural history of back pain show these responses, both those with acute and chronic symptoms. The fact that different patients show preferences for different movements should be considered in the construction of future trials. In the past, individual assessment of suitability for exercise regimes has rarely been conducted.

The importance of directional preference in management strategies has been recognised in other classification systems: Fritz and George (2000) include a flexion and an extension syndrome, Sikorski (1985) includes an anterior and a posterior element category, Wilson *et al.* (1999) also include patterns that are based on directional preferences or antipathies. One pattern is worse with flexion, another worse with extension. The largest group were those made worse by flexion activities, which represented about 65% of the population sample. The other classification systems categorised 36% to 50% of their samples as having directional preferences for extension or flexion (Fritz and George 2000; Sikorski 1985).

As different mechanical back pain problems display different directional preferences, all back pain cannot be viewed as a homogeneous entity, nor can it be presumed that all patients will respond in the same way to the same exercises.

Reliability studies

Certain studies have sought to evaluate the reliability of the McKenzie system as a whole, whereas other studies have examined the reliability of components of the whole approach. The Kappa coefficient is commonly used in reliability studies (see Glossary). Principle findings are summarised in Table 11.5.

Kilby *et al.* (1990) developed a clinical algorithm to test out the reliability of the syndrome classification system. The behaviour of pain with repeated movements and sustained positions was the key factor in the determination of the syndrome. Two clinicians, with limited attendance on McKenzie courses, assessed forty-one patients. One assessed the patient while the other one observed; no communication was allowed. Inter-clinician agreement was assessed by Kappa, with percentage agreement being used where numbers were insufficient for Kappa analysis. The answers were within 10% of perfect agreement in all but three questions. There was perfect or near perfect agreement on questions about centralisation (Kappa 0.51), constant pain, referred pain, pain on static loading and central or symmetrical pain. There was poorer agreement about the presence of a kyphotic and lateral shift deformity and pain at end-range. Agreement was less good by diagnosis, with less than 60% agreement on the classification recorded, although this improved to 74% if derangements three and four, and five and six were amalgamated (McKenzie 1981).

The strong point of the system revealed by this study is the level of agreement on interpreting pain behaviour on repeated movements. Centralisation, reduction or abolition of pain may be reliably interpreted. Visual observation, such as the presence of a lateral shift, has a weaker level of agreement. When this decision-making process was taken out of the equation, and derangement three and four and five and six amalgamated, agreement on derangement classification increased substantially. In thirteen of the forty-one (32%) of the sample, the diagnosis was uncertain or the problem had resolved.

Riddle and Rothstein (1993) conducted a multi-centred study involving 363 patients and forty-nine clinicians evaluating the reliability of the classification system. Information for the clinicians on the criteria for classification into syndromes was summarised by the authors. Only sixteen of the clinicians had attended at least one postgraduate course in the use of the McKenzie approach, so for most of them this four-page pamphlet, which contained inaccuracies, was the only information available. Patients were assessed first by one clinician and then within fifteen minutes by the second clinician, meaning that patients were put through two lengthy assessments that may have had the effect of changing symptoms. For all clinicians, agreement on classification was 39% (Kappa 0.26) and ranged from 22% to 60% in the different clinics (Kappa 0.02 to 0.48). Agreement was even less in those with some training at 27% (Kappa 0.15).

This study did not assess any component parts of the assessment procedure, but only the final mechanical syndrome classification. The study reveals a considerable lack of understanding of factors involved in this classification process by the participating clinicians. For instance, the different derangements, one and two, three and four, and five and six, are differentiated by the site of the pain. However, pain that one clinician reported to be referred to the knee or foot was reported in another area on 50% or more of occasions. Classification of postural, dysfunction and derangements syndromes was completely muddled – of the thirty-eight patients, one clinician reported postural syndrome, the other clinician reported 29% dysfunction and 29% derangement. Of twenty-eight patients that one clinician reported to be derangement five, the other clinician reported 25% dysfunction, 18% derangement one and two and 21% derangement three and four. The study certainly shows that in the hands of untrained clinicians, the system cannot be reliably used as basic errors in interpretation of pain site and pain behaviour are being made.

Razmjou *et al.* (2000b) reformulated some of the data reported by Riddle and Rothstein (1993) to compare the effect of education. When it comes to differentiating between the different syndromes, although percentage agreements are not much better between the untrained and the partially trained clinicians, there is far less variability. In particular, there is no disagreement between postural and derangement categories, and the most common mistake is between dysfunction and derangement syndromes.

The patient population studied were a very chronic group, with a mean duration of symptoms of seventy-four weeks. In the instructions given to clinicians, only ten of each repeated movement was allowed. Despite this, rather surprisingly in a group that would be expected to require lengthier periods of testing, clinicians failed to give a diagnosis in only sixteen (4%) patients. The study reveals the importance of experience and education in the use of a classification system, which allows interpreters to gain an understanding of the significance of different aspects of the assessment. Lack of experience permits multiple erroneous decisions during the diagnostic process.

Donahue *et al.* (1996) evaluated the reliability of the identification of a lateral shift and relevant lateral component. Forty-nine patients were examined separately by two clinicians drawn from a pool of ten clinicians, all with no postgraduate McKenzie training. Reliability was studied for a two-step process – first the agreement on presence of a lateral shift using a spirit level, second on the relevance of the lateral component by performing repeated movements. Relevance was determined by a change in the location or intensity of pain during or immediately following side glide testing. Overall there was 47% agreement (Kappa = 0.16). However, when the two steps of the process were evaluated separately, the results were very different. The inter-tester reliability of the presence and direction of lateral shifts using the spirit level was 43% agreement (Kappa = 0.00). The inter-tester reliability of the relevance of the lateral component as determined by symptom response to repeated movements was 94% agreement (Kappa 0.74).

Another study demonstrated that larger lateral shifts could be reliably observed. Tenhula *et al.* (1990) examined twenty-four patients with 'an observable lateral shift', with apparently those with an equivocal shift not being admitted to the study. However, an operational definition of what is 'an observable lateral shift' was not given. One clinician judged the presence and direction of a shift while the second determined the same factors from a slide image of the patients. Perfect agreement (Kappa 1.00) was found. This study also found a statistically significant relationship between the shift and a positive side bending movement when it was seen to alter symptoms. This indicates the usefulness of repeated movements to identify the presence of a lateral shift.

Razmjou *et al.* (2000a) examined components of the assessment as well as the classification system itself. One clinician examined forty-five patients while a second clinician observed the interaction; both had considerable postgraduate McKenzie training. Various elements of the assessment process were shown to have good to excellent reliability, including the relevance of the lateral component and lateral shift, the presence of a sagittal plane deformity, syndrome identification and derangement sub-classification. The presence of a lateral shift had moderate reliability. There were three disagreements over classification; one clinician classified these patients as 'other', and one clinician as dysfunction and derangement.

It is interesting to contrast the proportion of syndrome classification made by these experienced McKenzie practitioners with the untrained and partially trained clinicians in Riddle and Rothstein (1993). While Razmjou *et al.* (2000a) diagnosed derangement in about 88% of patients, dysfunction in about 7% and posture in 2%, in the other study classification was respectively about 55%, 35% and 10%. Clinicians unfamiliar with the system do not recognise the preponderance of derangements in clinical practice and overestimate the prevalence of the other two mechanical syndromes.

Fritz *et al.* (2000a) used a different method to evaluate the inter-tester reliability of centralisation involving video footage of patient assessments. This was then shown to forty clinicians and forty student clinicians, who were also given clear operational definitions of centralisation, peripheralisation and status quo. Agreement over symptomatic response among all clinicians was 88% (Kappa 0.79), with students only slightly less reliable than qualified clinicians.

Werneke *et al.* (1999), as part of a descriptive study of centralisation, carried out a reliability check. Clinicians had near perfect agreement both in location of most distal pain and in categorisation of patients into centralisation, partial centralisation or non-centralisation groups (Kappa 0.917 to 1.00).

Kilpikoski *et al.* (2002) evaluated two clinicians and thirty-nine patients on inter-tester agreement on certain aspects of a McKenzie assessment. One examiner questioned the patient with the other examiner present; they then took it in turns to examine the patient independently. As in other studies, observation of the presence (Kappa 0.2) and direction (Kappa 0.4) of a lateral shift was less reliable than the relevance of the shift (Kappa 0.7). Reliability of classification into McKenzie main syndromes (Kappa 0.6), sub-classification (Kappa 0.7), centralisation (Kappa 0.7) and directional preference (Kappa 0.9) were all good to very good.

Some other studies examining the reliability of different aspects of spinal assessment include evaluations of relevant tests, and these are included in the table below (11.5). Nelson *et al.* (1979) and Strender *et al.* (1997) examined lateral tilt or sagittal configuration. Strender *et al.* (1997) and McCombe *et al.* (1989) examined pain production during single sagittal plane test movements, and Spratt *et al.* (1990) examined repeated movements and pain location and aggravation.

In summary, several studies attest to the good reliability of assessment of symptomatic response, including centralisation (Kilby *et al.* 1990; Fritz *et al.* 2000a; Donahue *et al.* 1996; Razmjou *et al.* 2000a; Werneke *et al.* 1999). Decision-making based on observation, such as the presence or not of a lateral shift, has a tendency to be less reliable (Kilby *et al.* 1990; Donahue *et al.* 1996); however, it can be reliable in substantial shifts (Tenhula *et al.* 1990). Although the McKenzie classification system has been shown to be very unreliable when used by clinicians who are naïve to it (Riddle and Rothstein 1993), the system has been shown to have very good reliability in those who are experienced in the approach (Razmjou *et al.* 2000a).

Table 11.5 Studies evaluating the reliability of different aspects of the McKenzie system (see text for more detail)

Component	Agreement	Kappa	Reference
Centralisation	90–100%	0.51	Kilby *et al.* 1990
	88%	0.79	Fritz *et al.* 2000a
	94%		Sufka *et al.* 1998
		0.96	Werneke *et al.* 1999
	95%	0.7	Kilpikoski 2002
Relevant lateral component – by symptom response	94%	0.74	Donahue *et al.* 1996
	98%	0.85–0.95	Razmjou *et al.* 2000
	89%	0.6	Kilpikoski 2002
Directional preference	90%	0.9	Kilpikoski 2002
Constant pain	95%		Kilby *et al.* 1990
Site of pain	93–100%		Kilby *et al.* 1990
		0.92–1.0	Werneke *et al.* 1999
Kyphotic deformity	80%		Kilby *et al.* 1990
	100%	1.0	Razmjou *et al.* 2000
Lateral shift – by observation	55%		Kilby *et al.* 1990
	43%	0.0	Donahue *et al.* 1996
		1.0	Tenhula *et al.* 1990
	78%	0.52	Razmjou *et al.* 2000
	76%	0.39	Strender *et al.* 1997
	70%		Nelson *et al.* 1979
Presence	76%	0.2	Kilpikoski 2002
Direction	78%	0.5	
Classification	58–74%		Kilby *et al.* 1990
	39%	0.26	Riddle and Rothstein 1993
	93–97%	0.7–0.96	Razmjou *et al.* 2000
	74–95%	0.6–0.7	Kilpikoski 2002
Pain production: – single test movements	82–88%	0.63–0.76	Strender *et al.* 1997
		0.31–0.57	McCombe *et al.* 1989
Repeated movements:			Spratt *et al.* 1990
– pain location	100%		
– pain aggravation	53–59%		

Comparison with other classification systems and assessment procedures

It may be instructive at this point to compare the reliability of the McKenzie approach, which has been reviewed above, with examples of other systems of classification and also other assessment procedures that are commonly used in physical therapy.

Wilson *et al.* (1999) investigated the inter-tester reliability of a classification system for back pain that has similarities with the McKenzie approach, as it uses pain patterns and response to movement testing and posture. For instance, one group is worse with flexion, another worse with extension. Overall agreement on classification was moderately good at 79% (Kappa = 0.61). Fritz and George (2000) investigated a classification system based upon a mixture of history, findings from physical examination and pain response to extension and flexion. Overall reliability was again moderately good (Kappa value 0.56).

Reliability of palpation studies

Mechanical diagnosis and therapy primarily uses movement, pain responses and function for assessment purposes. In general, palpation adds very little to this interpretation. A key failing of tests that are dependent upon palpation or observation is their very poor history of reliability. Across a wide range of studies, as illustrated below (Table 11.6), these procedures have been shown to be of limited use in identifying objective or stable markers. Although frequently the same clinician is reasonably reliable in reaching the same conclusion on different occasions, the reliability of palpatory tests between clinicians is consistently poor. To use such insubstantial factors to predict treatment would seem to be unwise.

Most studies are performed on volunteers without symptoms; sometimes the study was conducted on a spinal model. Different statistical measures have often been used in these studies, which have also been conducted with different methods, so results are not always directly comparable. A number of studies have used Kappa values (see Glossary), but not all studies have used this statistical analysis. The conclusion of some studies can only be given in a qualitative judgement. Some studies use intraclass correlation coefficients (ICC), in which the maximum is 1.00, indicating perfect agreement. Mean values are given where possible, sometimes obtained by calculation from original data.

Included in the following tables are results from studies that have also investigated the reliability of tests using pain responses (indicated in bold). Although comparisons between diverse studies using dissimilar statistical analyses may be problematic, the results across different studies consistently reinforce the same conclusions. At a glance it can be seen that intra-tester reliability is considerably better than inter-tester reliability, which is consistently poor. However, procedures that use pain response are far more reliable than those using palpation.

Table 11.6   Reliability of palpation examination procedures in the lumbar spine compared to reliability of pain behaviours

Reference	Assessment procedure (mean)	Intra-tester reliability (mean)	Inter-tester reliability	Intra-/Inter-tester reliability of pain behaviour
Mootz *et al.* 1989	Fixations, present or absent	K 0.17*	K 0.00	
McKenzie and Taylor 1997	Spinal level	K 0.74*	K 0.28	
Lindsay *et al.* 1995	AM PIM		K -0.1* K 0.05*	
Binkley *et al.* 1995	AM Spinal level		K 0.09 K 0.30	
Carty *et al.* 1986	AM	K 0.58	K 0.30	
Gonnella *et al.* 1982	PIM	Dependable	Not dependable	
Billis *et al.* 1999	Spinal level	Good	Poor	
Simmonds *et al.* 1995	Grade of accessory motion on spinal model		Large force variability: e.g. 2 – 131 N, 16 – 259 N	
Hardy and Napier 1991	Grade of accessory motion on spinal model	Significant variability, P< 0.01	Significant variability, P < 0.001	
Maher and Adams 1995	Stiffness in human spines		ICC 0.19	

Continued next page

Reference	Assessment procedure (mean)	Intra-tester reliability (mean)	Inter-tester reliability	Intra-/Inter-tester reliability of pain behaviour
Maher and Adams 1994	Stiffness in human spines **Pain response**		ICC 0.17* ICC 0.66*	
Matyas and Bach 1985	Review: AM **Pain** on accessory movements **Pain** on SLR **Pain** on flexion	Reliability coefficients*: 0.30	Reliability coefficients*: 0.26	Reliability coefficients*: 0.78 / 0.68 0.96 / 0.86 0.96 / 0.73
Van Dillen *et al.* 1998	25 items – alignment and move-ment 28 items – pain response		K 0.46*	K 0.96*

SLR = straight leg raise
ICC = intraclass correlation coefficient
K = kappa
* = calculated from original data
AM = accessory movements
PIM = passive intervertebral movements

The overwhelming evidence from the table is that while intra-tester reliability can be good, inter-tester reliability is consistently poor, or at best fair. Experience does not particularly appear to affect clinicians' ability to be consistent with their peers. Studies that have used experienced clinicians (Vincent-Smith and Gibbons 1999; van Deursen *et al.* 1990; Mootz *et al.* 1989; Simmonds *et al.* 1995; Mior *et al.* 1990) have not shown better results than studies involving student physical clinicians or chiropractors (Carmichael 1987; Mior *et al.* 1990; Matyas and Bach 1985). The poor reliability of judgements about spinal mobility raises the possibility that *"this information provides a false impression of meaningfulness that hinders rather than helps treatment selection and patient management"* (Maher and Adams 1994, p. 807).

Furthermore, the clinical utility of basing treatment on stiffness levels may be unwarranted. *"The large amount of variability in spinal stiffness values between subjects, or at different levels within the one subject, makes the determination of areas of abnormally increased stiffness difficult. Increased stiffness may in fact be a normal variant and bear no relationship to the patient's presenting symptoms"* (Maher and Adams 1992, p. 259).

The other irresistible conclusion from these studies is that pain response is a more reliable indicator than perceptions of stiffness (Matyas and Bach 1985; Maher and Adams 1992, 1994). *"Studies have consistently shown that manual assessment of factors such as bony anomalies, tissue texture, muscle tension, joint compliance, and range of motion are unreliable whether performed by physioclinicians, physicians, or chiropractors. Tests which relied solely on patient response such as pain and tenderness were found to be more reliable"* (Maher and Adams 1992, p. 258).

It is instructional to compare the Kappa values given in Table 11.6 with those in Table 11.5 of studies evaluating the reliability of different aspects of the McKenzie system. These reinforce the same point: pain response is considerably more reliable than palpation or observation.

Studies into the prognostic and diagnostic utility of centralisation

One of the key symptomatic responses employed in mechanical diagnosis is centralisation. Several studies have investigated this phenomenon, and these will be outlined below. Centralisation is discussed in more depth in Chapter 8. In all of the following studies, the level of training in the McKenzie approach of the involved clinicians is at least considered and displays considerable variability. Main findings are summarised in Table 11.7.

Donelson *et al.* (1990) were the first to describe in the literature the phenomenon that had been observed initially by McKenzie in 1956 (McKenzie 1981). Out of 225 consecutive patients with back pain, eighty-seven patients with radiation of pain to the buttock, thigh or calf were included in this study. Patients had a range of acute and chronic symptoms. Mechanical evaluation and treatment using end-range repeated sagittal and frontal plane movements was conducted, using the movement that abolished distal pain. Outcomes, which were reviewed independently, were said to be excellent if there was complete relief of symptoms, and good if there was partial relief and improvement in three secondary criteria: patient satisfaction, improvement in physical examination and return to work. A fair result was defined as partial relief, but with failure to improve in some of the secondary criteria and a poor outcome defined as no relief.

Centralisation occurred mostly on the initial visit and sometimes in the subsequent few days. The opposite movement to the one that centralised symptoms always exacerbated them. Seventy-six (87%) patients reported centralisation and seventy-two (83%) reported good or excellent outcomes. In those who had an excellent or good outcome 100% and 77% had centralisation of symptoms, while in those with fair or poor outcomes centralisation occurred in 57% and 37%. Centralisation occurred regardless of the length of time symptoms had been present – 89% in those with symptoms of less than four weeks, 87% in those with symptoms for four to twelve weeks and 84% in those with symptoms for over twelve weeks.

Long (1995) looked at centralisation in a chronic low back pain population. Two hundred and twenty-three patients were classified as centralisers or non-centralisers depending on their response to an initial mechanical evaluation – the most distal, but not all lower limb symptoms had to be abolished. Patients were then entered into a work-hardening programme, after which outcome measures were collected by staff blind to classification. Both groups reported significant reductions in pain intensity measures, but centralisers reported a greater improvement and also a higher return to work rate (68% compared to 52%). There were significant improvements in lifting ability and Oswestry disability scores, but no differences between the groups.

Karas *et al.* (1997) studied a back pain population who were out of work and compared the predictive value of centralisation and Waddell's non-organic signs regarding return to work. One hundred and seventy-one patients were examined, of whom 126 were used in the final calculations. Centralisation was defined as proximal movement or decrease of symptoms in response to movements in one direction within two treatments. Treatment consisted of exercises in the patients' direction of preference, recovery of function and physical conditioning. Low Waddell score (P=0.006) and centralisation (P=0.038), both separately and together, were associated with higher return to work rates. Failure to centralise or abolish symptoms rapidly and high Waddell scores are both associated with a lack of response to mechanical therapy and predict a poor outcome.

Sufka *et al.* (1998) compared, in twenty-four patients, those who completely centralised symptoms within two weeks and those who did not. Poorer outcomes were found in those with chronic symptoms. Centralisation occurred more frequently in those with acute compared to chronic symptoms (83% vs 60%) and in those with back pain only compared to those with pain below the knee (80% vs 43%). Two functional outcome measures were used – both showed greater improvements in the centralisation group, one of which was significant.

Donelson *et al.* (1997) conducted a one-off mechanical evaluation on sixty-three chronic back patients and compared the clinicians' findings with those from diagnostic disc injections. Following the mechanical assessment, patients were classified as centralisers, peripheralisers or no change. Following discography, classification was made as to positive discogenic pain and competency of the annulus. The investigator performing the discogram studies was blinded to the findings from the mechanical assessment. In those in whom pain centralised or peripheralised, 74% and 69% had positive discogenic pain, compared to 12% in the no-change group (P<0.001). Ninety-one percent of those who centralised had a competent annulus, compared to 54% of those who peripheralised (P<0.042).

Werneke *et al.* (1999) conducted a study involving 289 acute back and neck patients. Patients were classified into three groups: centralisation, non-centralisation and partial reduction. Centralisation was defined much more strictly than previous studies, as a lasting abolition of pain from the initial assessment, with further proximal movements of pain on all subsequent visits until all pain is abolished. The partial reduction group allowed a more gradual decrease in distal pain over a period of time and between clinic visits. With this stricter definition centralisation occurred less frequently (31%) than other studies, but partial reduction also happened regularly (44%). The complete centralisation group averaged fewer visits than both other groups, four compared to eight (P<0.001). However, concerning outcomes of pain and function, both the centralisation and partial reduction groups had greater improvements than the non-centralisation group (P<0.001). Thus the partial centralisation took longer but achieved the same outcome; this happened in two distinct patterns. About a third demonstrated a proximal change in pain on the initial visit, which was maintained, while 71% showed no change on the initial visit, but gradually centralised over time. About half had showed this improvement by the third visit, 74% by the fifth visit and 93% by the seventh visit. The authors speculate that improvements in this group were due to the natural history of acute problems, although equally they could have resulted from the prescribed exercise therapy. If patients had not demonstrated an improvement by the seventh visit, no significant changes were noted.

Werneke and Hart (2001) looked at the power of centralisation and non-centralisation to predict outcomes one year after patients were recruited to the study above in the 223 patients with back pain; 84% were contacted. The centralisation and partial reduction group were analysed together and compared to the non-centralisation group. Other demographic, historical, work-related and psychosocial factors were also considered. These included factors previously found to be of important prognostic value, such as pain intensity, duration of symptoms, prior spinal pain, workers' compensation, work satisfaction, Waddell's non-organic signs, depressive symptoms, somatisation and fear–avoidance. The outcomes considered were pain intensity, return to work, sick leave, function at home and health care usage. Nine of the twenty-three independent variables had an individual prognostic influence on certain outcomes at one year. However, in a multivariate logistic regression analysis that included all the significant factors from the univariate analyses, only two factors remained significant. Only centralisation / non-centralisation classification and leg pain at outset were predictive, with pain pattern classification predicting four out of the five outcomes.

Skytte (2001) studied sixty patients who were classified into centralisers (twenty-five) and non-centralisers (thirty-five) and followed them for one year. Forty-six percent of the non-centralisation group received surgery, compared to 12% of the centralisation group (P=0.01). Significant differences were also seen in reported disability and leg pain favouring the centralisation group, but no differences were seen in medication use, sick leave or back pain.

In summary, centralisation is a common occurrence in acute and chronic spinal pain. Various studies have demonstrated that, compared to patients who fail to centralise, the phenomenon is associated with significantly better outcomes relating to pain, function and return to work (Donelson *et al.* 1990; Long 1995; Karas *et al.*

1997; Sufka *et al.* 1998; Werneke *et al.* 1999). The converse is also very apparent from these studies; non-centralisation is significantly associated with a poor outcome. The study by Werneke *et al.* (1999) suggests that if a decrease in pain location score is not apparent by the seventh visit, no improvements are likely. Werneke and Hart (2001) further investigated the predictive value of centralisation or partial reduction compared to non-centralisation along with twenty-three other psychosocial, somatic and demographic variables. Non-centralisation was the most powerful independent predictor of poor outcomes. This is the first study in which a clinical variable has been shown to be of more significance than psychosocial factors in predicting chronic pain and disability.

Studies addressing the reliability of assessment of centralisation are summarised in a section above. Williams *et al.* (1991) demonstrated the use of the lordotic sitting posture to bring about centralisation, and this study is also summarised above in the section on directional preference. The data from the study by Donelson *et al.* (1997) has been re-analysed to determine the diagnostic utility of mechanical diagnosis and assessment (Delaney and Hubka 1999). They determined that using the McKenzie system assessment for discogenic pain had a sensitivity of 94% and specificity of 82%, while assessment for an incompetent annulus had a sensitivity of 100% and specificity of 86%. Compared to nine other tests used in assessment of low back pain, none were more sensitive, but three were more specific.

Table 11.7 Studies investigating centralisation (see text for detail)

Reference	N	Patient description	% C	Outcomes relative to centralisation (Significant differences)
Donelson et al. 1990	87	Acute 61%, sub-acute 17%, chronic 22% Symptoms below knee 51%	87%	*Correlation between centralisation and good/ excellent outcome (P<0.001), non-centralisation and poor/fair outcome (P<0.001)*
Long 1995	223	Chronic 100% Symptoms below knee 49% Out of work 100%	47%	*Greater reduction in pain intensity (<0.05), higher return to work rate (P=0.034)*

Continued next page

Reference	N	Patient description	% C	Outcomes relative to centralisation (Significant differences)
Karas et al. 1997	126/171	Acute and chronic Out of work 100%	73%	More frequent return to work (P=0.038)
Donelson et al. 1997	63	Chronic 100% Majority pain below the knee Not working 70%	49%	74% positive discogram (P<0.007), of whom 91% competent annular wall (P<0.001)
Sufka et al. 1998	36/48	Acute 16%, sub-acute 42%, chronic 42% Symptoms below the knee 39%	69%	Greater functional improvement (P=0.015)
Werneke et al. 1999	289	Back pain 77% Acute 100% Symptoms below knee/ elbow 31% Not working 37%	1: 31% 2: 44%	1: Fewer visits (P<0.001) 1+2: Greater improvements in pain (P<0.001), and function (P<0.001)
Werneke and Hart 2001	187	Acute 100%, reviewed at one year	77%	Non-centralisation predicted work status, function, health care use (P<0.001) and pain intensity (P=0.004)

% C = proportion in which centralisation occurred.

Werneke et al. 1999: 1 = centralisation, 2 = partial centralisation (see text).

Conclusions

This chapter has presented the current literature that is relevant to the McKenzie approach. New research is continuously being conducted, and no doubt some new studies will have been missed in this review. The literature has been described by intervention studies, by directional preference, by reliability studies and by studies investigating centralisation.

Intervention studies in the shape of RCTs are deemed to be the 'gold standard' measurement of effective treatment. To date, several studies attest to the efficacy of the McKenzie approach, but more high-quality studies are needed. In particular, there is the suggestion from several studies that patients with chronic back pain may find the approach especially helpful, and yet this is an area that has been little explored. Most studies have been conducted with patients with acute/sub-acute back pain, a group who often have a good prognosis whatever is done to them.

In most of the literature to date there has been no attempt to classify patients before treatment. It is assumed that all patients respond equally to extension or flexion exercises regardless of their problem. However, back pain is a symptom, not a diagnosis. Several studies attest to the fact that all back pain does not respond equally to the same exercise, but that individual patients have directional preferences for particular exercises (Donelson *et al.* 1990, 1991; Wilson *et al.* 1999; Fritz and George 2000). Some of this work has been done by different groups of clinicians who have, independently of the McKenzie classification system, identified specific sub-groups based upon directional preference. Failure to incorporate this into intervention studies could produce a situation in which some patients improve with, for instance, extension exercises, some worsen, and the net result for the group *as a whole* is no change.

Reliability studies show that a core component of the system of mechanical diagnosis and therapy, evaluation based upon symptomatic response, generally has good to excellent reliability. By way of comparison a section also looks at the reliability of palpation techniques, which the literature shows to be a far less reliable means of examination. The classification system as a whole has been shown to be reliable in the hands of experts, but not when tested by clinicians who are naïve to the system. Centralisation can both be reliably evaluated and has been shown to be a significant prognostic factor; its presence strongly associated with good outcomes and its absence strongly associated with poor outcomes. Several studies suggest that failure to achieve this symptomatic change within seven treatment sessions indicates a failure to respond.

12: Serious Spinal Pathology

Introduction

Other chapters give descriptions of the mechanical syndromes as described by McKenzie (1981, 1990). These will encompass the majority of back pain patients, most of whom will have derangements, a few dysfunction, and even fewer present with pain of postural origin. Only a small number of patients are not grouped in one of the mechanical syndromes. This includes a few patients who have serious spinal pathology, which is the subject of this chapter. The next chapter deals with other conditions.

Within specific conditions that must be considered are the serious spinal conditions that need early identification and onward referral. A brief description is given here of cancer, infection, fractures, cauda equina and cord signs; these are given as the most common examples of serious spinal pathology. Identification of these patients is also considered in the section about *'red flags'* in the chapter on history-taking (14). A brief description is also given here of ankylosing spondylitis, as an example of one of the inflammatory arthropathies that affect spinal joints. Again, patients who are suspected of having this condition need appropriate referral so diagnosis can be clarified, although this is not the referral emergency represented by cauda equina and similar spinal problems.

It is always important to have an index of suspicion concerning specific serious spinal pathology and to use the initial assessment to triage patients (CSAG 1994; AHCPR 1994):

- serious spinal pathology

- nerve root problems

- non-specific 'mechanical' backache.

However, it must always be remembered that the vast majority of all patients fit into the latter category of non-specific, mechanical back pain. *Serious spinal pathology accounts for less than 1% of all back pain; inflammatory arthropathies also account for less than 1% of all back pain* (Waddell 1998; CSAG 1994). 'Red flag' conditions are very unusual; in a cohort of over 400 patients with acute back pain presenting to doctors in primary care, six (1.4%) had fractures or carcinomas (McGuirk *et al.* 2001).

The sections in this chapter are as follows:

- cancer * *RED FLAG*

- infections * *RED FLAG*

- fractures * *RED FLAG*

- osteoporosis

- cauda equina syndrome * *RED FLAG*

- cord signs * *RED FLAG*

- ankylosing spondylitis.

Cancer * *RED FLAG*

In a retrospective review of radiographs of 782 patients with back pain, 0.84% had metastatic disease (Scavone *et al.* 1981a). In over 400 patients with acute back pain in primary care, 0.7% had a carcinoma: one of the kidney, one of the liver and one of the prostate (McGuirk *et al.* 2001). In nearly 2,000 walk-in patients with a chief complaint of back pain, thirteen patients (0.66%) proved to have cancer as the cause of their back pain (Deyo and Diehl 1988b).

Tumours of the lumbar spine can be clinically silent, cause back pain only, or may cause neurological deficit as well (Macnab and McCulloch 1990; Findlay 1992). They may be either benign or malignant, with a high incidence of neurological involvement in both. Neurological damage may involve the spinal cord or nerve roots or plexus, thus producing upper or lower motor neurone signs and symptoms (Rodichok *et al.* 1986; Ruff and Lanska 1989).

Primary tumours are extremely rare in the spine, while secondary tumours are less so. The breast, lung and prostate are the most common sources of spinal metastases, being the origin of over 60% of spinal metastases (Schaberg and Gainor 1985; Rodichok *et al.* 1986; Bernat *et al.* 1983). The thoracic spine is the most common site of metastases (50% or more), and about 20 – 30% occur in the lumbar spine (Ruff and Lanska 1989; Bernat *et al.* 1983). Back pain may be the presenting finding in about 25% of patients with malignant lesions. However, back pain may be absent; in one profile of 179 patients with spinal metastases, 36% were free of back pain (Schaberg and Gainor 1985). Although all tumours become visible on radiographs, 30% of the bone mass may be destroyed before a lesion is evident.

If the vertebral body is affected, pain is generally produced by pressure on, and then destruction of, the richly innervated periosteum. As the tumour spreads, the vertebra may collapse and soft tissues become involved. Severe pain may be accompanied by paralysis as tumour invasion causes collapse of the vertebra, deformity and neural encroachment (DeWald et al. 1985). With intradural tumours back pain occurs later, and muscle spasm and neurological involvement are a more common presentation. As symptoms are the result of a space-occupying lesion, which will only continue to grow and will certainly not shrink or vary over time, once pain commences it will become progressively more severe and intractable.

Findlay (1992) describes the clinical presentation thus: a deep-seated, boring constant pain, which is persistent and worsens as the pathology progresses. Unlike normal musculoskeletal pain, there is a lack of variability over time, and frequently, especially in children, the pain is worse at night. Musculoskeletal pain can also occur at night, but is usually relieved by a change in position; cancer pain is much more severe, may drive the patient from bed and can lead to frequent disturbances all night long (Cadoux-Hudson 2000). Certain tumours trigger considerable paravertebral muscle spasm. Neurological deficit and radicular pain may accompany back pain or may follow it. Tumours may produce localised nerve root or cauda equina syndromes, cord signs, or multiple root level signs if the plexus is damaged (Findlay 1992; Rodichok et al. 1986; Ruff and Lanska 1989).

While none of the physical signs were significantly associated with cancer, various elements of the history were (Deyo and Diehl 1988b). Findings that were significantly more common in cancer patients: age fifty years or over, previous history of cancer, sought medical care in last month and not improving, duration of episode greater than one month (Table 12.1). Although not significant, unexplained weight loss was also associated with cancer. Various laboratory findings were also significantly associated with cancer: erythrocyte sedimentation rate (ESR) of more than 50mm/hour (likelihood ratio 19.2), ESR more than 100mm/hour (likelihood ratio 55.5), anaemia (likelihood ratio 4). Radiographic findings of lytic or blastic lesions were excellent discriminators of cancer patients (likelihood ratio 120).

The individual sensitivity and specificity of many of these factors was poor; thus, a constellation of warning factors and an algorithmic approach to diagnosis were proposed (Deyo and Diehl 1988b). Those patients with a history of previous cancer should undergo ESR and x-ray investigation; in this group the prevalence of cancer is 9%. Those aged over 50, or with failure to improve with conservative therapy or unexplained weight loss/systemic signs should undergo ESR tests, and an x-ray should be considered – in this group cancer prevalence is 2.3%. In the rest – 60% of the original sample – no testing strategy is necessary, and the prevalence rate of cancer is 0%.

Table 12.1 Significant history in identification of cancer

History	Sensitivity	Specificity	Likelihood ratio
> 50 years	0.77	0.71	2.7
Previous history of cancer	0.31	0.98	14.7
Unexplained weight loss	0.15	0.94	2.7
Failure to improve after one month of therapy	0.31	0.90	3.0
No relief with bed-rest	>0.90	0.46	
Duration of pain > one month	0.50	0.81	2.6

Source: Deyo et al. 1992

The importance of a previous history of cancer as a risk factor for back pain that is caused by metastases is amply illustrated by a series of known cancer patients investigated for spinal pain. In these patients, 54% and 68% were discovered to have epidural, vertebral or nerve root metastases (Ruff and Lanska 1989; Rodichok et al. 1986).

Infections * RED FLAG

Spinal infections are extremely rare causes of back pain (Macnab and McCulloch 1990). An estimation of incidence is one per 250,000 of population (Digby and Kersley 1979). A survey in Denmark found an incidence of five cases of acute vertebral osteomyelitis per million of population per year – a rate of 0.0005% (Krogsgaard et al. 1998). The lumbar spine was affected in 59% and the thoracic spine in 33%. The highest incidence of the disease was in the 60 – 69-year-old age group, with over two-thirds of cases occurring in those between 50 and 80. However, osteomyelitis can occur in adults or children. An impaired immune system is common, and risk factors include insulin-dependent diabetes mellitus, treatment with corticosteroids, chemotherapy, and renal or hepatic failure (Carragee 1997; Krogsgaard *et al.* 1998).

Back pain may be the main symptom in most patients (Carragee 1997). Patients have severe, progressive back pain of a non-mechanical nature, leading to spinal rigidity; tension signs are common (Macnab and McCulloch 1990). Patients are often unwell, with raised temperature, and suffer from general malaise, night pain, night sweats and raised erythrocyte sedimentation rate (Wainwright 2000). However, fever is not always present, varying between 27% and 83%, depending on the type of infection (Deyo *et al.* 1992).

Spinal infections are usually blood-borne from other sites. An unequivocal primary source of infection is found in about 40% of patients with osteomyelitis. The most common source is from the genitourinary tract, and secondly skin and respiratory infections; other relevant infections include spinal tuberculosis, brucellosis, epidural space infections and, reportedly, injections sites from illegal intravenous drug use (Deyo *et al.* 1992; Carragee 1997; Krogsgaard *et al.* 1998; Waldvogel and Vasey 1980).

A report on thirty patients with non-tuberculous pyogenic spinal infection found urinary tract infection to be the most common source of infection (30%), although in a few patients disease appeared to have been precipitated by spinal trauma (Digby and Kersley 1979). There was a preponderance of two age groups, adolescents and the elderly. Localised back pain was the predominant symptom; this was not always severe, but tended to be constant and unrelated to posture or movement. A febrile episode frequently preceded the onset of back pain, and the erythrocyte sedimentation rate was raised in all cases.

A case report documents a history of acute onset back pain with symptoms referred to the lateral border of the foot with lateral shift and kyphotic deformity, gross limitations of all movements, and limited straight leg raise who was found to have discitis (Greene 2001). He was unable to tolerate shift correction due to pain. Other features provoked suspicion of 'red flags'. The patient reported severe unremitting pain, for which no position of ease could be found, and the pain was getting worse. He was unable to sleep because of the pain and reported symptoms of nausea. He looked unwell and had a raised temperature. In another case report a previously healthy 51-year-old woman presented with acute back pain, restricted range of movement and loss of motor function in both lower extremities (Poyanli *et al.* 2001). She had a high fever and raised ESR, and in this instance a pneumococcal osteomyelitis led to impaired consciousness in a matter of days.

Table 12.2 Significant history in identification of spinal infection

- recent or present febrile episode
- systemically unwell
- severe constant unremitting pain, worsening
- no loading strategy reduces symptoms.

Fractures * *RED FLAG*

Fractures tend to occur in two groups of patients – those involved in major trauma of any age, more commonly men, and females over 70 years old involved in minor trauma (Scavone *et al.* 1981b). One retrospective review of over 700 radiographs identified acute fractures in less than 3% of patients (Scavone *et al.* 1981a). In over 400 patients with acute back pain in primary care attending their GP, 0.7% had a fracture: two osteoporotic fractures and one crush fracture (McGuirk *et al.* 2001).

A fracture of the transverse process typically leaves patients with a persistent grumbling backache and considerable loss of function in spite of relatively insignificant signs on x-ray. Compression or wedge fractures of the vertebral body may be caused by major traumatic events or by lesser trauma in those at risk of osteoporosis. Those at risk include older post-menopausal women, those who have had hysterectomies and those on long-term corticosteroid therapy. The most common site of such injuries is between T10 and L1 (Macnab and McCulloch 1990).

Table 12.3 Significant history in identification of compression fracture

History	Sensitivity	Specificity
Age >50	0.84	0.61
Age >70	0.22	0.96
Trauma	0.30	0.85
Corticosteroid use	0.06	0.995

Source: Deyo *et al.* 1992

Osteoporosis

Osteoporosis is the most common metabolic disorder affecting the spine. The suggested World Health Organisation definition is bone mineral density more than 2.5 standard deviations below the mean of normal young people (Melton 1997). According to this definition, approximately 30% of postmenopausal white women in the US have the condition, and 16% have osteoporosis of the lumbar spine. Prevalence is less in non-white populations. Bone density decline begins in both sexes around forty years of age, but accelerates after fifty, especially in women (Bennell *et al.* 2000).

Low bone density leads to increased risk of fracture with no trauma or minimal trauma. The most common fracture sites are the lumbar spine, femur and radius. Vertebral fractures affect about 25% of postmenopausal women; however, a substantial proportion of fractures are asymptomatic and never diagnosed, and so the true rate could be higher. Despite widespread belief that osteoporosis primarily affects women, recent data shows that in fact vertebral fractures are as common in men as women. Because women live longer, the lifetime risk of a vertebral fracture from 50 onwards is 16% in white women and only 5% in white men (Melton 1997; Andersson *et al.* 1997).

Although it occurs predominantly in the elderly and in postmenopausal women, there are important secondary causes of osteoporosis not related to age. These include history of anorexia nervosa, smoking, corticosteroid use, inadequate intake or absorption of calcium and vitamin D, amenorrhea, low levels of exercise, lack of oestrogen and coeliac disease (Smith 2000; Bennell *et al.* 2000).

Low bone mass (osteopenia) is in itself asymptomatic and individuals may be unaware that they have the condition until a fracture occurs. Although pain can be absent, it can be severe, localised and difficult to treat and take many weeks to settle; the fractures also cause a loss of height (Smith 2000).

The condition, or suspicion of it, is an absolute contraindication to manipulation and mobilisation techniques. However, exercise is not only not contraindicated, but should be included as part of the management strategy for primary and secondary prevention. The effects of exercise on skeletal strength vary at different ages (Bennell *et al.* 2000). Gains in bone mass are much greater in childhood and adolescence than in adulthood. The adult skeleton is very responsive to the adverse effects of stress deprivation and lack of exercise, which tends to exacerbate the natural decline in bone density that occurs with ageing. Trials of exercise have consistently shown that loss of bone mass is reduced, prevented or reversed in the lumbar spine and femur (Bennell *et al.* 2000; Wolff *et al.* 1999).

Exercise that has a higher ground impact is most effective at bone strengthening. Non-weight-bearing exercises such as cycling or swimming do not strengthen bones, whatever other benefits they may provide (Bennell *et al.* 2000). Exercise programmes have included stair-climbing, aerobics, skipping, jumping, dancing and jogging. More impact and loading is appropriate in primary prevention, but a less vigorous programme should be used in frailer groups. Programmes should be progressed in terms of intensity and impact, and maintained indefinitely, as the positive effects are reversed when regular exercise is stopped. Physiotherapy management and exercise guidelines have been recently reviewed in considerable detail (Bennell *et al.* 2000; Mitchell *et al.* 1999). Exercise therapy is complementary to but not a substitute for medical management, which includes hormone replacement therapy, calcium, vitamin D, calcitonin, biphosphonates and fluoride (Lane *et al.* 1996).

Posture is an important factor in osteoporosis. Flexion should be minimised as this can trigger damage to the vertebra; extension exercises and an extended posture should be encouraged. A group of fifty-nine women with postmenopausal osteoporosis were allocated to different exercise groups, performing extension, flexion, a combination of both or a no-exercise group. At follow-up at least sixteen months later the extent of further fractures in the different groups was compared. Further deterioration was significantly less in the extension group (16%) than the flexion group (89%), the combined group (53%) and the no-exercise group (67%) (Sinaki and Mikkelsen 1984).

Cauda equina syndrome * RED FLAG

Cauda equina syndrome results from compression of sacral nerve roots, although lumbar nerve roots are usually also involved. The most common causes are massive central or lateral disc herniations, sometimes associated with spinal stenosis or spinal tumours – each responsible for about half the total (Kramer 1990). It only occurs in about 1 – 2% of all lumbar disc herniations that come to surgery, so its estimated prevalence rate among all back pain patients is about 0.0004% (Deyo *et al.* 1992). In an earlier series of 930 disc protrusions, cauda equina occurred in 0.6% (O'Connell 1955). It has been reported that there will be one new case each year for every 50,000 patients seen in GP surgeries, an incidence of 0.002% (Bartley 2000).

Principal findings in the history and physical examination that should alert clinicians to the possibility of cauda equina syndrome are in Table 12.4.

Table 12.4   Significant history and examination findings in identification of cauda equina syndrome

- bladder dysfunction, such as altered urethral sensation, urinary retention, paralysis, overflow incontinence and difficulty in initiating micturation
- loss of anal sphincter tone or faecal incontinence
- 'saddle anaesthesia' about the anus, perineum or genitals, or other sensory loss (buttocks, posterior thigh)
- impairment of sexual function
- absence of Achilles tendon reflex on both sides
- foot drop, calf muscle or other motor weakness
- unilateral or bilateral sciatica
- reduced lumbar lordosis and lumbar mobility.

Source: Kramer 1990; Tay and Chacha 1979; Kostuik *et al.* 1986; Choudhury and Taylor 1980; Shapiro 2000; Fanciullacci *et al.* 1989; Gleave and Macfarlane 1990

The most consistent finding is urinary retention, with a sensitivity of 0.90; sciatica, abnormal straight leg raise, sensory (especially 'saddle anaesthesia') and motor deficits are all common, with sensitivities of over 0.80. Anal sphincter tone is diminished in 60% to 80% of cases (Deyo *et al.* 1992). However, not all these signs and symptoms are present in all cases. A combination of features is most pathognomonic, with the constellation of bowel and bladder disturbance, bilateral sciatica and neurological signs and symptoms, especially around the 'saddle area' being most characteristic.

Roach *et al.* (1995) evaluated the use of a series of questions to identify serious back problems and found that most had poor sensitivity, but that several had a high specificity. Questions about sleep disturbance and control of urination were very specific; combining questions improved sensitivity. However, urinary disturbance of frequency may be reported in cases of back and nerve root pain not due to cauda equina syndrome (Bartley 2000).

Two types of onset of cauda equina are described (Tay and Chacha 1979; Kostuik *et al.* 1986; Shapiro 2000). A sudden onset of cauda equina compression without previous symptoms or a history of recurrent back pain and sciatica, the latest episode resulting in or progressing to a cauda equina lesion. Trauma is only reported in a minority. The most common levels of disc herniations are generally reported to be L4 – L5 and L5 – S1 (> 90%), with the average age about 40 years old. However, in a review of over 300 patients disc herniations were reported at all lumbar levels, with 38% at the two lowest levels and 27% at L1 – 2 (Ahn *et al.* 2000a). Cauda equina compression caused by tumours tends to progress in a slower fashion.

Haldeman and Rubinstein (1992) tell a cautionary tale of cauda equina syndrome onset being associated with lumbar manipulation – with twenty-six cases of such being reported in the world literature between 1911 and 1989. The most disturbing aspect was the failure to recognise the classic features of the syndrome by treating chiropractors and initial medical contacts, leading ultimately to delayed diagnosis. *A delay in diagnosing cauda equina syndrome may have alarming implications.*

Those who have surgery delayed more than forty-eight hours are significantly more likely to have persistent bladder and bowel incontinence, severe motor deficit, sexual dysfunction and persistent pain (Shapiro 2000). Ahn *et al.* (2000a) conducted a met-analysis of 322 patients from forty-two surgical series and confirmed this. Significant differences were found in resolution of urinary and rectal function, and sensory and motor deficits in patients treated within forty-eight hours compared to those treated after forty-eight hours from the onset of symptoms. *The bottom line is, suspicion of cauda equina syndrome demands urgent referral.*

Cord signs * *RED FLAG*

In the upper lumbar region whether a large disc herniation or other space-occupying lesion causes cauda equina syndrome or cord signs and symptoms is a product of variable anatomy. The spinal cord terminates in general at about the level of the L1 – L2 intervertebral disc, but individual differences range from termination at about T12

– L1 to L2 – L3 (Bogduk 1997). Below these levels the lumbar, sacral and coccygial nerve roots run freely in the cauda equina. If the cauda equina is compressed, a lower motor neurone lesion is produced as described above; if the spinal cord is involved, an upper motor neurone lesion is produced.

With a lower motor neurone lesion signs and symptoms are essentially segmental, although several segments can be involved. This involves the combination of dermatomal pain patterns and areas of sensory deficit, myotomal weakness and absent or reduced reflexes that have been listed under cauda equina syndrome and disc problems reviewed in the relevant chapter. Upper motor neurone lesions involve the central nervous system and thus signs and symptoms are extra-segmental.

Spinal cord compression can result from bony or discal protrusions into the spinal canal, especially in those with congenitally narrow spinal canals, or can result from spinal neoplasms (Berkow *et al.* 1987). There may be gradual or rapid progress from back pain to signs and symptoms of corticospinal tract involvement (Table 12.5). These patients should be referred to the appropriate specialist.

Table 12.5 Significant history and examination findings in identification of upper motor neurone lesions

- non-dermatomal sensory loss (for instance, bilateral 'stocking' paraesthesia)
- non-myotomal muscle weakness (for instance, several segments)
- hyper-reflexia
- positive Babinski sign or extensor plantar response
- ankle clonus
- positive Lhermitte sign – neck flexion produces a generalised 'electric shock'
- generalised hypertonicity
- generalised flaccidity
- bladder and/or bowel dysfunction.

Source: Butler 1991; Berkow *et al.* 1987

Ankylosing spondylitis

Ankylosing spondylitis (AS) is one of the inflammatory arthropathies that may affect the spine. These are systemic, multi-system diseases that include a primary musculoskeletal component. AS is characterised by chronic inflammation and tissue damage affecting principally the spine and sacro-iliac joints, but also peripheral joints and entheses, and non-articular structures such as the uvea (Goodacre *et al.* 1991; Berkow *et al.* 1987). Onset is usually insidious between the ages of 20 and 35, and rare after 40 (Macnab and McCulloch 1990). The disease, as with many conditions, represents a continuum of involvement from mild to severe. In later stages the disease process leads to ossification of spinal ligaments; the characteristic changes are clearly visible on radiographs, and severe restriction of movements and spinal deformity may occur.

Early in the disease there may be little to see, and a diagnosis of AS may be missed. Many people with ankylosing spondylitis remain unaware of their diagnosis, their symptoms of early morning stiffness and backache accepted as 'normal' and no investigations or health care are sought (Little 1988; Gran *et al.* 1985). Recognition of the disease has improved so that diagnosis has come to be made more quickly, although still involving several years' delay (Calin *et al.* 1988).

Prevalence

It has been estimated that AS is ten times more common in men than women (Calin and Fries 1975); however, in the latter the disease may present in a milder form and therefore not be recognised. Population-based epidemiological studies with definite diagnosis based on radiographic findings estimated overall prevalence as around 1%, with higher rates in men and lower rates in the older population (Gran *et al.* 1985; Carter *et al.* 1979; Braun *et al.* 1998). It is estimated that about 10 – 15% of ankylosing spondylitis cases begin during childhood years, with symptoms commencing in lower limb peripheral joints in about half of this group (Schaller 1979).

The antigen HLA-B27 is present in about 95% of patients with the condition, and this antigen is present in about 7% of the healthy white population. The disease is rare among black populations. Possibly about 10% of HLA-B27 positive adults have AS, but probably nearer 2% (van der Linden and Khan 1984). Higher prevalence rates have been suggested (Calin and Fries 1975), but this idea has been rejected (Rigby 1991). However, it is suggested that up to 5% of back pain sufferers in primary care may represent a non-specific or mild form of inflammatory joint pain (Underwood and Dawes 1995; Dougados *et al.* 1991; Braun *et al.* 1998).

Natural history

From several reviews of large numbers of patients with ankylosing spondylitis published in the 1950s, the following statements were derived concerning the natural history of the disease (Carette *et al.* 1983):

- onset is insidious

- it progresses with a series of exacerbations and remissions

- limitation of spinal movements and spinal deformity increase with time

- if peripheral joints are involved, this usually occurs early

- iritis develops early and tends to re-occur

- functional disability is usually mild

- the course is more severe if onset is during childhood or adolescence

- the disease has a milder form in women than in men.

Back and/or thigh pain is the presenting feature in over 70%, with peripheral joint disease in about 20% (Wordsworth and Mowat 1986). Pain and stiffness in the back becomes universal. The course of the disease tends to be a series of exacerbations and remissions (Goodacre *et al.* 1991; Mau *et al.* 1988). Radiological verification of sacro-iliitis or spinal involvement may not be present for ten years (Mau *et al.* 1987, 1988).

Carette *et al.* (1983) reported a long-term study of fifty-one patients with ankylosing spondylitis with mean disease duration of thirty-eight years. The average age at onset was 24 years old. About a third of patients denied any pain, another third described it as mild, 26% as moderate and only 4% as severe. Pain was generally most severe in the first ten years and then gradually decreased. Over the forty years only five deteriorated, and fourteen improved. Nearly all were working or had been working and were now retired due to age rather than the disease. Spinal restriction was mild in 41%, moderate in 18% and severe in 41%; deformity was mild in 67%, moderate in 15% and severe in 18%. A quarter of those with moderate or severe loss of mobility had little or no deformity. Peripheral joint involvement was noted in 36% in order of frequency: shoulders, hips, knees, ankles and metatarsophalangeals. Peripheral joint involvement and iritis, present in 24% of this sample, were both associated with more severe disease. Most had sacro-iliitis and spondylitis according to radiography.

In summary, for most individuals with this disease it takes a benign course with minimal pain, loss of mobility or functional disability (Mau *et al.* 1987). Less than 20% of patients with adult onset ankylosing spondylitis progress to significant disability, with early peripheral involvement suggesting more severe disease. In most the pattern of disease is established in the first ten years.

Diagnostic criteria

Recognition of patients with more advanced disease may be possible on radiography. Early disease is less easily detected. Diagnostic criteria for ankylosing spondylitis were specified at the Rome conference in 1963 and modified in New York in 1966. These were a combination of clinical and radiological criteria. Further modifications have been proposed that merge the two sets of criteria (Table 12.6).

Table 12.6 Modified New York criteria for diagnosis of ankylosing spondylitis

A.   DIAGNOSIS

    1.   Clinical criteria:

        a)   Low back pain and stiffness for more than three months, which improves with exercise, and is not relieved by rest.

        b)   Limitation of motion of the lumbar spine in both sagittal and frontal planes.

        c)   Limitation of chest expansion relative to normal values corrected for age and sex.

    2.   Radiological criterion:

        a)   Sacro-iliitis grade 2 or more bilaterally or grade 3 – 4 unilaterally.

B.   GRADING

    1.   Definite ankylosing spondylitis if the radiological criterion is associated with at least one clinical criterion.

    2.   Probable ankylosing spondylitis if:

        a)   Three clinical criteria present.

        b)   The radiological criterion is present without any clinical criteria.

Source: van der Linden *et al.* 1984

Symptoms said to be suggestive of back pain of an inflammatory nature are: back pain at night enough to leave the bed, early morning stiffness for more than half an hour, pain and stiffness made worse by rest, improvement with exercise, association with other joint problems and an absence of nerve root signs (Calin and Fries 1975; Gran 1985). Many patients also have a positive family history. These characteristic clinical features led to the proposal for solely clinical criteria as a screening test for ankylosing spondylitis (Calin *et al.* 1977). Five features were found to best discriminate back pain due to ankylosing spondylitis from back pain of other causes (Table 12.7). The authors stated 95% sensitivity and 85% specificity against the control group for four or more of these features. However, when the same criteria were applied to other samples, a sensitivity of only 23% or 38% was found (Gran 1985; van der Linden *et al.* 1984).

Table 12.7 The clinical history as a screening test for ankylosing spondylitis

- onset of back pain before the age of 40
- insidious onset
- persisting for at least three months
- associated with morning stiffness
- improved with exercise.

Source: Calin *et al.* 1977

Tests purporting to identify involvement of the sacro-iliac joint (SIJ) suffer from poor reliability and unproven validity (see section on SIJ, Chapter 13). SIJ tests have been examined in ankylosing spondylitis patients; one study found little correlation between different tests (Rantanen and Airaksinen 1989). Commonly used tests have been shown to be unhelpful in distinguishing ankylosing spondylitis patients from those with other sources of back pain (Russell *et al.* 1981; Gran 1985). However, Blower and Griffin (1984) found two tests significantly associated with patients with ankylosing spondylitis – pain on pressure over the anterior superior iliac spine and local sacral pressure. These tests were not positive in every patient, and they were not always both positive in the same patient. In clinical practice some patients can experience significant exacerbation of symptoms in response to Cyriax's (Cyriax 1982) three pain provocation tests, which can last several days. Many such patients have gone on to be proven to have AS.

The sensitivity and specificity of individual criterion is low, but items related to the history perform better than items of physical examination (van den Hoogen *et al.* 1995). The prevalence of diseases has a profound effect on the value of a test. The study by Calin *et al.* (1977) was performed in a hospital population, in which with higher prevalence rates the positive predictive value of a test will be greater.

In primary care, when screening for a rare disease such as ankylosing spondylitis, the positive predictive value of a positive test is extremely low, but the negative predictive value of a negative test is high (Streiner and Norman 1996).

In summary, specific inflammatory conditions such as AS, as well as non-specific spondylarthropathies, are diseases that run a chronic course. Earlier and milder forms may often be undiagnosed and may be more common than previously imagined. As in other conditions, a clinical reasoning process and combination of features is likely to be most helpful in identifying patients with presumed ankylosing spondylitis or a non-specific inflammatory joint condition who will need further investigation to confirm this diagnosis. Such patients also respond to a mechanical evaluation in an atypical way. Patients who are suspected to have this pathology should be referred to a rheumatologist.

Conclusions

This chapter has considered some of the most common specific and serious pathologies that may affect the lumbar spine. These conditions are rarely encountered in clinical practice, but occasionally patients with these problems may appear, despite being screened by GPs or physicians. It is thus vital, in terms of safe practice, that clinicians are aware of these entities and the 'red flags' that might indicate their presence, as well as the atypical responses to mechanical evaluation that may accompany them.

Some of these conditions are absolute contraindications to mechanical therapy – cauda equina syndrome, fractures, cord signs and spinal infection. *If it is suspected that patients have any of these pathologies, urgent referral is essential.* If suspicion is supported by several factors in the history and physical examination, it is always better to be safe than sorry – get the patient to a specialist as soon as possible. In the presence of ankylosing spondylitis, osteoporosis or even cancer, if a mechanical problem is also present, cautious and appropriate management can be offered. If these pathologies are suspected, but not diagnosed, then appropriate referral is necessary.

The detail provided in this chapter is summarised in the form of criteria and operational definitions contained in the Appendix – these are essential for identification of the different pathologies.

13: Other Diagnostic and Management Considerations

Introduction

The majority of patients with back pain will be included in the mechanical syndromes (see Chapter 8). From time to time consideration of other diagnoses may have to be made. In this chapter certain specific conditions are described, as well as certain non-specific entities whose existence is controversial.

Specific conditions, such as spinal stenosis, hip joint problems and spondylolisthesis are described in this chapter. These are differential diagnoses that will have to be considered on some occasions. Other management issues are considered here, such as back pain in pregnancy, surgery, post-surgery and chronic back pain. Other entities are also described in this chapter whose existence or clinical recognition is somewhat more contentious, such as zygapophyseal joint disorders and instability. Conditions are briefly described, and key features and suggested management approaches are mentioned.

A normal mechanical evaluation, as outlined in Chapters 14 and 15, is always conducted first. These conditions only need to be considered with a failure to identify a mechanical syndrome. As will be made clear, putative recognition of these problems is often difficult and can only be done once a thorough mechanical evaluation has excluded one of the more common mechanical syndromes. *Only after the completion of a thorough mechanical evaluation, possibly over several days and/or generation of an atypical response, should these differential diagnoses be considered.*

The following sections are presented in this chapter:

- spinal stenosis
- hip problems
- sacro-iliac joint problems
- low back pain in pregnancy
- zygapophyseal joint problems
- spondylolysis and spondylolisthesis
- post-surgical status

- chronic pain

- mechanically inconclusive

- surgery

- post-surgical status

- chronic pain

- Waddell's non-organic signs and symptoms

- treating chronic backs – the McKenzie Institute International Reabilitation Programme.

Source: McKenzie Institute International Rehabilitation Programme

The detail provided in this chapter is summarised in the form of criteria and operational definitions contained in the Appendix – these are essential for identification of the different syndromes.

Spinal stenosis

Patients who have spinal stenosis that has been confirmed objectively by imaging studies may benefit from mechanical evaluation or generalised physiotherapy advice. With an ageing population it is highly likely that patients with undiagnosed stenosis will be encountered in physiotherapy clinics. In hospital populations an annual incidence of fifty per million inhabitants has been estimated, but many patients with minor symptoms do not seek medical attention, so its prevalence in the general community is unknown (Johnsson 1995). Although spinal stenosis can frequently be suspected by clinical information, objective investigations are needed to make the diagnosis. Imaging studies are essential for the definitive diagnosis of lumbar spinal stenosis (Yoshizawa 1999).

Pathophysiology

Stenosis is a condition associated with extensive degenerative changes of the disc and zygapophyseal joints at multiple levels, which may include degenerative spondylolisthesis (Amundsen *et al.* 1995). However, stenosis has both a structural and a dynamic component. The postural nature of the patient's pain is partly related to the narrowing effect that extension has on the spinal canal and the intervertebral foramen. The more the canal is structurally narrowed by the degenerative process, the more easily slight extension motion causes compression of the nerves (Penning and Wilmink 1987;

Penning 1992; Willen *et al.* 1997). Extension also causes an increase in epidural pressure, which is raised anyway in individuals with stenosis (Takahashi *et al.* 1995a, 1995b). Flexed postures have the reverse effects, widening the canal and foramen and reducing the epidural pressure, which explains why temporary relief can be gained in sitting or leaning forward.

Clinical presentation

Two types of stenosis are described depending upon whether the degenerative changes affect the nerve roots in the spinal canal or in the intervertebral foramen (Porter 1993; Heggeness and Esses 1991; Getty 1990). Laterally the root may be entrapped by bony changes, giving unremitting radicular pain from which there is no relief even at night, and which is made worse on walking. With central stenosis there is little or no leg pain at rest. This is brought on in one or both legs with walking a limited distance, termed neurogenic claudication, and is relieved with flexed postures (Porter *et al.* 1984; Porter 1993). In practice, the distinction between the two types of stenosis may be less clear (Amundsen *et al.* 1995). To further confuse diagnosis, stenosis and disc herniation may occur together (Sanderson and Getty 1996). Central stenosis can also produce signs and symptoms of cauda equina syndrome, with considerable variability in the reported prevalence of this condition (Johnsson 1995; Oda *et al.* 1999).

There has often been a long history of back pain with subsequent development of leg pain, and the condition is rarely found in those under fifty (Getty 1990; Heggeness and Esses 1991). The distinguishing feature of the condition is the postural nature of the patient's pain, with aggravation of leg symptoms when standing, and especially when walking. Leg pain is likely to be worse than back pain. Conversely, patients report relief of symptoms when they adopt positions of flexion, such as sitting or leaning forward. Walking distances can be severely impaired because of neurogenic claudication. Extension is often very limited and may provoke leg symptoms if sustained, while flexion may be maintained. Signs and symptoms of motor, sensory and reflex deficit and root tension signs are less common than with disc herniations, occurring in about 50% of patients (Heggeness and Esses 1991; Amundsen *et al.* 1995; Getty 1990; Fritz *et al.* 1998; Jonsson *et al.* 1997a; Onel *et al.* 1993; Hall *et al.* 1985; Zanoli *et al.* 2001).

There are, however, no clear clinical presentations that distinguish the different nerve root compression syndromes of lateral and central stenosis and disc herniation (Jonsson and Stromqvist 1993). One study found that history findings most strongly associated with the diagnosis of spinal stenosis are greater age, severe lower limb pain and the absence of pain when sitting. Physical examination findings most strongly associated with the diagnosis were wide-based gait, abnormal Romberg test, thigh pain with thirty seconds of lumbar extension and neuromuscular deficits (Katz *et al.* 1995). Differential diagnosis between stenosis and derangement is considered in Table 13.2 (from original idea Young 1995).

As part of their previous study, Iversen and Katz (2001) examined forty-three patients with radiographically confirmed structural evidence of spinal stenosis. The correlation between radiological changes and severity of symptoms was poor. The mean age was 72, the mean duration of symptoms three years. The prevalence of certain findings is presented in Table 13.1. Walking and standing were the most common aggravating factors, but getting up from a chair made pain worse in 43%, and sitting and leaning forward in about 25%; bending forward only made 15% better. Reduced or absent lordosis and minimal extension were common features, and if extension was maintained pain tended to radiate further down the leg. About 60% of subjects reported numbness or tingling and weakness, and findings of sensory or muscle impairment were common.

Table 13.1   Features of history and examination in spinal stenosis

Clinical feature	Prevalence rate in sample of 43
History	
Severe difficulties with walking	63%
Worse walking uphill	78%
Worse walking on flat ground	72%
Worse standing for 5 minutes	65%
Better side lying	68%
Better / worse seated	52% / 24%
Physical examination	
Wide-based stance	43%
Romberg test positive	39%
Reduced lumbar lordosis	65%
Lumbar extension < 10 degrees	65%
Pain on flexion	79%

Continued next page

Clinical feature	Prevalence rate in sample of 43
Pain on 5 sec extension in back	67%
Pain on 30 sec extension in back / thigh / calf	77% / 51% / 28%
Absent or reduced pinprick	60 – 79%
Weakness extensor hallucis longus	79%

Source: Iversen and Katz 2001

Differential diagnosis – derangement or stenosis

Table 13.2 Distinguishing spinal stenosis from derangement with leg pain

Clinical presentation	Derangement	Spinal stenosis
Age	20 – 55	>> 50
History	Sudden / gradual onset Episodes	Long history LBP Gradual onset leg pain
Status	Improving Unchanging Spontaneous resolution more likely	Unchanging Worsening Spontaneous resolution unlikely
Symptom behaviour	Variable Centralisation / peripheralisation	Consistent pattern Walking distance limited
Aggravating factors	Variable Often flexion activities – bending, sitting, driving, etc. Sometimes flexion and extension activities	Consistent Always walking Sometimes standing Activities of extension
Relieving factors	Variable Often walking, moving about, lying	Consistent Always flexion activities Bending, sitting, stooping often relieves pain temporarily
Radiography	Variable Clinically insignificant	Extensive degenerative changes Degenerative spondylolisthesis
Mobility	Major losses flexion and extension common	Extension always limited or absent Flexion well maintained
Neurological presentation	Variable sensory and motor deficit Positive tension test	Sensory and motor deficit less common Negative tension test
Response to repeated movement testing	Better / worse Centralisation / peripheralisation Obstruction to curve reversal Variable mechanical presentation	Extension produces no worse Flexion reduces no better Consistent response Mechanical presentation unchanging

Source: adapted from Young 1995

Spencer (1990) discusses the essential difference between a disc herniation and spinal stenosis as relating to the mechanism of insult to the nerve root. The latter, being due to compression, occurs without nerve tension signs in the older patient, with spontaneous resolution less likely; there is pain during walking and relief with sitting. In contrast, symptoms from a disc herniation are due to tension or compression on the nerve root, the patient is younger, with nerve tension signs, is made worse by flexion and better with extension and has a good chance of spontaneous resolution. These two clinical presentations represent extremes at either end of a continuum; in clinical practice combinations of the different mechanisms of symptom production may be found.

Management

Computed tomography, myelography and magnetic resonance imaging (MRI) are the most important imaging studies for evaluating and quantifying the degree of forminal stenosis and making the diagnosis (Jenis and An 2000; Yoshizawa 1999). However, studies into these technologies lack methodological rigour and do not permit strong conclusions about the relative diagnostic accuracies of the different procedures (Kent *et al.* 1992). Furthermore, degenerative changes are not closely correlated with symptoms (Iversen and Katz 2001; Amundsen *et al.* 2000). Abnormal findings occur in the asymptomatic population; in those over 60 years of age, 21% had spinal stenosis (Boden *et al.* 1990).

In the US in the previous two decades, surgery for spinal stenosis has more than quadrupled (Taylor *et al.* 1994). However, the long-term effects of surgical intervention are uncertain and deteriorate with time, and over a third of patients have only fair to poor outcomes (Katz *et al.* 1991,1996; Jonsson *et al.* 1997b; Tuite *et al.* 1994; Turner *et al.* 1992). In one of the latest reviews on surgical interventions for back pain, the authors concluded that there is no acceptable evidence for the efficacy of any form of decompression for spinal stenosis or for any form of fusion (Gibson *et al.* 1999).

Even when the long-term result is more favourable compared to conservative treatment, failure to improve with surgery is still common. After four years, about 30% of one surgical cohort were the same or worse, compared to about 50% of those who had been treated conservatively (Atlas *et al.* 2000). In the most recent comparison of surgical and conservative management of stenosis, in which a subgroup of patients was randomised to different treatment groups, the outcome was most favourable for surgically treated patients, especially those with very severe symptoms. However, many improved with conservative management also, especially those with milder symptoms, and those who had an unsatisfactory result treated later with surgery still had a good outcome. Results were entirely independent of the radiological degree of degeneration, which could not be used to predict the outcome of treatment (Amundsen *et al.* 2000).

Despite being a degenerative condition, the natural history of spinal stenosis is frequently non-progressive and conservative management is thus a valid alternative (Porter *et al.* 1984; Johnsson *et al.* 1991,1992; Atlas *et al.* 1996c). Patients followed up over five to ten years have reported an improvement in symptoms (15 – 20%) and symptoms unchanged (60 – 70%), as well as a worsening of symptoms (15 – 20%) (Johnsson *et al.* 1992; Oda *et al.* 1999).

Various conservative treatments have been proposed, usually involving multiple and vigorous therapies, although none have been adequately evaluated (Fritz *et al.* 1997,1998; Onel *et al.* 1993; Heggeness and Esses 1991; Oda *et al.* 1999; Simotas *et al.* 2000). Reviewing some of these programmes, which typically include exercises and drug therapy or epidural steroid injections, it is reported with follow-up between one and five years that 15% to 43% of patients will have continued improvement after conservative treatment (Simotas 2001). A mechanical evaluation is worth undertaking to see if any element of the condition is reversible. These patients may benefit from advice to avoid positions of extension and use of flexion exercises. Failure to change the level of symptoms and disability is likely to be common in this group.

Table 13.3 Significant history and examination findings in identification of spinal stenosis

- history of leg symptoms when walking
- may be eased when sitting or leaning forward
- absence of directional preference
- no lasting change in symptoms in response to therapeutic loading strategies
- loss of extension
- possible provocation of symptoms in sustained extension, with relief on flexion
- age greater than 50

- possible nerve root signs and symptoms
- extensive degenerative changes on x-ray
- confirmation by CT or MRI.

Hip problems

Although not a condition of the lumbar spine, hip problems should be considered in the differential diagnosis as the referral of pain pattern can be similar in both. The history in hip problems is generally distinctive, and the lumbar spine is often excluded from the outset. Generally the pain pattern and the aggravating and relieving factors sound like the hip, and this is confirmed by the finding of restricted movement and/or reproduction of pain with hip tests. If the hip proves to be negative, then look at the lumbar spine.

Wroblewski (1978) has described the location of pain in eighty-nine patients (102 hips) with primary osteoarthritis (OA) who were awaiting hip surgery (Table 13.4). None of the sites featured alone; all patients described pain in several locations, with the most frequent combination including the greater trochanter, anterior thigh and knee. In 108 patients with less severe OA, who had minimal limitation of activities, pain in the anterior thigh was experienced by over half, and smaller proportions had pain in the posterior and lateral aspect of the thigh and in the knee (Jorring 1980). These pain patterns are not unique to the hip joint.

Table 13.4 Pain sites in hip osteoarthritis

Site[1]	Proportion of hips affected Wroblewski 1978	Jorring 1980
Greater trochanter	70%	17%
Knee	69%	18%
Anterior thigh	62%	56%
Groin	46%	8%
Shin	39%	
Buttock	39%	

[1]More than one site affected in most individuals.
Source: Wroblewski 1978; Jorring 1980

The pain is usually associated with weight-bearing, especially early in the course of the disease, but may become more constant as it progresses. Often patients will report an easing of or no pain when sitting, in contrast to many spinal problems. Morning stiffness, pain on first weight-bearing, pain on movement of the limb and during weight-bearing are common but not universal findings (Jorring 1980).

Symptomatic hip OA occurs in about 5% of adults, most commonly in those over fifty, while over 20% of those over 55 display radiographic changes of hip OA (Felson 1988; Lawrence *et al.* 1998). Younger individuals may show no radiographic signs of involvement of the hip, and non-specific conditions may cause the joint to be symptomatic.

In OA fibrosis, thickening and contracture of the capsule produces stiffness, reduced mobility and pain at end range of movements (McCarthy *et al.* 1994). Different patterns of radiological and pathological changes have been observed (Cameron and Macnab 1975). While in 60% of the patients studied capsular restrictions were minimal until there were gross degenerative changes, in 40% there were early and marked capsular restrictions without major radiological changes. Movements commonly implicated, and which need to be included in the physical examination of the hip, are flexion, medial rotation, abduction and extension (Dieppe 1995). The hip quadrant (a combination of flexion / adduction) is also a useful test movement (Maitland 1991). Resisted tests should also be conducted, a common cause of groin pain being adductor strains. When a symptomatic hip is present, some or all of these tests should provoke the patient's pain and may form a useful part of treatment. If these tests are negative, attention focuses on the lumbar spine.

Table 13.5 Significant history and examination findings in hip joint problems

- pain worsened by weight-bearing, eased by rest
- worse with first few steps after rest
- pain pattern – groin, anterior thigh, knee, anterior shin, lateral thigh, possibly buttock
- positive pain provocation tests (reproduction of patient's pain) using passive or resisted movements.

For management considerations of hip joint problems, see *The Human Extremities: Mechanical Diagnosis and Therapy (McKenzie and May 2000)*.

Sacro-iliac joint problems

The role of the sacro-iliac joint (SIJ) in spinal problems is one of the more controversial issues in back pain. While some authorities claim a predominance of SIJ disorders among back pain patients (Don Tigny 1990), others state it has a negligible role (Cyriax 1982). It is instructive to be aware that the issues of reliability and validity of 'SIJ tests' dominate the literature on SIJ. In other words, the debate is, at this stage, is this a recognisable entity? This is a necessary, but as yet incomplete, preliminary process before it can be decided which is the best way to manage the problem.

Several studies using SIJ blocks have shown that the joint is a definite if minor source of back pain. Schwarzer *et al.* (1995) found that 13% of 100 consecutive chronic back pain patients had a positive response to a single SIJ intra-articular injection of anaesthetic. In a sample of eighty-five patients chosen with suspicion of SIJ involvement due to the area of pain, 53% were positive to a single joint block (Dreyfuss *et al.* 1996). However, a positive response to a single intra-articular injection cannot be seen as a 'gold standard' test. Zygapophyseal joint injections in the cervical and lumbar spine have revealed a placebo response to a single injection of 27% and 38% (Barnsley *et al.* 1993; Schwarzer *et al.* 1994a). Likewise, in the SIJ when double injections have been used, 53% demonstrate a placebo response; that is, relief on the first injection, but failure to gain relief on the second (Maigne *et al.* 1996). In a sample that was carefully selected as likely to have SIJ problems, 18% of fifty-four patients responded to double joint blocks.

Diagnosis
All these studies compared clinical features, pain patterns and responses to commonly used 'SIJ tests' in those who responded to the injections and those who did not (Schwarzer *et al.* 1995; Dreyfuss *et al.* 1996; Maigne *et al.* 1996). *No historical features nor physical examination procedures, nor constellation of such demonstrated worthwhile and consistent diagnostic value.*

Before consideration is given to the SIJ as a possible source of symptoms, it is essential first to exclude the lumbar spine and hip joints, otherwise tests for SIJ will generate many false-positive responses. In a population of 202 chronic back pain patients, 60% had at least one positive SIJ pain provocation test (Laslett 1997). However, once lumbar and hip joint pathology were excluded, only 17% were left with at least one SIJ positive test. When a criterion of at least three and preferably four positive tests was used to distinguish SIJ pathology, only 6.5% and 3.5% were truly positive. Lumbar problems were detected using the following criteria: McKenzie mechanical evaluation to detect centralisation, pressure on lumbar spinous processes to provoke familiar pain and the presence of acute lateral shifts. Hip problems were excluded using pain provocation tests – passive medial rotation and abduction, and resisted lateral rotation.

The ability of non-SIJ problems to mimic true SIJ problems is further supported by another study (Slipman *et al.* 1998). Fifty patients were selected who had pain over the SIJ area and who were positive to three SIJ pain provocation tests. Only thirty patients had a positive response to a single intra-articular anaesthetic block (60%), which meant that at least 40% of those positive to pain provocation tests are false-positives. As only a single joint block was used, the proportion of those mimicking SIJ is likely to be considerably higher.

It is thus apparent that SIJ problems are not easy to differentiate. The most common site of pain is over the buttock and posterior thigh (Slipman *et al.* 2000), but the pain pattern has no clear distinguishing characteristics. Asymptomatic volunteers who allowed SIJ injections to provoke pain described an area of pain just inferior to the posterior inferior iliac spine, with some also describing referral into the lateral buttock and thigh (Fortin *et al.* 1994). Other studies have demonstrated referral down the full length of the limb, both anteriorly and posteriorly. Two studies (Schwarzer *et al.* 1995a; Dreyfuss *et al.* 1996) that attempted to differentiate subjects with SIJ pathology from those without it by using SIJ injections found that referral of pain below the knee was as common in both groups. Groin and anterior thigh and leg pain were more common, and pain above L5 was rare in the SIJ groups. These were not exclusive characteristics, and one study found lower lumbar pain to be common and pain patterns to be highly variable (Slipman *et al.* 2000). These studies show that SIJ pathology cannot be recognised by pain patterns alone.

One study has tried to compare findings from the history and mechanical assessment in a group of chronic patients who responded to SIJ, facet injections or discography (Young and Aprill 2000). Findings from the facet and SIJ groups were similar, both showing lack of obstruction or movement loss after repeated movements, lack of centralisation or peripheralisation, and sometimes abolition of distal symptoms without centralisation. The entire SIJ group had three or more SIJ pain provocation tests positive, compared to 25% or 30% in the other two groups, and all but one had no pain at or above L5.

Pain provoked on rising from sitting was present in most of both disc and SIJ groups.

There exist numerous test manoeuvres that are said to diagnose SIJ disorders. These have been widely investigated and found wanting on many counts. Two sorts of test exist, those that attempt to provoke the patient's pain by 'stressing' the SIJ mechanically and those that seek to implicate the SIJ by trying to observe or palpate a difference in mobility or alignment with the asymptomatic side. Generally pain provocation tests are much more reliable between testers than tests that are based upon palpation or observation, which are frequently unreliable (Potter and Rothstein 1985; Lindsay *et al.* 1995; Laslett and Williams 1994; Carmichael 1987; van Deursen *et al.* 1990). Although pain provocation tests have also been found not to be reliable (McCombe *et al.* 1989; Strender *et al.* 1997), these tests generally perform much better than tests based on palpation or observation.

A selection of these studies is presented in Table 13.6. Mostly trials have been included that reported the Kappa statistic (see Glossary). As in palpatory procedures for the lumbar spine, intra-tester comparisons are more reliable, with poor to moderate reliability, than inter-tester ones, with only poor reliability. Overall tests that use pain provocation (shown in bold) have considerably better reliability than tests based upon palpation (shown in ordinary text).

Table 13.6 Reliability of examination procedures of the sacro-iliac joint (SIJ)

Reference	Assessment procedure	Intra-tester reliability (mean Kappa)	Inter-tester reliability (mean Kappa)
Carmichael 1987	Gillet test	0.18	0.02
Meijne *et al.* 1999	Gillet test	0.055*	-0.025*
Van Deursen *et al.* 1990	6 palpatory tests		0.04*
Mior *et al.* 1990	Mobility testing • Students • Chiropractors	} 0.50* }	0.09* 0.08*
Vincent-Smith and Gibbons 1999	Standing flexion test	0.46	0.05

Continued next page

Reference	Assessment procedure	Intra-tester reliability (mean Kappa)	Inter-tester reliability (mean Kappa)
O'Haire and Gibbons 2000	Palpation and observation of SIJ anatomy	0.26*	0.06*
Freburger and Riddle 1999	Instrumented SIJ alignment		0.18
Lindsay et al. 1995	Mobility and positional tests **Pain provocation** tests		0.16* 0.33*
Dreyfuss et al. 1996	Gillet test 4 **pain provocation** tests	0.22	0.54*
Laslett and Williams 1994	7 **pain provocation** tests		0.70*
Strender et al. 1997	SIJ compression – **pain provocation**		0.26
McCombe et al. 1989	3 **pain provocation** tests		0.23*
			Agreement
Potter and Rothstein 1985	11 palpatory tests 2 **pain provocation** tests		39% 85%
Mann et al. 1984	Iliac crest heights		Mean 6.6 out of 11

K = kappa
* = calculated from original data

A systematic review considered the reliability of clinical tests for the SIJ (van der Wurff et al. 2000a). They found no evidence of reliable outcomes for mobility tests, while some studies demonstrated reliability for some pain provocation tests.

Multiple tests perform better, and single positive tests should be viewed as irrelevant (Laslett 1997; Cibulka et al. 1988; Osterbauer et al. 1993; Cibulka and Koldehoff 1999; Broadhurst and Bond 1998). A multi-test regime using five pain provocation tests has been found to have good reliability, Kappa value 0.70 (Kokmeyer et al. 2002). The authors recommended three positive tests out of five be conducted.

Various palpation or mobility tests have been examined on 'normal' volunteers with 'positive' findings in significant numbers (Dreyfuss et al. 1994; Egan et al. 1996; Levangie 1999a). These tests cannot be said to diagnose SIJ problems as the asymmetrical mobility that they rely on is found in the asymptomatic population. No substantive positive association between pelvic asymmetry and back pain was found in a study of over 100 patients and controls (Levangie 1999b).

Attempts to palpate movement abnormalities should be further cautioned against due to the minimal movement that occurs at the joint – a review of sixteen in vitro and in vivo studies found this to be less than four degrees of rotation and about 3mm of translatory motion (Walker 1992). Recent high-quality studies using implanted tantalum balls and radiography have found no significant difference in mobility between symptomatic and asymptomatic joints in patients with unilateral symptoms (Sturesson 1997). The amount of movement found was minimal, less than two degrees, and during the Gillet test is *"so minute that external detection by manual methods is virtually impossible"* (Sturesson *et al.* 2000a, 2000b).

Two studies (Maigne *et al.* 1996; Dreyfuss *et al.* 1996) have tested the diagnostic validity of twelve commonly used SIJ tests against the results of double or single anaesthetic blocks of the joint. Neither pain provocation nor palpatory tests were useful predictors of a positive response to injection. Thus none of these tests, either singly or in combination, demonstrated worthwhile diagnostic value when compared with SIJ pathology identified by intra-articular blocks. However, the results may have differed if pathology was related to para-articular structures, such as ligaments. A systematic review of the validity of clinical tests for the SIJ concluded that there is no evidence to support the diagnostic value of either mobility or pain provocation tests (van der Wurff *et al.* 2000b).

A recent review of the published evidence to guide examination of the SIJ reached the following conclusions (Freburger and Riddle 2001). A combination of positive pain provocation tests and pain pattern may be useful for considi`ing a diagnosis of SIJ. The most useful tests appear to be Patrick's test, pressure over sacral sulcus, thigh thrust / posterior shear, resisted hip abduction, and iliac compression and gapping. The most useful indicators in the pain pattern are absence of pain in the lumbar area, pain below L5, around the posterior superior iliac spine and in the groin area. Movement and symmetry tests appear to be of little value.

Attempting to detect a SIJ problem is thus extremely problematical, and a staged differential diagnostic process should always be used (Table 13.7). Given the likelihood of false-positive test results, without care, it is very likely that SIJ problems are needlessly overdiagnosed.

Table 13.7 The staged differential diagnosis for SIJ problems

1. Exclusion of more common causes of buttock, thigh and groin pain, namely lumbar and hip problems. A normal mechanical evaluation should be conducted and the patient may be given a trial of exercises over a twenty-four-hour period to further test out responses. There is no value in conducting a barrage of SIJ tests on day one, as there will be a large number of false-positive responses. A relevant lateral shift is produced by lumbar problems, to which the treatment should be directed. Centralisation, reduction or abolition of pain with repeated lumbar movements confirms a mechanical syndrome and further testing becomes irrelevant.

2. Clinicians may be alerted by failure to respond, atypical responses to repeated movements and lack of directional preference.

3. The hip joint should first be discounted using pain provocation testing (see appropriate section).

4. Pain must be present over the buttock, but may radiate anteriorly and posteriorly.

5. Multiple pain provocation tests (Laslett and Williams 1994; Kokmeyer *et al.* 2002) should be undertaken and at least three and preferably four should provoke the patient's pain for a positive identification of a SIJ problem.

    a. Distraction*

    b. Compression*

    c. Posterior shear or thigh thrust or posterior pelvic pain provocation test* (see section below: Back pain in pregnancy)

    d. Pelvic torsion or Gaenslen's test* (both sides)

    e. Sacral thrust

    f. Cranial glide

    g. Patrick sign or Faber test*

*Five tests used by Kokmeyer *et al.* 2002

Using such a clinical reasoning process with a patient history, dynamic mechanical evaluation and pain provocation testing of first the hip and then the SIJ has been compared to double anaesthetic joint blocks (Young *et al.* 1998). Agreement between the physical examination and the injection was 91%, with a Kappa value of 0.82.

Table 13.8 Significant examination findings in identification of SIJ problems

•   exclusion of lumbar spine by extended mechanical evaluation

•   exclusion of hip joint by mechanical testing

•   negative response to mobilisation of lumbar spine

•   positive pain provocation tests (reproduction of patient's pain) – at least three tests.

Management

A wide range of interventions has been proposed for the treatment of SIJ syndrome. This includes exercise, manipulation, injections of corticosteroid and local anaesthetic, injections of sclerosing agents, and even surgical arthrodesis (Bernard 1997). Within the field of physical therapy, there are some ornate classification systems of SIJ syndromes based upon pathological models of innominate subluxations and fixations (such as Lee 1997; Don Tigny 1997). Palpation and mobility testing are used to discern these, but there is little evidence of reliability or validity, as already noted. With the problems involved in recognising true SIJ pathology and the difficulty of assembling such a cohort, scientifically testing out specific interventions has never been satisfactorily achieved. Thus no evidence exists as to the efficacy of any proposed interventions for the SIJ.

There is an incomplete understanding of the pathology of the SIJ and the reason for pain, although various theoretical models exist. It is not known if the source of symptoms is articular or para-articular – if it is the latter, then the injection studies mentioned earlier may not expose it. Pain may be due to a mechanical articular lesion and sometimes responds to repeated end-range exercises or clinician techniques. If pain appears to be mechanical – intermittent, twinges, unilateral, activity-related – it is worth exploring symptom response to repeated end-range anterior and posterior pelvic rotation. On the other hand, pain may be due to soft tissue insufficiency around the pelvis and require stabilising with a belt – see next section on back pain in pregnancy.

It has also been suggested that SIJ pathology is primarily inflammatory – in such a case pain would be a constant, dull aching, aggravated by mechanical therapy. Bone scanning with quantitative sacro-iliac scintigraphy has provided evidence of inflammation in women with chronic non-specific back pain (Davis and Lentle 1978; Rothwell *et al*. 1981). Inflammatory sacro-iliac disease, not related to ankylosing spondylitis, was diagnosed in this way in twenty-two of fifty patients, compared to two of sixty-six controls (Davis and Lentle 1978). If such pathology is the root of symptoms, mechanical therapy will be unhelpful.

If, having performed the staged differential diagnostic process outlined above, mechanical SIJ involvement is suspected, management will be determined by response to repeated movements. These movements need to focus on rotation of the pelvis. With the present uncertain understanding of pathology and lack of clearly evaluated practice, a degree of experimentation may be warranted, but failure to respond is common. For SIJ problems related to pregnancy, see the following section.

Low back pain in pregnancy

Prevalence

Back pain is a common although not universal experience for many women during pregnancy. As in other types of back pain, there are still ambiguities inherent in the terminology, diagnosis and classification (Heiberg and Aarseth 1997). This section draws together some of the evidence relating prevalence and classification as well as making some suggestions concerning management.

Following large cohorts of women through pregnancy with repeated questionnaires and a good response rate (over 85%) is the best way of establishing incidence and prevalence. Those studies that have done this have found prevalence rates of between 47% and 76% (Mantle *et al.* 1977; Berg *et al.* 1988; Ostgaard *et al.* 1991, 1994a; Kristiansson 1996a; Sturesson *et al.* 1997). The mean rate across multiple studies thus gives a prevalence of back pain of just over 50% of pregnant women. This compares to a one-year prevalence rate in the general population of about 40% (see Chapter 1).

Natural history

Back pain during pregnancy is not a static entity, but changes during trimesters. Onset is most common during the third to seventh months of pregnancy (Fast *et al.* 1987; Mantle *et al.* 1977), and there is an increase of back pain as the pregnancy proceeds (Ostgaard *et al.* 1997a; Kristiansson *et al.* 1996a). In those who had back pain prior to pregnancy, there is in fact a decreased rate of back pain during the pregnancy, and following the birth there is a rapid decline in back pain. The incidence of back pain during pregnancy is considerably greater and accounts for the cumulative increase in total back pain (Figure 13.1). Ostgaard *et al.* (1997a), in 362 women, found 18% had back pain before pregnancy, 71% during and 16% six years later.

There is also a variability of impact and severity of back pain during pregnancy. Less than 20% appear to have constant pain, and intermittent symptoms are much more common (Berg *et al.* 1988; Fast *et al.* 1987). Ten to 15% of pregnant women suffer severe back pain that interferes with daily activities, and may need time off work, while far more women suffer troublesome, but not severe pain (Mantle *et al.* 1977; Berg *et al.* 1988; Fast *et al.* 1990; Heiberg and Aarseth 1997). In general there is a tendency for increasing severity of pain as the pregnancy proceeds. On a 0 – 10 visual analogue scale, average pain intensity before the pregnancy and at weeks twelve and thirty was respectively 1.3, 3.9 and 4.5 (Ostgaard and Andersson 1991).

Figure 13.1 Back pain during pregnancy

Weeks of pregnancy: 12, 24, 36, pp

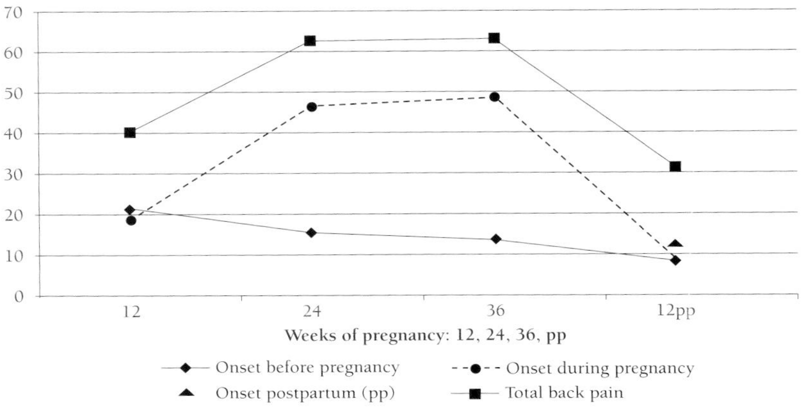

Source: Kristiansson *et al.* 1996a

Multiple variables that may be risk factors for back pain in pregnancy have been investigated. The strongest and most consistent associations with back pain during pregnancy are a prior history of back pain, mechanical and psychosocial stresses at work, the hormonal effects of pregnancy and method of birth.

Classification of back pain in pregnancy

The site of symptoms has been used as a means of classifying back pain during pregnancy. Although these groups are distinguished by pain distribution and appear to behave differently, definitely established pathological models have not been proven. *"Pregnant women with 'back pain' can be separated into two groups with different pain patterns – one group with pain in the back and one group with pain in the posterior pelvis"* (Ostgaard *et al.* 1994a).

Posterior pelvis pain (PPP) is felt over the buttock and sacro-iliac area and back pain is felt in the lumbar region. PPP appears to be more common during pregnancy (range 24 – 48%) than low back pain (range 10 – 32%); combinations of the two types of pain are also common (Ostgaard *et al.* 1991, 1994a, 1996; Kristiansson *et al.* 1996a; Noren *et al.* 1997; Sturesson *et al.* 1997).

During the pregnancy these different symptoms behave differently. Low back pain is more common both before and after pregnancy, but remains relatively stable or even declines in prevalence during the pregnancy. PPP, which increases dramatically during pregnancy, is probably the most common form of back pain (Ostgaard *et al.* 1991, 1994a, 1994b, 1996; Mens *et al.* 1996; Kristiansson *et al.* 1996a, Kristiansson and Svardsudd 1996). One study found the point prevalence of back pain to remain stable at about 7%, while PPP increased from 10 – 30% during the early part of the pregnancy (Ostgaard *et al.* 1994a). 'Normal' low back pain and PPP are differentiated by pain patterns and by certain other features of history and physical examination (Table 13.9).

Table 13.9 Distinguishing features of low back pain and posterior pelvic pain

Low back pain (LBP)	Posterior pelvic pain (PPP)
History of back pain prior to pregnancy	No previous history of back pain
Pain – lumbar region Nerve root pain unusual (1% all women)	Pain – buttock, SIJ area, radiation into thigh, also possibly pubic area, groin, coccyx and pelvis No nerve root pain
Lumbar flexion aggravates	Pain aggravated by weight-bearing
Loss lumbar range of movement	Lumbar range of movement normal
Pain on lumbar pressure	Pain-free intervals
Negative PPP provocation test	Positive PPP provocation test

PPP provocation test – patient lies supine with hip flexed to 90 degrees, clinician stabilises pelvis and pushes posteriorly through femur. Positive test reproduces concordant pain with gentle pressure (Ostgaard *et al.* 1994b). Also known as thigh thrust or posterior shear test.

Source: Ostgaard *et al.* 1991, 1996; Kristiansson and Svardsudd 1996; Mens *et al.* 1996

The thigh thrust or PPP provocation test was evaluated in a consecutive group of seventy-two pregnant women (Ostgaard *et al.* 1994b). One clinician took the history and one performed the test, blind to whether the women had pain or what type of pain. Twenty-seven women had PPP, twelve had LBP or thoracic pain and thirty-three had no pain. The sensitivity of the test in identifying PPP was 81%, its specificity in excluding those who did not have PPP was 80%, and positive and negative predictive values were 71% and 88% respectively.

It is postulated that low back pain is 'normal' back pain as experienced by the non-pregnant population, while PPP is specific to the pregnant condition (Ostgaard 1997b). It is suggested that the effect of hormones on the aetiology of PPP is significant, with serum relaxin – which is released during pregnancy – causing a softening of ligamentous restraint and producing ligamentous insufficiency or instability at the joints of the pelvis (Kristiansson 1997, 1998; MacLennan *et al.* 1986; Ostgaard 1997b). Significant correlations have been found between mean relaxin levels and back pain and, in those with pregnancy onset back pain, a positive PPP provocation test (Kristiansson *et al.* 1996b). Symptoms may derive from instability at one or both SIJ, the symphysis pubis, or all three articulations (Albert 1998).

Lordosis and pregnancy
Pregnancy produces altered mechanical stresses on the lumbar spine. Different studies suggest that biomechanical response to the pregnant state is different in different women, and at different times of the pregnancy. Ostgaard *et al.* (1993) found no change in lumbar lordosis between the twelfth and thirty-sixth week of pregnancy, but did find a significant correlation between a large lumbar lordosis and back pain. Bullock *et al.* (1987) found a significant increase in lordosis between about the eighteenth and thirty-eighth weeks. There was a mean increase of 7.2 degrees, but with considerable variety, with some women showing a marked increase – one woman's lordosis increased by 22.3 degrees. Increasing lordosis was associated with increased height and weight, but no correlation was found with back pain. Dumas *et al.* (1995) also found a significant increase in lordosis up to about thirty-two weeks. This increase continued in multigravidas after this point, but the lordosis decreased in primagravidas after thirty-two weeks.

Mechanical response to pregnancy may in fact be variable and individual. Of twenty-five women, about half showed a decrease in lordosis initially and about half stayed the same or increased (Moore *et al.* 1990). However, later in the pregnancy about half showed an increase in lordosis and about half stayed the same or showed a decrease in the lordosis. The tendency for the lordotic curve to increase with the progression of the pregnancy was associated with a greater likelihood of back pain.

Management of back pain during pregnancy

Evidence about management of back pain in pregnancy is rather thin; a Cochrane review only contained one trial that fulfilled their inclusion criteria (Young and Jewell 1999).

It is likely that women with PPP and ordinary lower back pain (LBP) will respond differently. Education and exercise programmes have produced better outcomes than control groups and have been found useful by the majority of women with LBP (Ostgaard *et al.* 1997a; Noren *et al.* 1997; Mantle *et al.* 1981). Women with PPP did not benefit from a programme of exercises and education, nor did they benefit from the protective effect of pre-pregnancy fitness, as did women with LBP (Ostgaard *et al.* 1994a). Women with PPP may worsen if treated with back strengthening exercises (Ostgaard 1997b). However, a study of women with persistent PPP after pregnancy showed no difference in outcome between groups randomised to education and refraining from exercise and those given exercises (Mens *et al.* 2000). Abdominal training was performed either focusing on diagonal or longitudinal trunk muscles, with the latter viewed as placebo. All groups could also use a pelvic belt. After eight weeks of intervention there was no significant difference between the groups, but 64% reported improvement.

Several investigators have found that women with PPP report a reduction of pain and disability, especially when walking, with the use of a non-elastic sacro-iliac or trochanteric belt (Ostgaard *et al.* 1994a; Berg *et al.* 1988; Mens *et al.* 1996).

Reports suggest variable mechanical responses to pregnancy, one of which is increased lordosis. These women may report themselves to be much worse when standing or walking, but better when sitting – such women may respond to the flexion principle (see Chapter 25 for details). Certain of the procedures may need to be adapted to cope with the pregnant abdomen, for instance by abduction at the hips. Alternatively, increased lordosis may cause postural strains and respond to postural correction in standing.

Other women may respond to the extension principle. Due to the pregnancy, certain procedures are ruled out. After a certain point in time it is not appropriate for women to lie prone; the exact time varies. When prone lying or extension in lying become impossible, extension in standing is usually still tolerated. From a four-point kneeling position, a certain amount of extension can also be gained by dropping the abdomen to the floor. Inability to reach end-range extension may limit the effectiveness of these procedures and full reduction may not be obtained.

If PPP, as defined above, is present, women should be offered a firm belt and advised about restricting weight-bearing activities. Overdoing activities may aggravate pain the following day. Keeping generally fit with activities such as swimming may help. Although pain may not recede during the pregnancy, prognosis post-partum is good. Some women present with a mixture of LBP and PPP.

Table 13.10 General guidelines on management of women with back pain during pregnancy

- A distinction must be made between LBP and PPP. In terms of natural history and response to interventions, these appear to be different entities, and therefore management must distinguish between the two.
- Women with PPP benefit less from educational and exercise programmes, but frequently get some benefit from a firm support belt.
- Women with LBP may be classified according to one of the mechanical syndromes:
    - Derangements commonly respond to the flexion principle, some to the extension principle
    - Postural syndrome should also be considered
- An educational and exercise programme appears to be beneficial in some women, especially those with LBP. Programmes involve the following (Ostgaard 1994a, 1997a; Noren et al. 1997):
    - individualised according to the type of back pain
    - no passive treatment
    - lifting/working techniques and discussion of vocational ergonomics
    - muscle training and general exercise involving back extensors, abdominals and pelvic floor
    - relaxation
    - didactic educational component
    - home programme

Zygapophyseal joint problems

Diagnosis

Zygapophyseal or 'facet' joints have long been assumed to be a cause of back pain; however, its prevalence rate or means of recognition is unclear. The most effective way to establish that a zygapophyseal joint is the source of a person's back pain is to inject the joint with anaesthetic. This should be done under fluoroscopic guidance to ensure that the injection is accurately located. Based on single diagnostic blocks of this type, the prevalence of zygapophyseal joint pain has been reported to range from 8 – 75% in sixteen different studies (Dreyer and Dreyfuss 1996).

Unfortunately, such intra-articular injections are associated with a high rate of false-positive findings. Substantial numbers have pain abolished by a placebo injection or respond to a first but not a second injection. Rates of such false-positive responses to single lumbar zygapophyseal joint blocks have been shown to occur in 32%, 38% and over 60% of individuals (Schwarzer et al. 1992, 1994a, 1994d). The positive predictive value of a single joint block has been rated at only 31% (Schwarzer et al. 1994a). Furthermore, the amount injected must respect the capsule of the joint, which will leak or tear if more than a few millilitres are injected, and thus may affect other structures (Raymond and Dumas 1984). These factors invalidate previous attempts to describe this entity using only single joint blocks, some with excessive quantities of contrast agent, saline or analgesic.

Prevalence

Using a rigorous research design involving two separate joint blocks, the prevalence of zygapophyseal joint pain has been estimated at 15% of 176 (Schwarzer et al. 1994b) and at 40% of sixty-three (Schwarzer et al. 1995b) patients with chronic back pain. In another study that used pain provocation and pain relief to make the diagnosis, 17% of fifty-four chronic back pain patients had the diagnosis confirmed (Moran et al. 1988). In another study involving ninety-two consecutive chronic back pain patients, both the zygapophyseal joints and the intervertebral disc were investigated as sources of pain (Schwarzer et al. 1994d). The latter were diagnosed by exact pain reproduction on discography, with abnormal image, provided no pain was reproduced at a control segmental level. Thirty-nine percent had positive discograms, while 9% were positive to double zygapophyseal joint blocks. Only 3% of the patients had a combination of zygapophyseal and discogenic pain.

Clinical features

Clinical features have not been found that could predict patients' response to such injections. Factors such as movement limitation, day or night pain, pain on certain movements, pain aggravated or relieved by certain activities, and area of pain referral could not distinguish those patients who responded to zygapophyseal joint injections from those who did not (Schwarzer *et al.* 1994b, 1995b; Jackson *et al.* 1988). For instance, features such as aggravation of pain by rotation, or extension and rotation, or referral of pain were poor discriminators of zygapophyseal pain. Two earlier studies (Fairbank *et al.* 1981; Helbig and Lee 1988) suggested certain features that were present in patients who responded to zygapophyseal joint injections. However, these criteria were later found to be unreliable in distinguishing this from other sources of pain (Schwarzer 1994c).

Direct stimulation of facet joints has produced mostly local or buttock pain (Marks 1989). However, those responding to double joint blocks are as likely to have symptoms radiating into the thigh and lower leg as those who do not respond (Schwarzer *et al.* 1994b). The only pain pattern that appears to differentiate between responders and non-responders is central pain, which was never found in those responding to double joint blocks (Schwarzer *et al.* 1994b, 1994d). Computed tomography was unable to distinguish painful joints either (Schwarzer *et al.* 1995c).

One small study has demonstrated the accuracy of diagnosis by manual examination when compared to zygapophyseal joint blocks in the cervical spine (Jull *et al.* 1988). In twenty patients, manual therapy showed 100% sensitivity and specificity in diagnosing cervical zygapophyseal joint pain. Such a study has not been reproduced, nor has it been replicated in the lumbar spine.

Recently a new set of criteria to identify patients with painful zygapophyseal joints has been identified and proposed through studying responders and non-responders to joint injections (Revel *et al.* 1992, 1998). Pain should always be relieved by recumbency, and four of the following variables also had to be present:

- age greater than 65 years

- pain not exacerbated by coughing

- pain not worsened by hyperextension

- pain not worsened by flexion

- pain not worsened rising from flexion

- pain not worsened by rotation-extension.

If the patient has five of these seven criteria, has not had spinal surgery, does not have true sciatica, does not have upper lumbar or sacro-iliac joint pain, there is a greater than 90% chance that they will respond to an injection. These characteristics should not be considered diagnostic for zygapophyseal joint pain, but only indicative of a patient who will respond to a zygapophyseal joint injection.

One study has tried to compare findings from the history and physical examination in a group of chronic patients who responded to SIJ, facet injections or discography (Young and Aprill 2000). Findings from the facet and SIJ groups were similar, both showing lack of obstruction or movement loss after repeated movements, lack of centralisation or peripheralisation, and abolition of distal symptoms without centralisation.

Management
Not only is the identification of this group problematical, but no effective treatment has been identified. Open uncontrolled studies evaluating the value of intra-articular steroid injections report relief in 18 – 63% of subjects in ten studies; however, such study designs are inherently biased and are likely to report favourable outcomes (Dreyer and Dreyfuss 1996). Corticosteroid injections into zygapophyseal joints when evaluated under randomised, controlled study design are no more effective than injections of saline (Lilius *et al.* 1989; Carette *et al.* 1991).

Radiofrequency facet joint denervation is a recent treatment option that appeared to have positive short-term effects in two small studies (Gallagher *et al.* 1994; van Kleef *et al.* 1999). However, a larger, more recent study found the intervention to lack treatment effect at twelve weeks (Leclaire *et al.* 2001).

In summary, zygapophyseal joints can be a source of pain, but identification through a normal clinical examination appears to be unlikely. At this stage there is no clinical benefit in identifying them as a separate group. Such patients may respond mechanically.

Spondylolysis and spondylolisthesis

Definitions and classification
Spondylolysis is a defect in the pars interarticularis. Spondylolisthesis denotes a forward displacement of a vertebral body, which can occur if there are defects in both neural arches.

Spondylolysis and spondylolisthesis have been classified according to origin. The commonly accepted classification is as follows (Macnab and McCulloch 1990):

- dysplastic

- isthmic

- degenerative

- traumatic

- pathological.

This classification refers largely to onset – dysplastic being due to a congenital deficiency, isthmic occurring in childhood. In essence, the first two are 'developmental', the other categories being 'acquired' in later life (Smith and Hu 1999). Developmental defects and those that occur as a result of disc degeneration are the categories that are most likely to be seen clinically, and so are considered here. The incidence of spondylolisthesis due to trauma or bone disease is unknown, but clinically should be considered a 'red flag' condition unsuitable for mechanical therapy.

Isthmic spondylolisthesis is further categorised as follows (Stinson 1993):

- fatigue fracture of the pars interarticularis with slippage

- an intact, but elongated, pars interarticularis

- acute fracture.

The degree of the slip has been graded according to two methods. The Meyerding classification divides the top of the sacrum into four equal sections. A slip in the first quarter is grade I, a slip in the last quarter is grade IV. A more accurate measurement can be given in percentage terms (Hensinger 1989).

The majority of individuals with spondylolisthesis have low-grade slippages. In a population survey, which found sixty-nine cases in a sample of 1,147 subjects (6% prevalence), the degree of slip was grade I in 79%, grade II in 20% and grade III in 1% (Osterman *et al.* 1993). In over 300 patients, nearly 90% were classified as grade 0, I or II (Danielson *et al.* 1991).

Relevance to symptoms

Despite the alarming nature of the abnormality, spondylolisthesis is not inevitably a source of back pain. Van Tulder *et al.* (1997c) conducted a systematic review of radiographic findings and back pain. Six studies investigated spondylolysis or spondylolisthesis, of which five concluded there was no association between these findings and back pain. One study of middle-aged patients found the association between spondylolisthesis and back pain to be weak and only present in women (Virta and Ronnemaa 1993). *"Roughly half of patients with this finding do not have back pain, so finding may be unrelated"* to symptoms (Roland and van Tulder 1998).

The prevalence rate of isthmic spondylolysis in the general adult population and in the back pain population is generally about the same, around 6%. If such defects were a common source of back pain, these findings would be much more common in the latter (Porter and Hibbert 1984; Micheli and Yancey 1996; Macnab and McCulloch 1990).

The role of disc pathology as a confounding factor in the presence of spondylolisthesis has been demonstrated in several studies (Macnab and McCulloch 1990; Henson *et al.* 1987; Deutman *et al.* 1995). These are reminders that the finding of spondylolisthesis may be irrelevant to symptoms, and that a mechanical evaluation should always be attempted.

Prevalence

There is no evidence that the defect exists at birth; it most commonly appears between the ages of 5 and 7, with a subsequent increase during adolescence, after which prevalence rates remain relatively static during adulthood (Ciullo and Jackson 1985; Johnson 1993). Defects of the pars interarticularis are strongly associated with spina bifida occulta (Fredrickson *et al.* 1984). Isthmic spondylolysis and spondylolisthesis occur predominantly at L5 – S1.

In 500 school children, the incidence of spondylolysis was 1.8% and isthmic spondylolisthesis 2.6%; this increased to 2% and 4% respectively in young adulthood (Fredrickson *et al.* 1984). Osterman *et al.* (1993) reported an incidence of 6% of isthmic spondylolisthesis in a random population survey of adults. Macnab and McCulloch (1990) found the incidence of spondylolisthesis in nearly a thousand patients to be 7.6%, but in those under 25 it was 19%, in those between 26 and 39 it was 7.6% and in those over 40 it was 5.2%.

They concluded that in the younger patient it was more likely that the defect was the cause of their symptoms.

Numerous reports have suggested that the prevalence rate is greater, sometimes up to 50%, in the young athletic population (Jackson *et al.* 1976; Micheli and Wood 1995; Johnson 1993; Morita *et al.* 1995; Jackson 1979; Foster *et al.* 1989; Hardcastle *et al.* 1992; Hollenberg *et al.* 2002). Association suggests there may be a causal relationship between some sports and symptomatic spondylolysis. However, an awareness of risk in this group should be tempered by several factors: the high prevalence of back pain in all adolescents, the uncertain nature of sport as a risk factor for back pain and the biased study designs that have been used to look at this question.

Backache is commonly reported by school children and rises linearly during teenage years (Duggleby and Kumar 1997; Leboeuf-Yde and Kyvik 1998; Taimela *et al.* 1997; Burton *et al.* 1996). According to one study, the one-year period prevalence of back pain is about 10% in 12-year-olds, rising to over 40% in 20-year-olds (Leboeuf-Yde and Kyvik 1998). By early adulthood, the high prevalence rates of back symptoms are already well established, after which the steep increase flattens out (Leboeuf-Yde and Kyvik 1998; Burton *et al.* 1996).

In fact, both physical inactivity and sporting activity have been associated with adolescent back pain (Burton *et al.* 1996; Taimela *et al.* 1997; Prendeville and Dockrell 1998). Participation in sport is not clearly a risk factor for juvenile non-specific back pain, while hours of television watching has been significantly associated with back pain (Duggleby and Kumar 1997).

Most studies in sporting groups have been conducted in limited populations in which the diagnosis has been sought – such a study design may produce a biased sample. In a population study of over 3,000 élite, adult Spanish athletes, the general prevalence of spondylolysis was 8%, although certain sports demonstrated much higher rates (Soler and Calderon 2000). This would suggest that sport itself is not a risk factor in adults, but that *certain* sports may be more associated with the defect.

In adolescents, only infrequently is spondylolysis or spondylolisthesis the cause of back pain, but, especially in athletes, this diagnosis should be considered. Micheli and Wood (1995) compared the final diagnosis after investigations in 100 randomly selected adolescent patients with back pain from a sports medicine clinic and 100 randomly selected adult patients with acute back pain. Average age in the two groups were 16 and 32. A stress fracture of the pars interarticularis was found in 47% of the adolescents, but only 5% of the adults. The authors recommend that the index of suspicion should be raised if there has been a history of repetitive hyperextension training, such as gymnastics, cricket or baseball, and pain is provoked on hyperextension.

Aetiology

Isthmic spondylolysis does not exist at birth. It is acquired during growth caused by a stress fracture of the pars interarticularis. Its acquisition is thought to be related to weight-bearing (Rosenberg *et al.* 1981).

Cadaveric experiments have induced fractures of the neural arch with repetitive cyclical loading, especially implicating extension forces (Cyron *et al.* 1976). However, mechanical fatigue of the pars is possible during any strenuous activity that generates sufficient force and number of cycles, especially in young people, since their intervertebral discs are more elastic and their neural arch may not be completely ossified (Cyron and Hutton 1978). It is thought that the defect is a fatigue fracture due to repeated minor trauma or stress rather than the result of one traumatic incident (Wiltse *et al.* 1975).

Besides mechanical factors, a familial tendency also exists for the development of pars interarticularis defects (Wiltse *et al.* 1975). Prevalence of 33% has been reported among those with a family history of spondylolysis (Johnson 1993).

Unlike other stress fractures, defects of the pars interarticularis frequently persist and fail to heal (Wiltse *et al.* 1975). A possible cause for this persistence is the formation of a pseudo-arthrosis at the site of the defect because of communication with adjacent zygapophyseal joints. Synovial cells and tissue and loose fibrous tissue similar to a joint capsule have been commonly found at these sites (Shipley and Beukes 1998). Furthermore, neural elements have been identified within the pars defect and in the 'ligament' associated with it, and thus it is a feasible source of back pain in some (Schneiderman *et al.* 1995; Eisenstein *et al.* 1994).

Progression and natural history

Not all spondylolysis progresses to spondylolisthesis. Progression of the slip occurs most commonly in a short period and during the adolescent growth spurt between eight and fourteen years of age, after which it tends to remain stable (Comstock *et al.* 1994; Lonstein 1999; Fredrickson *et al.* 1984). During the growth period, a stress fracture or slippage triggered by excessive exertion may become symptomatic (Hensinger 1989; Micheli and Yancey 1996). Progression is said to be rare once individuals reach adulthood (Danielson *et al.* 1991; Fredrickson *et al.* 1984), but may occur. This is more likely in the case of a spondylolisthesis than a spondylolysis (Ohmori *et al.* 1995). Progression of the slip is not prevented by surgical intervention (Seitsalo *et al.* 1991).

Progression of isthmic spondylolisthesis during adulthood has been reported and is said to be a possibility in about 20% of individuals with this finding (Floman 2000). Thus, an incidental and irrelevant finding can become a source of symptoms; the average age in a set of eighteen patients was forty-four. The individuals had incapacitating low back and leg pain, with most reporting radicular pain due to local spinal stenosis brought about by the narrowing and the increased slip (Floman 2000).

Degenerative spondylolisthesis occurs most frequently at L4 – L5, in those over fifty, and is more common in women, especially those who have had multiple pregnancies (Grobler *et al.* 1994; Herkowitz 1995; Sanderson and Fraser 1996). Vertebral displacement with an intact neural arch can critically narrow a small spinal canal (Porter 1993). Clinical findings are thus those of spinal stenosis (see section on spinal stenosis) from other degenerative causes – leg pain brought on by walking, relieved by flexion, low prevalence of neurological signs and symptoms and restricted range of extension (Herkowitz 1995). A long history of back pain is usual and radiographs should display considerable degenerative changes.

Clinical presentation

As has been stressed before, both pars fractures and spondylolisthesis can be asymptomatic and incidental findings in the normal population, or an individual can have these abnormalities as well as unrelated back pain (van Tulder *et al.* 1997c).

In patients with a finding of spondylolysis the main symptom is back pain, with or without radiation into the thigh (Porter and Hibbert 1984). The pain is localised around L5; patients are said to be able to point to the site of pain (Ciullo and Jackson 1985; Johnson 1993). In patients with a symptomatic spondylolisthesis, back and radicular pain may be present; neurological signs and symptoms are also found less commonly (Frennered *et al.* 1991; Seitsalo 1990; Seitsalo *et al.* 1990; Boxall *et al.* 1979; Kaneda *et al.* 1985).

The adolescent group should be assessed with a greater index of suspicion concerning this diagnosis, especially those involved in vigorous sport. It is suggested that a number of different sports are risk factors for developing spondylolysis (Duggleby and Kumar 1997). Those that involve repetitive hyperextension may involve the greatest risk, such as gymnastics, baseball and bowling in cricket. Trauma is not often involved and in many instances symptoms have an insidious onset, but may coincide with the adolescent growth spurt (Micheli and Yancey 1996).

In some individuals the degree and angle of slippage increases when they move from lying to standing (Boxall *et al.* 1979; Lowe *et al.* 1976), thus sustained weight-bearing is likely to be a cause of aggravation and recumbency a cause of relief. Prolonged standing, walking or sitting may bring on symptoms, which are relieved by lying. Symptoms may be initiated or aggravated by strenuous activity in the adolescent group, such as sporting participation, and decreased by rest.

Physical findings are likely to vary depending on the grade or stage of the defect. Very often there is full range of movement. Extension of the spine is often painful and exacerbates or produces the patient's symptoms (Balderston and Bradford 1985; Micheli and Yancey 1996; Hardcastle 1993; Hollenberg *et al.* 2002; Micheli and Wood 1995). This will be a consistent and unchanging response, which does not get easier, as might occur in derangement. Both repeated flexion and extension might worsen symptoms (Payne and Oglive 1996).

In more extreme cases, signs may be more pronounced. Distortion of the pelvis and trunk, tight hamstrings with a waddling gait, a prominent step-off at the level of the slippage, and folds and protrusion in the abdominal wall have been reported (Balderston and Bradford 1985; Hensinger 1989; Harris and Weinstein 1987).

McKenzie (1981) recommends a simple clinical test to help determine if a spondylolisthesis is responsible for the presenting symptoms, as it often reduces or abolishes pain in the presence of this condition. With the patient standing, place one hand across their sacrum and the other firmly against their abdomen. With further compression from both hands, pain arising from spondylolisthesis is markedly reduced or abolished. On sudden release of pressure, which must be maximal, there may be a sharp return of pain of short duration. The test should be repeated three times, and if pain is experienced on release of pressure each time, it is likely that pain is from the spondylolisthesis. Pain from derangement is usually worsened, and that from other mechanical syndromes unaffected. Another provocative manoeuvre is the one-leg lumbar hyperextension test, in which the patient stands on the ipsilateral leg and bends backwards in an attempt to reproduce their familiar symptoms (Ciullo and Jackson 1985). Neither test has been formally evaluated.

A comparison has been made of 111 adult patients with isthmic spondylolisthesis with at least one year of back pain and/or sciatica to thirty-nine chronic patients prior to surgery (Moller *et al.* 2000). Most of the slippages were grade I or II; symptoms were mostly constant, worsened by sitting and walking, woke patients at night and were associated with moderately restricted function. Sciatica was present in 70%, but positive signs were unusual, with tight hamstrings, positive straight leg raising and sensory disturbance present in 20% or less. The profile of functional disturbance, aggravating factors, and signs and symptoms were strikingly similar for both spondylolisthesis and non-specific chronic back pain groups. *This study shows that in adults at least there is no clear clinical presentation that distinguishes back pain patients with spondylolisthesis from those with non-specific back pain.*

Diagnosis
Ultimately, to make the diagnosis of spondylolysis or spondylolisthesis, imaging studies are required. Radiographs can be insensitive tools in the detection of the defect (Congeni *et al.* 1997). If the defect is large it may be visible on ordinary lumbar radiographs, while a spondylolysis or minimal slippage may only be revealed on oblique radiography (Hensinger 1989). Different radiographic views have different sensitivity to the lesion, with lateral and oblique views picking up over 75% and anterior-posterior views detecting 50% or less (Amato *et al.* 1984).

Various specialist imaging techniques are also used. Computed tomography scans with reverse gantry angle technique and scintigraphy or single photon emission computed tomography (SPECT) are more sensitive than radiographs (Saifuddin *et al.* 1998; Harvey *et al.* 1998; Bodner *et al.* 1988; Bellah *et al.* 1991; Collier *et al.* 1985). SPECT may be particularly useful in the identification of early lesions, when fractures are still metabolically active and x-rays may be normal (Lowe *et al.* 1984; Harvey *et al.* 1998). Later, when the lesion is well established, radiography is more specific (Papanicolaou *et al.* 1985).

Identification of a lyses defect by imaging, *let alone* any attempt to establish a causal link with the patient's pain through such means, clearly requires sophisticated techniques in the hands of a specialist.

Management
The literature is dominated by surgical interventions. Comparisons between surgical and conservative treatment of spondylolisthesis are rare; a convincing case for the superiority of surgery, even in more severe slippages, has not been previously made (Seitsalo *et al.* 1991; Seitsalo 1990; Harris and Weinstein 1987). However, in the first randomised trial comparing conservative and surgical treatments ever to be done, and including a two-year follow-up, the superiority of the surgical treatment was clear (Moller and Hedlund 2000). While function improved by 19% and pain by 26% in the surgery group, the comparative changes in the conservative treatment group were 0% and 9%. The exercise programme consisted of back and abdominal strength training conducted over at least one year, two or three times a week.

Conservative treatment of symptomatic spondylolisthesis does not favour any particular approach; rather, the literature consists of a few contradictory interventions. In one trial involving patients with a radiographic diagnosis of spondylolysis or spondylolisthesis, mostly with a minimal or absent slip, normal management was compared to specific stabilising exercises. Only the intervention group showed a statistically significant reduction in pain and disability, which was maintained at thirty months (O'Sullivan *et al.* 1997).

Both flexion and extension exercises have been used in patients with spondylolisthesis, and both have been found superior. One trial compared the effect of abdominal or back strengthening exercises, although details of the duration and number of sessions were not given. The overall recovery rate in the active extension group at three months was 6% and at three years was 0%, compared to 58% and 62% in the active flexion group (Sinaki *et al.* 1989). The authors state their belief that flexion exercises are preferred and that extension exercise should be avoided. This is based on the putative role of lumbar extension in causing fractures of the pars interarticularis.

Although this opinion is common, an extension programme has also been shown to be beneficial. A group of patients classified by their translational findings as spondylolisthesis, retrolisthesis or no defect were randomised to extension, flexion or control treatments. The exercise groups performed exercises and used a lumbar brace to maintain the appropriate posture. At one-month follow-up only the extension group patients showed a significant improvement across time, and this occurred in all translation subgroups (Spratt *et al.* 1993). The authors suggest that the favourable response to extension treatment, despite spondylolisthesis or retrolisthesis, may be because these findings are secondary to underlying disc pathology. The opinion that extension exercises should be contraindicated in the presence of a spondylolisthesis is not borne out by this study.

Most fatigue fractures mend with time, and spondylolysis are unusual in that this normal healing process does not always occur. However, healing can happen, and this is more likely when the fracture is still at a relatively acute stage (Hardcastle 1993). When 185 adolescents with spondylolysis were classified into early, progressive and late stage defects, according to computer tomography (CT) findings, their response to conservative management was significantly different. While 73% of those in the early stage achieved bony union according to radiography and/or CT three to six months later, only 38% of those in the progressive stage and 0% of those in the final stage did so (Morita *et al.* 1995). These findings make clear the importance of early detection of the fracture to ensure appropriate management, which in this case entailed absence from sport and use of a lumbar corset for three to six months.

In the young sporting population, reduction or cessation of the aggravating activities and stretching and strengthening programmes are recommended, with a gradual return to sport as symptoms allow (Johnson 1993). Some recommend the use of a brace to facilitate healing, although this is not universally required. While the results of a series of sixty-seven patients were good or excellent in 78% fitted with an anti-lordotic Boston brace, the intrusiveness of the intervention was extreme. It was to be worn twenty-three hours out of twenty-four for six months, and then reduced over a further six months (Steiner and Micheli 1985).

Summary

The finding of spondylolysis or spondylolisthesis on a radiographic report may be quite unrelated to a patient's symptoms, with even quite severe slippages present in individuals without back pain. A full mechanical evaluation may be safely conducted, and many such patients respond in a normal mechanical fashion. Atypical responses may imply that the defect has significance. Furthermore, certain items during history-taking and physical examination may alert the clinician to the possibility of this diagnosis.

Symptomatic isthmic spondylolysis should be suspected in adolescent sporting participants with a gradual onset of low back pain that is sports-related. Those involved in repetitive flexion/extension and/or ipsilateral side bending or rotation movements may be at particular risk. Extension is likely to increase symptoms, although not necessarily worsen them, and tight hamstrings may be present. This is a stress fracture, and referral to a sports physician is most appropriate; relative rest is the best management and mechanical therapy is contraindicated. However, only a minority of back pain in adolescents is due to spondylolysis. Mostly they present with symptoms from either postural or derangement syndromes.

Instability

Lumbar segmental instabilities have been categorised by cause as being due to fractures, infections, neoplasms, spondylolisthesis or degeneration. Degenerative lumbar instabilities are either primary or secondary, with the latter resulting from surgical destruction of some kind (Bogduk 1997). Primary instabilities are defined by their direction; for instance, translational instability, characterised by excessive anterior translation of one vertebra on another during flexion.

Primary instability has been variously defined as loss of motion segment stiffness, an increase in mobility or an increase of segmental rotations or translations (Richardson et al. 1999). Definite instability is indicated by more than 4 – 5mm of translation on a flexion–extension radiograph (Fordyce *et al.* 1995) and is traditionally associated with degenerative disc disease. More recently, clinical instability has been defined as *"a significant decrease in the capacity of the stabilizing system of the spine to maintain the intervertebral neutral zones within physiological limits which results in pain and disability"* (Panjabi, in Richardson *et al.* 1999, p. 13). The neutral zone is the area where movement of a motion segment occurs with minimal resistance from ligamentous structures, which offer restraint in the elastic zone to limit end-range movement. The stabilising system is comprised of three components: the passive system of the spinal column, the active system of the muscles and a neural control system. Back pain is said to occur when there is a deficit in any of the three components, resulting in abnormally large segmental motions that cause compression or stretch on pain-sensitive structures (Richardson *et al.* 1999).

Despite much discussion and considerable theoretical work that has elaborated the concept of primary instability, there are still numerous problems concerning definition, criteria, relationship to a pain state and clinical identification (Porter 1993; Spratt *et al.* 1993; Dupuis *et al.* 1985). Most definitions of instability involve increased or abnormal segmental motion. Some studies have shown large amounts of translation are more common in those with back pain compared to the general population (Spratt *et al.* 1993; Lehmann and Brand 1983; Sihvonen *et al.* 1997). However, 4mm and more of anterior translation has also been found in 10% to 20% of asymptomatic populations (Woody *et al.* 1983; Hayes *et al.* 1989). Only one study has demonstrated a link between the amount of translation and the degree of symptoms (Friberg 1987). In fact, all these studies have involved individuals with a diagnosis of spondylolisthesis or retrolisthesis. Various methods have been used to try to expose abnormal segmental motion during dynamic radiographic studies: centrode patterns, dynamic traction-compression and flexion-extension radiography.

All these techniques have flaws. Centrode patterns, the locus of successive positions of instantaneous centres of rotation, have been studied in vitro and in vivo (Gertzbein *et al.* 1984, 1985; Pearcy and Bogduk 1988). The group that developed centrode patterns found them to be associated with a high degree of error and inaccuracy, and they subsequently abandoned the technique as a clinical investigative tool (Weiler *et al.* 1990). A study using dynamic traction–compression radiography found that the severity of symptoms related to the amount of translation at the level of the spondylolisthesis

(Friberg 1987). Mean movement in the asymptomatic, moderate and severe pain groups were 0.7mm, 5.2mm and 7.5mm respectively. However, the technique was found to have a poor correlation with the results of dynamic flexion-extension radiography, which is the traditional method of diagnosis. By traction–compression, 8% of a cohort of patients were diagnosed with instability, compared to 96% by flexion–extension radiography (Pitkanen *et al.* 1997).

Flexion–extension radiography was the original method used to reveal instability. The technique was unable to expose abnormal or erratic motion during movement, but only at end-range (Stokes and Frymoyer 1987). There can be inconsistencies and inaccuracies in flexion-extension radiography, errors in classification and lack of definition about what is normal and what is pathological (Shaffer *et al.* 1990; Spratt *et al.* 1993). As a consequence of these failings, there is no gold standard method of diagnosing or measuring instability, nor is it a morphological abnormality that is correlated with back pain.

"Difficulties lie, particularly in vivo, in gaining a definition of instability that would indicate a relationship to a pain state and that would generate a method of quantification to demonstrate its presence. As a consequence, there is currently neither a gold-standard definition of clinical instability nor a gold-standard measure" (Richardson *et al.* 1999, p. 12).

"Various clinical criteria have been proclaimed as indicative or diagnostic of lumbar instability. At best, these constitute fancy. To be valid, clinical signs have to be validated against a criterion standard. The only available criterion standard for instability is offered by radiographic signs, but the radiographic signs of instability are themselves beset with difficulties. Consequently, no studies have yet validated any of the proclaimed clinical signs of instability" (Bogduk 1997, p. 224).

Degenerated discs have been correlated with higher levels of instability factor, which is a combination of translation and angulation (Weiler *et al.* 1990), and with an increasing spread of axes of movement (Penning and Blickman 1980). It has been suggested that instability may need to be considered an irrelevant product of disc pathology rather than a distinct clinical syndrome (Spratt *et al.* 1993). This is supported by some studies that have found radiographic instability persisting after symptoms have resolved. Radiographic instability has been shown both to improve spontaneously over time and to persist when symptoms have resolved (Sato and Kikuchi 1993; Lindgren *et al.* 1993).

The evidence does not prove that an excessive amount of translation at a lumbar segment is a source of symptoms, although it does suggest that there are serious difficulties in measuring this. If a gross abnormality such as a spondylolisthesis is not always directly related to symptoms, the role of lesser 'instabilities' in back pain awaits further elucidation. Furthermore, with the lack of 'gold standard' diagnosis, there are no clinical criteria that have been validated as being sensitive and specific in the recognition of this entity.

Mechanically inconclusive

There is a small group of patients whose symptoms are influenced by postures and movements, and yet who do not fit one of the three mechanical syndromes. Symptoms are affected by loading strategies, but in an unrecognisable or inconsistent pattern. This group does not display a mechanical presentation – range of movement is preserved, and there is no obstruction to movement. Pain may be constant or intermittent, and is frequently produced or increased at end-ranges. Repeated end-range movements in all planes may produce a worsening of symptoms, but no obstruction of extension or flexion by loading in the opposite direction. Thus, no directional preference is indicated.

There may be variations on a similar theme; for instance, catches of pain during movement, or initially there is a favourable response to repeated movement in one direction, which then becomes inconsistent or causes a worsening of symptoms if continued or if force progressions are included. The key to this mechanically inconclusive group, who nonetheless have symptoms that respond to loading strategies, is that a consistent directional preference cannot be found.

Criteria for mechanically inconclusive group are:

- symptoms affected by spinal movements

- no loading strategy consistently decreases, abolishes or centralises symptoms, nor increases or peripheralises symptoms

- inconsistent response to loading strategies.

This group sometimes responds to mid-range postures rather than end-range movements. Maintenance of posture correction, use of mid-range movements, especially slouch-overcorrect, avoidance of end-range postures and movements and interruption of painful positions may be helpful for this group.

Surgery

Lumbar disc herniation is one of the few clear occasions when surgery or other invasive treatment might be considered. Because many will improve if treated conservatively, early surgery should generally be avoided. The only specific indicators for early surgery are cauda equina syndrome and progressive or profound neurological deficit (Saal 1996). Otherwise if surgery is to be considered, certain strict criteria are necessary (see Table 5.1), as well as the failure of six weeks of attempted conservative therapy (see Table 5.4 for characteristic presentation of extrusions and sequestrations). Patients with these more severe disc herniations may do better with surgery than patients with protrusions (Hoffman *et al.* 1993).

Scheer *et al.* (1996) reviewed thirteen randomised controlled trials for sciatica and discogenic back pain, concentrating on the outcome of return to work. Chemonucleolysis, discectomy and epidural steroid injections were included in the review. For all interventions they found the evidence to be equivocal. In particular, they could not infer that surgery was better than conservative therapy in the long-term. Hoffman *et al.* (1993), in a literature synthesis, concluded that standard discectomy appears to offer better short-term outcomes than conservative treatment, but long-term outcomes are similar.

In a recent Cochrane review of surgery for lumbar disc prolapse, twenty-six randomised controlled trials were identified (Gibson *et al.* 1999). Meta-analyses showed that chemonucleolysis was clearly better than placebo, and discectomy was better than chemonucleolysis, and therefore discectomy is better than placebo. There was no difference in outcomes between microdiscectomy and standard discectomy, although both produced better results than percutaneous discectomy. Only one trial compared surgical with conservative treatment (Weber 1983). There were significant differences in favour of surgery at one year, but not at four or ten years. These reviewers concluded that there was considerable evidence for the clinical effectiveness of discectomy for *carefully selected* patients with sciatica who fail to improve with conservative care. All reviews comment on the poor quality of design methodology and reporting.

The trial by Weber (1983) is a randomised comparison between conservative and surgical treatment of disc herniations; such comparisons are rare, and so it is given considerable importance. In fact, it suffers from certain design faults that limit its implications. Critical defects include the large number of crossovers, the inadequate sample size and insensitive outcome measures (Bessette *et al.* 1996). It was a prospective study in which eighty-seven patients with mild symptoms were treated conservatively, sixty-seven patients with severe symptoms underwent surgery and 126 patients with uncertain indications for surgery were randomised. All but five of the latter group were followed up at one, four and ten years. At one year 92% of the surgery group were satisfied, compared to 79% in the conservatively treated group. Seventeen patients allocated to conservative treatment were operated on, and one patient allocated to surgery refused the operation. At four and ten years in those patients who were located, satisfaction in those allocated and treated surgically was 86% and 93%; and in those allocated and treated conservatively, 90% and 92%. Only at one year were there significant differences favouring the surgical group.

In a non-randomised study with over 500 patients treated either surgically or conservatively, follow-up was performed at one year (Atlas *et al.* 1996b). Surgical patients tended to have more severe symptoms and few patients with severe symptoms were treated conservatively, but about half of each treatment group had symptoms that were categorised as moderate. For the predominant symptom, 71% of the surgery group and 43% of the non-surgery group reported definite improvement. Those undergoing surgery saw quicker and more dramatic improvement in symptoms.

Although it seems fairly clear that appropriately selected patients will make quicker improvements with surgery, many patients will have satisfactory outcomes with conservative treatment, especially those with mild or moderate symptoms. Some of the drawbacks of surgery should also be remembered. The long-term follow-up of some surgical series shows high levels of persisting or recurring symptoms, unsatisfactory outcomes, further operations and a deterioration of results over time (Loupasis *et al.* 1999). Four to seventeen years after operation in a partial follow-up of over 500 patients, 70% complained of back pain, 45% of sciatica, 35% were still receiving some kind of treatment and 17% had undergone repeat operations (Dvorak *et al.* 1988). In another study with a minimum of ten years follow-up, 75% reported back pain and 56% leg pain (Yorimitsu *et al.* 2001). Hoffman *et al.* (1993) estimated that 5 – 15% of all operations lead to poor outcomes and further surgery.

Although certain clinical and morphological factors are significant in outcomes from lumbar discectomy, psychosocial and work-related factors can be as significant or more so (Schade *et al.* 1999). In this prospective study of forty-six patients, the size of herniation, nerve root compression, depression, occupational mental stress and support from the spouse were associated with post-surgical pain relief. However, only psychosocial factors were associated with return to work. Careful patient selection for surgery is clearly crucial.

Epidural steroid injection for sciatica
A less invasive medical intervention sometimes considered for sciatica is epidural steroid injection. Although there is limited evidence that this intervention may offer short-term pain relief, convincing proof of its therapeutic value is missing. In 1995 two systematic reviews of this intervention were published (Watts and Silagy 1995; Koes *et al.* 1995). Rather alarmingly, they came to different conclusions despite reviewing mostly the same studies. Ten papers were common to both, one extra paper was exclusive to one review and two additional papers were exclusive to the other review. According to Watts and Silagy (1995), epidural corticosteroid is effective in the management of lumbosacral radicular pain. However, the conclusion of Koes *et al.* (1995) was that the best studies showed inconsistent results, and the efficacy of steroid injections is as yet unproven. Given that such reviews are supposed to be based on a rigorous and objective analysis of the evidence, their conflicting conclusions attest to the qualitative judgements that may occur in this process (Hopayian and Mugford 1999).

Since then a further systematic review into injection therapy in general has been published (Nelemans *et al.* 2001). This included twenty-one papers, including one (Carette *et al.* 1997) published since the previous reviews. They considered studies as being either explanatory or pragmatic, where comparison with a placebo injection was termed an explanatory trial. They located four explanatory trials into the efficacy of epidural injections for sciatica. Although all four reported greater pain relief short-term in the experimental group, this was not statistically significant. More than six weeks after the intervention, there was no difference. Six pragmatic trials looked at the effects of epidural injections in a range of conditions, including sciatica. Four showed a non-significant positive effect short-term, and neither of the two that reported on long-term pain relief found any significant difference. Their overall conclusion was that convincing evidence about the efficacy of injection therapy is lacking (Nelemans *et al.* 2001).

Recent studies have tended to confirm the lack of efficacy of epidural corticosteroid injections. The placebo controlled study by Carette *et al.* (1997) is a recent high-quality paper examining the effects of methylprednisolone acetate compared to saline in 158 patients with sciatica due to a disc herniation. Improvements in function were better, but not significantly in the active treatment group at three weeks, and just significantly better regarding leg pain at six weeks. At three months there were no differences between groups, and at one year the incidence of surgery was the same in both groups. They conclude epidural injection may provide short-term pain relief only.

This same short-term result was produced in a similar recent study (Karppinen *et al.* 2001a) in which leg pain was significantly better in the active treatment group at two weeks. However, there later appeared to be a 'rebound' effect, with back pain less in the placebo group at three months and leg pain less at six months. Use of steroid did not obviate the need for surgery, rates being similar in both groups. However, sub-group analysis suggested that for contained herniations, the steroid injection produced significantly better results than for extrusions (Karppinen *et al.* 2001b). Buchner *et al.* (2000) found no significant difference in pain or function in conservatively treated groups, one of which received steroid injections, at two or six weeks and at six months.

Only one recent study, which used fluoroscopic imaging to ensure the steroid injection was delivered precisely to its target site, has shown results that clearly favour this intervention (Vad *et al.* 2002). However, in the study patients were not blinded to the intervention and a true placebo comparison was not used.

Post-surgical status

Those with symptoms may be those who have had successful surgery, but in whom pain has re-occurred, or else those who are surgical failures in whom the original symptoms may be reduced, but still remaining. Reoccurrence of symptoms may be due to a second disc herniation or perineural fibrosis (Spitzer *et al.* 1987).

Mechanical evaluation should always be offered to post-surgical patients. If symptoms have re-occurred, it is important to distinguish whether the cause is derangement or post-surgical adhesions – the latter presents as a flexion dysfunction or an adherent nerve root. These presentations should be treated in the normal manner described in the relevant chapters.

Early active rehabilitation has an important role post-surgery. The evidence suggests better outcomes can be gained if patients are put through a dynamic exercise programme after surgery than with surgery alone. Early active training involving extension, flexion and active straight leg raising instigated immediately post-surgery resulted in significantly less leg pain for at least three months compared to a less active control group, although at one year results were about the same (Kjellby-Wendt and Styf 1998). Dynamic exercise programmes have also been instigated at about one month following surgery, again producing better outcomes than a lighter exercise comparison treatment, especially at six months (Manniche *et al.* 1993a; Danielsen *et al.* 2000). In another study, six weeks after microdiscectomy patients were entered into an exercise or control group and followed up at one year (Dolan *et al.* 2000). The exercises consisted of a four-week programme of general mobility and strengthening exercises. The exercise group showed further improvements in pain and function that were maintained at one year, whereas the control group made no further improvements except those made by surgery. The post-surgical programme is clearly important in an early restoration of confidence and function.

One aspect of post-surgical rehabilitation that has been shown *not* to be beneficial is neural mobilisation, using initially passive and then active movements, such as straight leg raise and neck flexion (Scrimshaw and Maher 2001). The neural mobilisation group had worse outcomes, although the differences were not statistically significant. Both groups performed active strengthening exercises. *"This randomized controlled trial demonstrates not only that neural mobilization after spinal surgery is of no benefit to patients but it suggests that this physical regimen may in fact be harmful"* (Fraser 2001).

The value of an active exercise approach for those more than six months after surgery is also apparent (Manniche *et al.* 1993b; Timm 1994). Following a twelve-week course of dynamic extension exercises, there was a significant improvement of pain in 70% of those who completed the programme (Manniche *et al.* 1993). Timm (1994) compared passive modalities, manipulative therapy and low- and high-tech exercises for chronic back pain following an L5 laminectomy, with the low-tech group using extension and stabilisation exercises. Both exercise groups had significant and lasting improvements in mobility and function, and reduced disability. The passive treatment group was no better than a no-treatment control group, and the manipulative therapy group also produced minimal changes.

The above studies make clear that outcomes from surgical procedures can be significantly improved with the application of a dynamic exercise programme during the rehabilitation period.

Chronic pain

Chronic pain has traditionally been defined by pain duration; for instance, symptoms that have persisted for more than three to six months. However, timescale alone is now generally considered to be an inadequate definition for chronic pain. Other factors are considered important in the chronic pain experience. Psychosocial and behavioural factors complicate the clinical problem, and pain is disassociated from tissue damage. Patients may experience widespread pains, and the problem is more likely to prove difficult to treat (Spitzer *et al.* 1987; Adams 1997).

From the review of the epidemiology of back pain in Chapter 1, it is apparent that many individuals have persistent symptoms, but that in this group severity and disability are often minimal. Waddell (1998) estimates that while 6 – 10% of all adults may have persistent or recurrent back pain, most lead relatively normal lives, are working, do not seek health care and have little disability. Categorisation of chronic patients should not be determined simply by pain duration. Of those who have persistent symptoms, many demonstrate mechanical responses, although sometimes response may be slower.

The length of time that symptoms have been present should never be seen as a deciding factor in the application of therapy. Many of those with chronic symptoms can benefit from a mechanical assessment. *Patients who have long-standing low back pain should not be denied a mechanical assessment.* Many patients with long-term problems display directional preference for certain repeated movements (Donelson *et al.* 1990, 1991, 1997; Long 1995; Rath and Rath 1996). Not all will resolve their problems, but many patients with chronic symptoms improve their ability to manage their condition. Because of the length of time the problem has been present, a slower and more ambivalent response may occur. However, also within this group it should be recognised that alternative approaches may be appropriate.

Within the group with chronic pain are also found those who demonstrate multiple 'yellow flags', inappropriate pain behaviours, widespread pain and aggravation of symptoms with all activity. Just 1 – 2% of the adult population has chronic, intractable pain with major disability. They have been off work for months or years, and they absorb considerable health care resources (Waddell 1998). Those most severely disabled by pain are likely to exhibit some or all of the features listed (Table 13.11); those who are moderately distressed may only show one or two features.

Table 13.11 Possible characteristics of patients with chronic intractable pain

- persistent pain
- interruption of work, social and other activities of daily living
- depressed
- distressed
- unhelpful beliefs
- multiple health care interventions
- multiple treatment failures
- anger.

Source: Waddell 1998

Symptoms may become complicated and persist due to non-mechanical problems. These are considered in more detail in Chapter 3, but in brief these consist of psychosocial or neurophysiological factors that act as barriers to resolution and obscure a mechanical problem. Psychosocial and cognitive factors are closely related to the development of chronic back disability. Depression, anxiety, passive coping and attitudes about pain are associated with chronic pain and disability. Catastrophising, hyper-vigilance about symptoms and fear–avoidance behaviour are some of the attitudes and beliefs that have been highlighted as being significant in this context (Linton 2000).

The timescale when these factors may become active modulators of patients' pain experience may be in the first few weeks (Philips and Grant 1991; Burton *et al.* 1995; Fritz *et al.* 2001). This further discounts the significance of pain duration for categorisation. It is also highlights the prominence of psychosocial factors at an early time in the natural history of back pain. It suggests that at no time, whether the patient is in the acute or chronic stage, can we afford to ignore these potential modulators of the pain experience.

Furthermore, persistent peripheral nociceptive input can induce changes in the central nervous system (Woolf 1991; Melzack and Wall 1988). This may lead to the sensitisation of neurones in the dorsal horn – a state characterised by reduced thresholds and increased responses to afferent input, such that normal mechanical stimuli is interpreted as pain. In this situation pain, aching and tenderness are likely to be widespread, and most normal activity is perceived as painful.

Thus a chronic pain state is not simply related to the time that symptoms have been present. These are patients in whom a mechanical response to loading strategies is obscured by non-mechanical factors, which may be psychosocial or neurophysiological in origin. Symptoms are likely to have been present for a prolonged period, but this may not always be so. Interruption of their normal lifestyle has usually occurred. Multiple or widespread pain sites are common. All activity increases symptoms, at least initially. There is no obvious directional preference, nor clear mechanical response; again, at least not initially. Often these patients display exaggerated pain behaviours and vocalisation. They nearly always hold mistaken beliefs and attitudes about pain and movement, and in particular are fearful of movement. Depression, anxiety and distress are all commonly found. They may display multiple Waddell's non-organic signs and symptoms, but other features may be more revealing.

Table 13.12 Key factors in identification of chronic pain patients

- no lasting change in pain location or pain intensity in response to therapeutic loading strategies
- persistent widespread symptoms
- all activity increases symptoms
- exaggerated pain behaviour
- mistaken beliefs and attitudes about pain and movement.

Waddell's non-organic signs and symptoms

For a further review of this topic, see Scalzitti (1997). Waddell *et al.* (1980) developed a collection of eight signs that are said to be indicative of non-organic pathology. Individual signs are not considered significant, and a cut-off point of three or more is recommended. In the original study, three positive signs were found in 33% and 50% of chronic problem backs, 12% of acute backs and 0% of normal subjects.

Table 13.13 Inappropriate signs

- superficial tenderness
- non-anatomical tenderness
- back pain on axial loading
- back pain on simulated rotation
- distraction test, such as straight leg raise
- regional, non-dermatomal weakness
- regional, non-dermatomal sensory disturbance
- over-reaction to examination / overt pain behaviour.

Waddell *et al.* (1984) have also described a series of seven inappropriate symptoms, in which patients offer descriptions that do not fit with normal clinical experience, again with the inference that they are related to psychological rather than physical features. Isolated symptoms are not relevant, and as some can occur in serious spinal pathology, they are only appropriate to non-specific back pain in which specific pathology has been excluded. Such symptoms were reported by an average of 36% of problem patients, 18% of referrals from primary care and 7% of normal subjects.

Table 13.14 Inappropriate symptoms

- tailbone pain
- whole leg pain
- whole leg numbness
- whole leg giving way
- no pain-free spells
- intolerance of treatments
- self-admission to hospital emergency department with back pain.

The aim of these behavioural signs and symptoms is to try to distinguish between physical and non-organic complaints, to assist in the identification of patients in whom there was a behavioural component to disability, and to prevent the administration of inappropriate treatment. Their presence does not indicate faking or simulated incapacity; rather, the authors see them as a form of communication between the patient and the clinician indicating distress and the need for more detailed psychological assessment (Main and Waddell 1998).

In the original study, agreement over the detection of non-organic signs was high (86%) between two examiners (Waddell *et al.* 1980). In a later report, Kappa values were given for inappropriate symptoms and signs of between 0.55 and 0.71 (Waddell *et al.* 1982). McCombe *et al.* (1989) found poor reliability in detecting individual signs, with a mean Kappa score of 0.15. This finding should further warn against the importance of individual non-organic signs.

Furthermore, as indicators of distress the signs may not be stable over time, but reflect the patient's attitude towards their back problem and their treatment. Clinically it has been found that whereas on initial assessment signs may be positive, several days later they no longer are. This may be a display of patient's initial distress, which is reduced a few days later when they have gained confidence in the clinician and the way that they are being managed. Werneke *et al.* (1993) found the presence of the signs reflected the success or failure of a rehabilitation programme to return patients to work. There was a significant reduction in their presence in those who returned to work, but no change in those who did not.

There is conflicting evidence about the clinical utility of non-organic signs to predict outcomes. Studies have found them useful in predicting poorer results in lumbar spinal surgery (Dzioba and Doxey

1984; Waddell *et al.* 1986) and correlated signs with poorer treatment outcomes in conservative management (Lehmann *et al.* 1983; Karas *et al.* 1997). In acute back pain patients, the presence of signs has been associated with poorer return to work, more treatment and the use of more imaging technology (Gaines and Hegmann 1999). Other studies have found no correlation between signs and return to work, health care use and later outcomes in acute and chronic patients (Fritz *et al.* 2000b; Polatin *et al.* 1997; Bradish *et al.* 1988; Werneke *et al.* 1993).

These signs and symptoms clearly need to be used with a certain amount of caution, and used in the context of the whole clinical picture, but may be useful on occasions when mechanical response is unclear. Other 'yellow flag' indicators are likely to be present; for instance, the patient displaying exaggerated pain behaviour and mistaken beliefs and attitudes about pain, activity and/or work. To be of significance, at least three signs should be present when tested, with the presence of multiple signs and symptoms being more compelling evidence of inappropriate behaviour. This does not indicate that the patient is malingering or in some way 'faking it'; rather, they have an inappropriate behavioural response to back pain, as well as possibly as a physical problem, and may need further psychological assessment. Such signs may vanish if the patient's anxieties and distress is moderated and their back pain is managed in a way that is satisfactory to them. However, attempting to treat their physical problem may not be successful if the behavioural problem is not also addressed. A multi-disciplinary pain management or cognitive behavioural functional rehabilitation programme may be more appropriate in some patients.

Management of chronic pain patients

So-called 'yellow flags' are not, however, a diagnostic category, but rather they are a confounding factor that may be a barrier to recovery. If these psychosocial concerns can be dealt with, then treatment may proceed straightforwardly. If they are not addressed, then these factors often prevent successful management.

This may be a difficult group to treat, but it is apparent that the emphasis should be on improved function, coping and self-management rather than resolution of pain. Foremost in the clinician's mind when assessing the patient should be the importance of focusing on functional changes rather than highlighting the effects of repeated movements on pain. The confounding effect that non-mechanical factors can have on the efficacy of purely mechanical interventions should be recognised.

For chronic musculoskeletal problems, it is recommended that a cognitive-behavioural framework be used for interaction with the patient (Turner 1996). This requires:

- awareness of and enquiries into psychological 'yellow flags' that suggest inappropriate pain behaviours and beliefs about pain and can be risk factors for the development of persistent pain

- appropriate information provision – the importance of the self-management principle for ongoing health problems, activity for musculoskeletal conditions and reassurance that pain on movement does not mean an exacerbation of the problem

- encouragement of a graduated, systematic resumption of activities.

Gifford (1998b) offers a useful approach to this small, but difficult patient group. *"On-going pain states are best explained to patients in terms of an altered sensitivity state as a result of altered information processing throughout the system, and not solely a result of damaged and degenerating tissues. This helps patients accept the notion that hurt does not necessarily equate with harm – which leads on to the positive message that carefully graded increases in physical activity mean stronger and healthier tissues. By contrast, continued focus on a tissue as the pain source reinforces fear of movement and activity, the need to be constantly vigilant for pain and the desire for increasingly expensive passive therapeutic interventions that are yet to demonstrate convincing efficacy"* (p. 33).

Failure to improve after a time-limited period of individual therapy should lead to recommendation for a chronic pain management, general exercise, functional restoration programme or behavioural therapy approach (Flor *et al.* 1992; Cutler *et al.* 1994; van Tulder *et al.* 1997b, Bendix *et al.* 1998; van Tulder *et al.* 2000c). Within the framework of the biopsychosocial model of pain is the proposal for active, behavioural therapy and exercise-based management (Wheeler and Hanley 1995; Rose *et al.* 1997; Frost *et al.* 1995, 1998).

Common features of successful programmes for chronic back problems have been identified (Linton 1998):

- use a multidimensional view of the problem, including psychosocial aspects

- conduct a thorough 'low-tech' examination

- communicate the findings of examination to the patient and an explanation of why it hurts and how to best manage it

- emphasise self-care, and explain that the way the patient behaves is integral to the recovery process

- reduce any unfounded fears or anxiety about the pain and movement ('hurt does not mean harm')

- make clear recommendations about starting normal activities and a graded approach to exercises

- do not medicalise the problem: avoid 'high-tech' investigations, long-term sick leave and advising the patient to 'take it easy'.

Treating chronic backs – the McKenzie Institute International Rehabilitation Programme

In New Zealand, the Accident Rehabilitation and Compensation Insurance Corporation (ACC) evaluated the effectiveness of four treatment programmes for chronic compensated back pain patients (Borrows and Herbison 1995b). All programmes used different exercise and rehabilitation regimes, one of which was a McKenzie regime. Nearly 800 patients, with an average of twenty months on compensation, were allocated, not randomised, to the different programmes.

The outcomes from the McKenzie programme are summarised in Chapter 11. In summary, the results show that not all functional rehabilitation programmes are the same. While two programmes produced significant improvements in a range of outcomes, the other two programmes hardly had any impact at all. 'Fitness to work' was the primary goal; this improved by 35% in the McKenzie programme, 20% in the next best intervention and by less than 4% in the other two. Functional disability and depression also improved markedly in the two best programmes, but minimally in the least effective two (Borrows and Herbison 1995b).

The timescale for providing these outcomes was very different. The average duration of the three other programmes was from 103 to 127 days, with all exceeding their initial estimated duration by nearly

50%. In comparison, although the McKenzie programme was residential, it had a finite duration of only fourteen days. The cost implications of this are not calculated in the original report, but could be considerable.

The authors of the report comment on the characteristics of the successful programmes (Borrows and Herbison 1995b):

- passing the responsibility for improvement to the patient

- ignoring or downplaying the significance of pain

- individual biomechanical assessment

- individual exercise programme

- pleasurable recreational activities.

The background of the ACC

In the 1980s the ACC was the sole provider of insurance cover for injuries arising from an accident at work, irrespective of fault. Part of their responsibility was to provide treatment and physical rehabilitation to restore 'injured' workers to 'workability'. Ultimately the scheme was discontinued as financially insolvent, as it was unable to cope with the escalating costs of providing compensation and rehabilitation. In an attempt to reduce costs, the organisation cut funding for rehabilitation and simply paid long-term earnings-related compensation. The situation arose in 1990 that almost 14,000 individuals with work-related 'injuries' were receiving earnings-related compensation. They had been off work for up to two years and no attempt was being made to rehabilitate them back to work.

In order to try to reinvigorate the rehabilitation process that had been put in abeyance, the McKenzie Institute International approached the government agency responsible for the ACC, who eventually were instructed to fund the trial mentioned above.

All participants had been on earnings-related compensation for at least three months and were willing to participate. The McKenzie programme excluded patients in whom specific pathology was diagnosed, scored high on psychometric questionnaires, if they refused to be compliant with the programme or if no movement reduced, abolished or centralised symptoms. Of those included some responded to extension, a few to flexion and some just responded to movement and reactivation in general. After two days' testing, 219 patients were accepted onto the programme from 252 referred by the ACC (87%). On the other programmes acceptance levels were 70%, 74% and 89%.

Patients were assessed independently by an ACC representative. This was done according to a standardised protocol, and a battery of functional and psychometric tests were applied that allowed independent verification of the outcome data. This was done prior to a full history-taking and mechanical evaluation, as well as further questionnaires, by programme personnel. Following this, patients were classified according to their mechanical syndrome.

The details of the McKenzie ACC programme

Many patients with a directional preference for extension were then assigned to repeated sessions on the REPEX machine. The Repeated End Range Passive Exercise (REPEX) machine causes repeated movements to end-range that are done while the patient lies on the equipment. These sessions were repeated for a maximum of ten minutes each hour on the first day, but according to the patient's tolerance. The machine allowed them to experience the sensation of movement without exertion, which was generally well tolerated. Following a session on the REPEX, the patient repeated extension in lying actively. REPEX was employed for up to the first seven days. The machine was important in extension responders, as most had very little range of movement and REPEX sped up the process of regaining this movement. It helped those who could not tolerate active extension exercises every hour to participate in regular movement. Many patients with gross losses of movement improved range dramatically, demonstrating what appeared to be the reduction of very stubborn lumbar derangements.

If patients demonstrated a preference for extension, as well as the hourly sessions on the REPEX, they were also given lumbar rolls, education on posture and introduced to the gym. There they undertook upper and lower body strengthening exercises and back extension exercises. They were also encouraged to take a short walk on an hourly basis.

Patients with a preference for flexion performed flexion in lying and in the gym performed exercises that promoted flexion. REPEX was generally unnecessary in this group as they were achieving end-range flexion effectively in their exercise programme.

If patients had no clear directional preference, they were assigned to the flexion group as a provocative regime. Unless patients developed a clear derangement, they were kept on unidirectional exercises for the first few days, with frequency and load gradually increased. Some patients responded positively to general mobilisation and reactivation.

In this deconditioned population, active participation, especially in the case of extension in lying, sometimes led to significant fatigue in the shoulders and arms. If this occurred, patients were advised to perform active sessions a little less frequently. To allow recovery from what for many was an excessive amount of exertion, they had twice daily sessions in the swimming pool. There the patients repeated their assigned exercises in a weight-relieving aquatic environment and also participated in water polo games, hydro-aerobics and unstructured fun activity. About an hour was allocated for lunch. The afternoon session repeated what had occurred in the morning, and the last two hours of each day were spent in 'play hardening' as opposed to 'work hardening' activity. This consisted of tennis, volleyball, table tennis, net ball, ten-pin bowling, horse riding, snooker, golf, jogging or brisk walking.

Day two largely repeated the format of the first day with REPEX, active exercise, gym, pool sessions and sporting participation. The number of sessions remained the same, but the passive and active repetitions were increased and the amount of participation in pool and sporting activity was increased where indicated.

By the second or third day, use of the REPEX was discontinued in many cases and active participation in gym activities was substituted. If it brought definite benefit, REPEX was used for longer periods. In the gym over the whole programme, the time spent on equipment, the number of equipment units utilised and the loading was progressively increased. Likewise, levels of self-applied end-range motion were progressed, with most attaining end-range by the fourth or fifth day. By day four or five the opposite movement was introduced – so, for instance, if a patient had been put on an extension regime, flexion and rotation exercises were started.

The remainder of the programme consisted of the same activities. Gym work on equipment and aerobics, active end-range movements, educational sessions, activities in the pool and 'play hardening'. Patients were individually assessed on a daily basis and their regime progressed accordingly. Group work could be somewhat challenging, depending on how the negative or positive attitude of the dominant personality affected group dynamics. The frequency of the pleasurable recreational activities was increased as it became apparent that patients would often forget their anxiety and fear about movement and their disability as they threw themselves vigorously into the spirit of the game. Games such as tennis and volleyball, which involved considerable flexion to retrieve the ball, were especially good at producing a return to normal function and overcoming individuals' fear of movement.

Patients' response to the programme varied. Some, with considerable disability or fearful behaviour, required more individualised education and instruction. In some their fear of activity was considerably worse than the effect of the activity itself. Once they had experienced that movement and activity could be tolerated, and especially when their enthusiasm for the recreational activities was stimulated, these fears were overcome.

Day four of the programme was often difficult, as the majority experienced an increased level of pain at about this point. Encouragement to persevere and focus on improving function, rather than pain, was especially important at this phase. A patient's belief systems were often a major part of the problem and had to be fully explored and dealt with. Mistaken beliefs and attitudes about pain and activity were often the result of iatrogenic advice. Patients had been told, for instance, 'don't move if it hurts', 'rest or you will do damage', or 'if you are in pain, take medication'. The programme appeared to alter the moods and attitudes of the patients. As they increased their activity, this was reflected in increased confidence and reduced disability and impairment. At the same time their depression and anxiety noticeably lessened.

While most of those who reported high rates of disability were consistent in their reporting and in their activities, a small number appeared to deliberately exaggerate their disability. These patients demonstrated multiple Waddell's non-organic signs and symptoms. They displayed exaggerated vocalisation and body language on testing and movement, but were able to play tennis, volleyball, snooker and other games with ease.

Those patients who reported no improvement on completion of the programme, those with the most intractable disability or psychological distress, may have received benefit from a multi-disciplinary pain management programme.

Conclusions

This chapter considers other categories of back pain besides the mechanical syndromes. If after a detailed and thorough mechanical evaluation conducted over a few sessions there has been a failure to classify the patient into one of the mechanical syndromes, only then should other diagnoses be considered. This occurs in only a minority of patients. Among those with specific pathology the group that is most important to recognise are those with serious spinal lesions. Recognition of these pathologies is gained largely from the history and is detailed in the previous chapter.

Appendix

Classification and operational definitions

Category *Mechanical syndrome*	Definition	Criteria** *Symptom response*
Reducible derangement	Internal disc displacement with competent annulus	Centralisation Abolition Decrease
Irreducible derangement	Disc displacement with incompetent or ruptured annular wall	Peripheralisation Increase in peripheral pain No centralisation, reduction or abolition
Dysfunction	Soft tissue structural impairment	Intermittent pain when loading restricted end-range
Adherent nerve root	Adhesions producing functional impairment of nerve root or dura	Intermittent pain at limited end-range flexion in standing and long sitting
Postural syndrome	Prolonged mechanical deformation of normal soft tissues	Pain only with prolonged loading Physical examination normal
OTHER	*Exclusion of above*	*Lack of above responses, plus the following*
Spinal stenosis	Bony or soft tissue narrowing of spinal or foraminal canal causing neurogenic claudication May be associated *with* degenerative spondylolisthesis	History – leg symptoms when walking, eased in flexion Minimal extension Sustained extension may provoke leg symptoms
Isthmic spondylolisthesis	Slippage of vertebral body	Sports-related injury in adolescence Worse with static loading
Hip	Pain-generating mechanism due to mechanical, inflammatory or degenerative changes in or around hip joint	History – pain on walking, eased on sitting Specific pain pattern Positive 'hip' tests
SIJ	Pain-generating mechanism due to mechanical, inflammatory or degenerative changes in or around SIJ	Three or more positive SIJ pain provocation tests
Mechanically inconclusive	Unknown intervertebral joint pathology	Inconsistent response to loading strategies No obstruction to movement

Continued next page

Category *Mechanical syndrome*	Definition	Criteria** *Symptom response*
Chronic pain	Pain-generating mechanism influenced by psychosocial factors or neurophysiological changes peripherally or centrally	Persistent widespread pain Aggravation with all activity Exaggerated pain behaviour Inappropriate beliefs and attitudes about pain

Serious spinal pathology – suspected	Definition	Criteria
Cauda equina	Compression of sacral nerves by disc herniation or tumour	Bladder / bowel involvement Especially urinary retention Saddle anaesthesia Sciatica
Cancer	Growth of malignant tumour in or near vertebrae	Age > 55 History of cancer Unexplained weight loss Constant, progressive pain unrelated to loading strategy, not relieved by rest
Fracture	Bony damage to vertebrae caused by trauma or weakness due to metabolic bone disease	Significant trauma Trivial trauma in individual with osteopenia
Spinal infection	Infection affecting vertebrae or disc	Systemically unwell Febrile episode Constant severe back pain unrelated to loading strategy
Ankylosing spondylitis	One of the systemic inflammatory arthropathies affecting spinal and other structures	Exacerbations and remissions Marked morning stiffness Persisting limitation all movements No directional preference, but better with exercise, not relieved by rest Systemic involvement Raised ESR, + HLA B27

** The operational definitions provided below present the criteria in more detail. These give the symptom responses and timescale by which classification should be recognised.

Classification algorithm

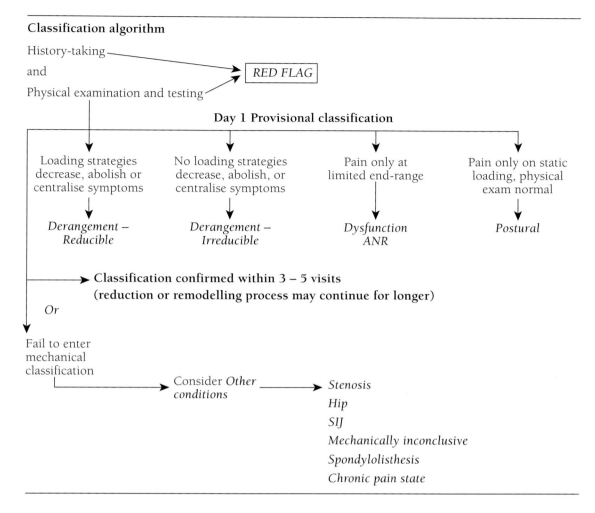

Operational definitions

The operational definitions describe the symptom and mechanical behaviours and the timescale needed to document each category.

Reducible Derangement

Centralisation: in response to therapeutic loading strategies, pain is progressively abolished in a distal to proximal direction, *and*

- each progressive abolition is retained over time until all symptoms are abolished, *and*
- if back pain only is present this moves from a widespread to a more central location and then is abolished *or*
- pain is decreased and then abolished during the application of therapeutic loading strategies
- the change in pain location, or decrease or abolition of pain, remain better, *and*

- should be accompanied or preceded by improvements in the mechanical presentation (range of movement and/or deformity).

Timescale

A derangement responder can be identified on day one, *or*

- a derangement responder will be suspected on day one and a provisional diagnosis made. This will be confirmed by a lasting change in symptoms after evaluating the response to a full mechanical evaluation within five visits

- decrease, abolition or centralisation of symptoms is occurring but the episode may not have completely resolved within five visits

- aggravating factors may precipitate a deterioration in symptoms and a longer recovery process.

Irreducible Derangement

Peripheralisation of symptoms: increase or worsening of distal symptoms in response to therapeutic loading strategies, *and/or*

- no decrease, abolition, or centralisation of pain.

Timescale

An irreducible derangement patient will be suspected on day one and a provisional diagnosis made; this will be confirmed after evaluating the response to a full mechanical evaluation within five visits.

Dysfunction

Spinal pain only, *and*

- intermittent pain, *and*

- at least one movement is restricted, and the restricted movement consistently produces concordant pain at end-range, *and*

- there is no rapid reduction or abolition of symptoms, *and*

- no lasting production and no peripheralisation of symptoms.

ANR

History of sciatica or surgery in the last few months that has improved, but is now unchanging, *and*

- symptoms are intermittent, *and*

- symptoms in the thigh and/or calf, including 'tightness', *and*

- flexion in standing, long sitting, and straight leg raise are clearly restricted and consistently produce concordant pain or tightness at end-range, *and*

- there is no rapid reduction or abolition of symptoms and no lasting production of distal symptoms.

Timescale
- a dysfunction/ANR category patient will be suspected on day one and a provisional diagnosis made; this will be confirmed after evaluating the response to a mechanical evaluation within five visits
- if the patient fails to fit all criteria another category must be considered
- rapid change will not occur in this syndrome, and symptoms will gradually reduce over many weeks, as range of movement gradually improves.

Postural

Spinal pain only, *and*
- concordant pain only with static loading, *and*
- abolition of pain with postural correction, *and*
- no pain with repeated movements, *and*
- no loss of range of movement, *and*
- no pain during movement.

Timescale
- a posture category patient will be suspected on day one and a provisional diagnosis made. This will be confirmed after evaluating the response to a mechanical evaluation within two to three visits
- if the patient fails to fit all criteria, another category must be considered.

'Other' categories are only considered on failure to enter a mechanical diagnosis within five treatment sessions. To be designated into 'Other' category, patients will fulfil:
- 'other' criteria, *and*
- criteria for specific other category as listed below.

'Other'

- no centralisation, peripheralisation, or abolition of symptoms, *or*
- does not fit derangement, dysfunction or posture criteria
- no lasting change in pain location or pain intensity in response to therapeutic loading strategies, *and*
- fulfils relevant criteria in suspected 'other' pathology listed below.

Indicators for possible 'Red Flags'

Cauda equina
- bladder dysfunction (urinary retention or overflow incontinence)
- loss of anal sphincter tone or faecal incontinence
- saddle anaesthesia about the anus, perineum or genitals
- global or progressive motor weakness in the lower limbs.

Possible cancer
- age greater than 55
- history of cancer
- unexplained weight loss
- constant, progressive pain not affected by loading strategies, worse at rest.

Other possible serious spinal pathology
One of the following:
- systemically unwell
- widespread neurology
- history of significant trauma enough to cause fracture or dislocation (x-rays will not always detect fractures)
- history of trivial trauma and severe pain in potential osteoporotic individual
- sudden and persistent extremes of pain causing patient to 'freeze'.

Possible inflammatory disorders
- gradual onset, *and*
- marked morning stiffness, *and*
- persisting limitation of movements in all directions
- peripheral joint involvement
- iritis, psoriasis, colitis, uretheral discharge
- family history.

Stenosis
- history of leg symptoms when walking upright
- may be eased when sitting or leaning forward
- loss of extension
- possible provocation of symptoms in sustained extension, with relief on flexion
- age greater than 50
- possible nerve root signs and symptoms
- extensive degenerative changes on x-ray
- diagnosis confirmed by CT or MRI.

Hip

- exclusion of lumbar spine by mechanical evaluation, *and*
- pain worsened by weight bearing, eased by rest or worse first few steps after rest, *and*
- pain pattern – groin, anterior thigh, knee, anterior shin, lateral thigh, possibly buttock, *and*
- positive hip pain provocation test(s) – (concordant pain).

Symptomatic SIJ

- exclusion of lumbar spine by extended mechanical evaluation, *and*
- exclusion of hip joint by mechanical testing, *and*
- positive pain provocation tests (concordant pain) – at least three tests.

Mechanically inconclusive

- symptoms affected by spinal movements
- no loading strategy consistently decreases, abolishes or centralises symptoms, nor increases or peripheralises symptoms
- inconsistent response to loading strategies.

Symptomatic spondylolisthesis

- suspect in young athletic person with back pain related to vigorous sporting activity
- worse with static loading.

Chronic pain state

- persistent widespread symptoms
- all activity increases symptoms
- exaggerated pain behaviour
- mistaken beliefs and attitudes about pain and movement.

Other definitions

Definition of centralisation

- in response to therapeutic loading strategies pain is progressively abolished in a distal to proximal direction with each progressive abolition being retained over time until all symptoms are abolished
- if back pain only is present, this is reduced and then abolished.

Criteria for a relevant lateral shift
- upper body is visibly and unmistakably shifted to one side
- onset of shift occurred with back pain
- patient is unable to correct shift voluntarily
- if patient is able to correct shift, they cannot maintain correction
- correction affects intensity of symptoms
- correction causes centralisation or worsening of peripheral symptoms.

Right and left lateral shift
- a right lateral shift exists when the vertebra above has laterally flexed to the right in relation to the vertebra below, carrying the trunk with it; the upper trunk and shoulders are displaced to the right
- a left lateral shift exists when the vertebra above has laterally flexed to the left in relation to the vertebra below, carrying the trunk with it; the upper trunk and shoulders are displaced to the left.

Contralateral and ipsilateral shift
- contralateral shift exists when the patient's symptoms are on one side and the shift is in the opposite direction; for instance, right back pain, with / without thigh / leg pain, and upper trunk and shoulders displaced to the left
- ipsilateral shift exists when the patient's symptoms are on one side and the shift is to the same side; for instance right back pain, with / without thigh / leg pain, with upper trunk and shoulders displaced to the right.

Criteria for a relevant lateral component
- acute lateral shift deformity OR loss of frontal plane movements *and / or*
- unilateral / asymmetrical symptoms affected by frontal plane movements
- symptoms fail to improve with sagittal plane forces *or*
- symptoms worsen with sagittal plane forces *and*
- symptoms improve with frontal plane forces.

References

Abdullah AF, Wolber PGH, Warfield JR, Gunadi IK (1988). Surgical management of extreme lateral lumbar disc herniations: review of 138 cases. Neurosurgery 22.648-653.

Abenhaim L, Rossignol M, Gobeille D, Bonvalot Y, Fines P, Scott S (1995). The prognostic consequences in the making of the initial medical diagnosis of work-related back injuries. Spine 20.791-795.

Adams MA, Hutton WC, Stott JRR (1980). The resistance to flexion of the lumbar intervertebral joint. Spine 5.245-253.

Adams MA, Hutton WC (1982). Prolapsed intervertebral disc. A hyperflexion injury. Spine 7.184-191.

Adams MA, Hutton WC (1983). The effect of fatigue on the lumbar intervertebral disc. JBJS 65B.199-203.

Adams MA, Hutton WC (1985a). Gradual disc prolapse. Spine 10.524-531.

Adams MA, Hutton WC (1985b). The effect of posture on the lumbar spine. JBJS 67B.625-629.

Adams MA, Dolan P, Hutton WC (1986). The stages of disc degeneration as revealed by discograms. JBJS 68B.36-41.

Adams MA, Dolan P, Hutton WC (1987). Diurnal variations in the stresses on the lumbar spine. Spine 12.130-137.

Adams MA, Dolan P, Hutton WC, Porter RW (1990). Diurnal changes in spinal mechanics and their clinical significance. JBJS 72B.266-270.

Adams MA (1994). Biomechanics of the lumbar motion segment. In: *Grieve's Modern Manual Therapy*. (2nd Ed). Eds. Boyling JD, Palastanga N. Churchill Livingstone, Edinburgh.

Adams MA, McNally DS, Chinn H, Dolan P (1994). Posture and the compressive strength of the lumbar spine. Clinical Biomechanics 9.5-14.

Adams MA, Dolan P (1995). Recent advances in lumbar spinal mechanics and their clinical significance. Clinical Biomechanics 10.3-19.

Adams MA, McNally DS, Dolan P (1996a). 'Stress' distribution inside intervertebral discs. JBJS 78B.965-972.

Adams MA, McMillan DW, Green TP, Dolan P (1996b). Sustained loading generates stress concentrations in lumbar intervertebral discs. Spine 21.434-438.

Adams MA, Dolan P (1997). Could sudden increases in physical activity cause degeneration of intervertebral discs? Lancet 350.734-735.

Adams MA, Mannion AF, Dolan P (1999). Personal risk factors for first-time low back pain. Spine 24.2497-2505.

Adams MA, May S, Freeman BJC, Morrison HP, Dolan P (2000a). Effects of backward bending on lumbar intervertebral discs. Spine 25.431-437.

Adams MA, Freeman BJC, Morrison HP, Nelson IW, Dolan P (2000b). Mechanical initiation of intervertebral disc degeneration. Spine 25.1625-1636.

Adams N (1993). Psychophysiological and neurochemical substrates of chronic low back pain and modulation by treatment. Physiotherapy abstracts 79.86.

Adams NBK, Ravey J, Bell AJ (1995). Psychological aspects of physical treatment intervention for chronic low back pain. *Proceedings 12th International Congress of World Confederation for Physical Therapy*. June 25-30, 1995, Washington DC, USA. Abstract 1093.

Adams N (1997). *The Psychophysiology of Low Back Pain*. Churchill Livingstone, New York.

AHCPR (1994). *Agency for Health Care Policy and Research – Acute Low Back Problems in Adults*. Eds. Bigos S, Bowyer O, Braen *et al*. Department of Health and Human Services, USA.

Ahlgren BD, Vasavada A, Brower RS, Lydon C, Herkowitz HN, Panjabi MM (1994). Anular incision technique on the strength and multi directional flexibility of the healing intervertebral disc. Spine 19.948-954.

Ahn SH, Ahn MW, Byun WM (2000b). Effect of the transligamentous extension of lumbar disc herniations on their regression and the clinical outcome of sciatica. Spine 25.475-480.

Ahn UM, Ahn NU, Buchowski JM, Garrett ES, Sieber AN, Kostuik JP (2000a). Cauda equina syndrome secondary to lumbar disc herniation. A meta-analysis of surgical outcomes. Spine 25.1515-1522.

Akeson WH, Amiel D, Abel MF, Garfin SR, Woo SLY (1987). Effects of immobilisation on joints. Clin Orth & Rel Res 219.28-37.

Albert H (1998). Pelvic pain in pregnancy. In: Eds Vleeming A, Mooney V, Tilscher H, Dorman T, Snijders C. *3rd Interdisciplinary World Congress on Low Back and pelvic pain*. November 19-21, 1998, Vienna, Austria.

Alexander AH, Jones AM, Rosenbaum DH (1991). Non-operative management of herniated nucleus pulposus: patient selection by the extension sign. Long-term follow-up. Orthop Trans 15.674.

Alexander H, Jones AM, Rosenbaum DH (1992). Nonoperative management of herniated nucleus pulposus: patient selction by the extension sign. Long-term follow-up. Orthopaedic Review 21.181-188.

Altman DG (1991). *Practical Statistics for Medical Research*. Chapman & Hall, London.

Amato M, Totty WG, Gilula LA (1984). Spondylolysis of the lumbar spine: demonstration of defects and laminal fragmentation. Radiology 153.627-629.

Amundsen T, Weber H, Lilleas F, Nordal HJ, Abdelnoor M, Magnaes B (1995). Lumbar spinal stenosis. Clinical and radiological features. Spine 20.1178-1186.

Amundsen T, Weber H, Nordal HJ, Magnaes B, Abdelnoor M, Lilleas F (2000). Lumbar spinal stenosis: conservative or surgical management? A prospective 10-year study. Spine 25.1424-1436.

Anderson R, Meeker WC, Wirick BE, Mootz RD, Kirk DH, Adams A (1992). A meta-analysis of clinical trials of spinal manipulation. J Manipulative & Physiological Therapeutics 15.181-194.

Andersson GBJ, Ortengren R, Nachemson AL, Elfstrom G, Broman H (1975). The sitting posture: an electromyographic and discometric study. Orth Clinics Nth Am 6.105-120.

Andersson GBJ, Murphy RW, Ortengren R, Nachemson AL (1979). The influence of backrest inclination and lumbar support on lumbar lordosis. Spine 4.52-58.

Andersson GBJ, Svensson HO, Oden A (1983). The intensity of work recovery in low back pain. Spine 8.880-884.

Andersson GBJ (1991). The epidemiology of spinal disorders. In: *The Adult Spine: Principles and Practice*. Ed. Frymoyer JW. Raven Press Ltd, New York.

Andersson GBJ, Deyo RA (1996). History and physical examination with herniated lumbar discs. Spine 21.24S. 10S-18S.

Andersson GBJ, Bostrom MPG, Eyre DR *et al.* (1997). Consensus summary on the diagnosis and treatment of osteoporosis. Spine 22.63S-65S.

Antti-Poika I, Soini J, Tallroth K, Yrjonen T, Konttinen YT (1990). Clinical relevance of discography combined with CT scanning. JBJS 72B.480-485.

Aprill C, Bogduk N (1992). High intensity zone: a diagnostic sign of painful lumbar disc on magnetic resonance imaging. Br J Rad 65.361-369.

Arem AJ, Madden JW (1976). Effects of stress on healing wounds. 1. Intermittent noncyclical tension. J Surg Res 20.93-102.

Arntz A, Dreessen L, Merckelbach H (1991). Attention, not anxiety, influences pain. Behav Res Ther 29.41-50.

Aronson HA, Dunsmore RH (1963). Herniated upper lumbar discs. JBJS 45A.311-317.

Ashton IK, Roberts S, Jaffray DC, Polak JM, Eisenstein SM (1994). Neuropeptides in the human intervertebral disc. J Orthop Res 12.186-192.

Assendelft WJJ, Koes BW, Knipschild PG, Bouter LM (1995). The relationship between methodological quality and conclusions in reviews of spinal manipulation. JAMA 274.1942-1948.

Assendelft WJJ, Koes BW, van der Heijden GJMG, Bouter LM (1996). The effectiveness of chiropractor for treatment of low back pain: an update and attempt at statistical pooling. J Manip Physio Thera 19.499-507.

Atlas SJ, Deyo RA, Patrick DL, Convery K, Keller RB, Singer DE (1996a). The Quebec Task Force Classification for spinal disorders and the severity, treatment, and outcomes of sciatica and lumbar spinal stenosis. Spine 21.2885-2892.

Atlas SJ, Deyo RA, Keller *et al.* (1996b). The Maine lumbar spine study, part ii. 1-year outcomes of surgical and nonsurgical management of sciatica. Spine 21.1777-1786.

Atlas SJ, Deyo RA, Keller *et al.* (1996c). The Maine lumbar spine study, part iii. 1-year outcomes of surgical and nonsurgical management of lumbar spinal stenosis. Spine 21.1787-1795.

Atlas SJ, Keller RB, Robson D, Deyo RA, Singer DE (2000). Surgical and nonsurgical management of lumbar spinal stenosis. 4-year outcomes from the Maine lumbar spine study. Spine 25.556-562.

Awerbuch M (1995). Different concepts of chronic musculoskeletal pain. Ann Rheum Dis 54.331-332.

Badley EM, Rasooly I, Webster GK (1994). Relative importance of musculoskeletal disorders as a cause of chronic health problems, disability, and health care utilisation: Findings from the 1990 Ontario health survey. J Rheumatol 21.505-514.

Bahnof R (2000). Intra-oral burns: rehabilitation of severe restriction of mouth opening. Case report. Physiotherapy 86.263-266.

Balague F, Nordin M, Sheikhzadeh A *et al.* (1999). Recovery of severe sciatica. Spine 24.2516-2524.

Balderston RA, Bradford DS (1985). Technique for achievement and maintenance of reduction for severe spondylolisthesis using spinous process traction wiring and external fixation of the pelvis. Spine 10.376-382.

Bandy WD, Irion JM (1994). The effect of time on static stretch on the flexibility of the hamstring muscles. Physical Therapy 74.845-852.

Bandy WD, Irion JM, Briggler M (1997). The effect of time and frequency of static stretching on flexibility of the hamstring muscles. Physical Therapy 77.1090-1096.

Bandy WD, Irion JM, Briggler M (1998). The effect of staic stretch and dynamic range of motion training on the flexibility of the hamstring muscles. JOSPT 27.295-300.

Bannerman N, Pentecost E, Rutter S, Willoughby S, Vujnovich A (1996). Increase in soleus muscle length: a comparison between two stretching techniques. NZ J Physio December 15-18.

Barlow Y, Willoughby J (1992). Pathophysiology of soft tissue repair. Br Med Bull 48.698-711.

Barnsley L, Lord S, Wallis B, Bogduk N (1993). False-positive rates of cervical zygapophyseal joint blocks. Clin J Pain 9.124-130.

Bartley R (2000). Nerve root compression and cauda equina syndrome. In: Eds: Bartley R, Coffey P. *Management of Low Back Pain in Primary Care*. Butterworth Heinemann, Oxford.

Battie MC, Cherkin DC, Dunn R, Ciol MA, Wheeler KJ (1994). Managing low back pain: Attitudes and treatment preferences of physical therapists. Physical Therapy 74.219-226.

Beattie P, Rothstein JM, Lamb RL (1987). Reliability of the attraction method for measuring lumbar spine backward bending. Physical Therapy 67.364-369.

Beattie PF, Brooks WM, Rothstein JM *et al.* (1994). Effect of lordosis on the position of the nucleus pulposus in supine subjects. A study using MRI. Spine 19.2096-2102.

Beattie P, Maher C (1997). The role of functional status questionnaires for low back pain. Physical Therapy 43.29-38.

Beattie PF, Meyers SP, Stratford P, Millard RW, Hollenberg GM (2000). Associations between patient report of symptoms and the anatomic impairment visible on lumbar magnetic resonance imaging. Spine 25.819-828.

Begg AC, Falconer MA, McGeorge M (1946). Myelography in lumbar intervertebral disk lesions. A correlation with operative findings. Br J Surg 34.141-157.

Belanger AY, Despres MC, Goulet H, Trottier F (1991). The McKenzie approach: how many clinical trials support its effectiveness? WCPT 11th International Congress Conference Proceedings 1334-1336.

Bellah RD, Summerville DA, Treves ST, Micheli LJ (1991). Low-back pain in adolescent athletes: detection of stress injury to the pars interarticularis with SPECT. Radiology 180.509-512.

BenDebba M, Torgerson WS, Long DM (2000). A validated, practical classification procedure for many persistent low back pain patients. Pain 87.89-97.

Bendix AF, Bendix T, Labriola M, Boekgaard P (1998). Functional restoration for chronic low back pain. Spine 23.717-725.

Bennell K, Khan K, McKay H (2000). The role of physiotherapy in the prevention and treatment of osteoporosis. Manual Therapy 5.198-213.

Bennett N, Jarvis L, Rowlands O, Singleton N, Haselden L (1995). *Results from the 1994 General Household Survey. OPCS.* HMSO, London.

Ben-Sira Z (1982). Lay evaluation of medical treatment and competence development of a model of the function of the physician's affective behavior. Soc Sci Med 16.1013-1019.

Benz RJ, Garfin SR (2000). Surgical treatment of spinal disorders. In: Eds: Mayer TG, Gatchel RJ, Polatin PB. *Occupational Musculoskeletal Disorders. Function, Outcomes & Evidence*. Lippincott Williams & Wilkins, Philadelphia.

Berg G, Hammar M, Moller-Nielsen J, Linden U, Thorblad J (1988). Low back pain during pregnancy. Obstet & Gynaecol 71.71-75.

Berkow R, Fletcher AJ, Bondy PK *et al.* (1987). *The Merck Manual of Diagnosis and Therapy (15th Ed)*. Merck & Co Inc, New Jersey.

Bernard TN (1990). Lumbar discography followed by computed tomography. Refining the diagnosis of low-back pain. Spine 15.690-707.

Bernard TN (1997). The role of the sacroiliac joints in low back pain: basic aspects, pathophysiology, and management. In: Eds Vleeming A, Mooney V, Dorman T, Snijders C, Stoeckart R. *Movement, Stability & Low Back Pain. The Essential Role of the Pelvis*. Churchill Livingstone, New York.

Bernat JL, Greenberg ER, Barrett J (1983). Suspected epidural compression of the spinal cord and cauda equina by metastatic carcinoma. Clinical diagnosis and survival. Cancer 51.1953-1957.

Bessette L, Liang MH, Lew RA, Weinstein JN (1996). Classics in *Spine*. Surgery literature revisited. Spine 21.259-263.

Beurskens AJ, de Vet HC, Koke AJ *et al.* (1995). Efficacy of traction for non-specific low back pain: a randomised clinical trial. Lancet 346.1596-1600.

Beurskens AJ, de Vet HC, Koke AJ *et al.* (1997). Efficacy of traction for nonspecific low back pain. 12-week and 6-month results of a randomized clinical trial. Spine 22.2756-2762.

Biering-Sorensen F (1983a). A prospective study of low back pain in a general population. 1. Occurrence, recurrence and aetiology. Scand J Rehab Med 15.71-79.

Biering-Sorensen F (1983b). A prospective study of low back pain in a general population. 2. Location, character, aggravating and relieving factors. Scand J Rehab Med 15.81-88.

Bigos SJ, Battie MC, Spengler DM *et al.* (1991). A prospective study of work perceptions and psychosocial factors affecting the report of back injury. Spine 16.1-6.

Billis EV, Foster NE, Wright CC (1999). Inter-tester and intra-tester reliability of three groups of physiotherapists in locating spinal levels by palpation. (Abstract) Physiotherapy 85.375.

Binkley J, Stratford PW, Gill C (1995). Interrater reliability of lumbar accessory motion mobility testing. Physical Therapy 75.786-795.

Black KM, McClure P, Polansky M (1996). The influence of different sitting positions on cervical and lumbar posture. Spine 21.65-70.

Bland JH (1993). Mechanisms of adaptation in the joint. In: Eds Crosbie J, McConnell J. *Key Issues in Musculoskeletal Physiotherapy*, 88-113. Butterworth Heinemann, Oxford.

Blikra G (1969). Intradural herniated lumbar disc. J Neurosurg 31.676-679.

Blower PW, Griffin AJ (1984). Clinical sacroiliac tests in ankylosing spondylitis and other causes of low back pain – 2 studies. Ann Rheum Dis 43.192-195.

Boden SD, Davis DO, Dina TS, Patronas NJ, Wiesel SW (1990). Abnormal magnetic-resonance scans of the lumbar spine in asymptomatic subjects. JBJS 72A.403-408.

Bodner RJ, Heyman S, Drummond DS, Gregg JR (1988). The use of single photon emission computer tomography (SPECT) in the diagnosis of low-back pain in young patients. Spine 13.1155-1160.

Bogduk N (1993). The anatomy and physiology of nociception. In: Eds Crosbie J, McConnell J. *Key Issues in Musculoskeletal Physiotherapy*. Butterworth-Heineman, Oxford.

Bogduk N (1994a). Innervation, pain patterns, and mechanism of pain production. In: Eds. Twomey LT, Taylor JR. *Physical Therapy of the Low Back*. Churchill Livingstone, New York.

Bogduk N (1994b). The innervation of the intervertebral discs. In: *Grieve's Modern Manual Therapy*. (2nd Ed). Eds Boyling JD, Palastanga N. Churchill Livingstone, Edinburgh.

Bogduk N, Derby R, Aprill C, Lord S, Schwarzer A (1996). Precision diagnosis of spinal pain. In: *Pain 1996 – An Updated Review*. Ed. Campbell JN. IASP, Seattle.

Bogduk N (1997). *Clinical Anatomy of the Lumbar Spine and Sacrum*. (3rd ed). Churchill Livingstone, New York.

Boissonnault W, Di Fabio RP (1996). Pain profile of patients with low back pain referred to physical therapy. J Orth Sports Physical Ther 24.180-191.

Bombardier C, Kerr MS, Shannon HS, Frank JW (1994). A guide to interpreting epidemiologic studies on the etiology of back pain. Spine 19.2047S-2056S.

Bongers PM, de Winter CR, Kompier MAJ, Hildebrandt VH (1993). Psychosocial factors at work and musculoskeletal disease. Scand J Work Environ Health 19.297-312.

Boos N, Rieder R, Schade V, Spratt KF, Semmer N, Aebi M (1995). The diagnostic accuracy of magnetic resonance imaging, work perception, and psychosocial factors in identifying symptomatic disc herniations. Spine 20.2613-2625.

Borkan J, Reis S, Hermoni D, Biderman A (1995). Talking about the pain: A patient-centred study of low back pain in primary care. Soc Sci Med 40.977-988.

Borrows JA, Herbison P (1995a). A comparative evaluation of four rehabilitation programmes for chronic back pain subjects in receipt of earnings compensation. *Proceedings 12th International Congress of World Confederation for Physical Therapy*. June 25-30, 1995, Washington DC, USA. Abstract 854.

Borrows J, Herbison P (1995b). *ACC Chronic Backs Study. Report of the Evaluation of Four Treatment Programmes*. ACC, New Zealand.

Boxall D, Bradford DS, Winter RB, Moe JH (1979). Management of severe spondylolisthesis in children and adolescents. JBJS 61A.479-495.

Bozzao A, Gallucci M, Masciocchi C, Aprile I, Barile A, Passariello R (1992). Lumbar disk herniation: MR imaging assessment of natural history in patients treated without surgery. Radiology 185.135-141.

Bradish CF, Lloyd GJ, Aldam CH *et al.* (1988). Do nonorganic signs help to predict the return to work of patients with low-back pain? Spine 13.557-560.

Brady TJ (1998). The patient's role in rheumatology care. Current Opinion in Rheum 10.146-151.

Brault JS, Driscoll DM, Laakso LL *et al.* (1997). Quantification of lumbar intradiscal deformation during flexion and extension, by mathematical analysis of MRI pixel intensity profiles. Spine 22.2066-2072.

Braun J, Bollow M, Remlinger G *et al.* (1998). Prevalence of spondylarthopathies in HLA-B27 positive and negative blood donors. Arth & Rheum 41.58-67.

Breig A (1961). *Biomechanics of the Central Nervous System*. Almqvist & Wiksell, Stockholm.

Brightbill TC, Pile N, Eichelberger RP, Whitman M (1994). Normal magnetic resonance imaging and abnormal discography in lumbar disc disruption. Spine 19.1075-1077.

Brinckmann P, Porter RW (1994). A laboratory model of lumbar disc protrusion. Fissure and fragment. Spine 19.228-235.

Brismar H, Vucetic N, Svensson O (1996). Pain patterns in lumbar disc hernia. Drawings compared to surgical findings in 159 patients. Acta Orthop Scand 67.470-472.

Broadhurst NA, Bond MJ (1998). Pain provocation tests for the assessment of sacroiliac joint dysfunction. J Spinal Dis 11.341-345.

Brock M, Patt S, Mayer HM (1992). The form and structure of the extruded disc. Spine 17.1457-1461.

Brodowicz GR, Welsh R, Wallis J (1996). Comparison of stretching with ice, stretching with heat, or stretching alone on hamstring flexibility. J Athletic Training 31.324-327.

Bronfort G (1999). Spinal manipulation. Current state of research and its indications. Neuro Clin Nth Am 17.91-111.

Brooks S, Dent AR, Thompson AG (1983). Anterior rupture of the lumbosacral disc. JBJS 65A.1186-1187.

Brown JB, Stewart M, McCracken E, McWhinney IR, Levenstein J (1986). The patient-centred clinical method.2. Definition and application. Family Practice 3.75-79.

Brown MF, Hukkanen MVJ, McCarthy ID *et al.* (1997). Sensory and sympathetic innervation of the vertebral endplate in patients with degenerative disc disease. JBJS 79B.147-153.

Brown JJ, Wells GA, Trottier AJ, Bonneau J, Ferris B (1998). Back pain in a large Canadian police force. Spine 23.821-827.

Buchner M, Zeifang F, Brocai DRC, Schiltenmolf M (2000). Epidural corticosteroid injection in the conservative management of sciatica. Clin Orth & Rel Res 375.149-156.

Buchwalter JA, Woo SLY, Goldberg VM *et al.* (1993). Soft-tissue aging and musculoskeletal function. JBJS 75A.1533-1548.

Buirski G (1992). Magnetic Resonance signal patterns of lumbar discs in patients with low back pain. Spine 17.1199-1204.

Buirski G, Silberstein M (1993). The symptomatic lumbar disc in patients with low-back pain. Magnetic resonance imaging appearances in both a symptomatic and control population. Spine 18.1808-1811.

Bullock JE, Jull GA, Bullock MI (1987). The relationship of low back pain to postural changes during pregnancy. Aus J Physio 33.10-17.

Burdorf A (1992). Exposure assessment of risk factors for disorders of the back in occupational epidemiology. Scand J Work Environ Health 18.1-9.

Burdorf A, Sorock G (1997). Positive and negative evidence of risk factors for back disorders. Scand J Work Environ Health 23.243-256.

Burgin R, Dromard S, Eaton D, Panter J, Swinkels A (2000). Variations in lumbar posture: risk factors for low back pain in asymptomatic adults. *Proceedings Congress and Exhibition of the Chartered Society of Physiotherpy*. Birmingham, UK, p64.

Burton AK, Tillotson KM, Troup JDG (1989). Prediction of low-back trouble frequency in a working population. Spine14.939-946.

Burton AK, Tillotson KM, Main CJ, Hollis S (1995). Psychosocial predictors of outcome in acute and subchronic low back trouble. Spine 20.722-728.

Burton AK, Clarke RD, McClune TD, Tillotson KM (1996). The natural history of low back pain in adolescents. Spine 21.2323-2328.

Burton AK, Waddell G, Tillotson KM, Summerton N (1999). Information and advice to patients with back pain can have a positive effect. A randomised controlled trial of a novel educational booklet in primary care. Spine 24.2484-2491.

Bush K, Cowan N, Katz DE, Gishen P (1992). The natural history of sciatica associated with disc pathology. A prospective study with clinical and independent radiologic follow-up. Spine 17.1205-1211.

Buswell J (1982). Low back pain: a comparison of two treatment programmes. NZ J Physio 10.13-17.

Butler DS (1991). *Mobilisation of the Nervous System*. Churchill Livingstone, Melbourne.

Bybee R, Mamantov J, Meekins W, Witt J (2001). Lumbar extension range of motion: a comparison of the effects of McKenzie advocated brief, frequent, and repeated stretching to static stretching. Proceedings 7th McKenzie Institute International Conference, 257-265. August 17-19, 2001, Ottawa.

Cadoux-Hudson T (2000). Neoplasms of the spine. In: Eds Bartley R, Coffey P. *Management of Low Back Pain in Primary Care*. Butterworth Heinemann, Oxford.

Calin A, Fries JF (1975). Striking prevalence of ankylosing spondylitis in "healthy" W27 positive males and females. New Eng J Med 293.835-839.

Calin A, Porta J, Fries JF, Schurman DJ (1977). Clinical history as a screening test for ankylosing spondylitis. JAMA 237.2613-2614.

Calin A, Elswood J, Rigg S, Skevington SM (1988). Ankylosing spondylitis – An analytical review of 1500 patients: the changing pattern of disease. J Rheum 15.1234-1238.

Cameron HU, Macnab I (1975). Observations on OA of the hip joint. Clin Orth & Rel Res 108.31-40.

Carette S, Graham D, Little H, Rubenstein J, Rosen P (1983). The natural disease course of ankylosing spondylitis. Arth & Rheum 26.186-190.

Carette S, Marcoux S, Truchon R *et al.* (1991). A controlled trial of corticosteroid injections into facet joints for chronic low back pain. New Eng J Med 325.1002-1007.

Carette S, Leclaire R, Marcoux S *et al.* (1997). Epidural corticosteroid injections for sciatica due to herniated nucleus pulposus. New Eng J Med 336.1634-1640.

Carey TS, Garrett J, Jackman A, McLaughlin C, Fryer J, Smucker DR (1995a). The outcomes and costs of care for acute low back pain among patients seen by primary care practitioners, chiropractors, and orthopaedic surgeons. New Eng J Med 333.913-917.

Carey TS, Evans A, Hadler N, Kalsbeek W, McLaughlin C, Fryer J (1995b). Care-seeking among individuals with chronic low back pain. Spine 20.312-317.

Carey TS, Evans AT, Hadler NM *et al.* (1996). Acute severe low back pain. A population-based study of prevalence and care-seeking. Spine 21.339-344.

Carey TS, Garrett JM, Jackman A *et al.* (1999). Recurrence and care seeking after acute back pain. Results of a long-term follow-up study. Medical Care 37.157-164.

Carey TS, Garrett JM, Jackman AM (2000). Beyond the good prognosis. Examination of an inception cohort of patients with chronic low back pain. Spine 25.115-120.

Carmichael JP (1987). Inter- and intra-examiner reliability of palpation for sacroiliac joint dysfunction. J Manip Physio Thera 10.164-171.

Carragee EJ (1997). Pyogenic vertebral osteomyelitis. JBJS 79A.874-880.

Carrico TJ, Mehrhof AI, Cohen IK (1984). Biology of wound healing. Surg Clinics Nth Am 64.721-733.

Carter ET, McKenna CH, Brian DD, Kurland LT (1979). Epidemiology of ankylosing spondylitis in Rochester, Minnesota, 1935-1973. Arth & Rheum 22.365-370.

Carter JT, Birrell LN (editors) (2000). *Occupational health guidelines for the management of low back pain at work. Evidence review and recommendations.* Faculty of Occupational Medicine, London.

Carty G, Matyas T, Collis-Brown G (1986). A comparison of the reliability of manual tests of compliance using accessory movements in peripheral and spinal joints. (Abstract) Aus J Physio 32.68.

Cassidy JD, Carroll LJ, Cote P (1998). The Saskatchewan health and back pain survey. The prevalence of low back pain and related disability in Saskatchewan adults. Spine 23.1860-1867.

Cavanaugh JM (1995). Neural mechanisms of lumbar pain. Spine 20.1804-1809.

Cedraschi C, Robert J, Goerg D, Perrin E, Fischer W, Vischer TL (1999). Is chronic non-specific low back pain chronic? Definitions of a problem and problems of a definition. Br J GP 49.358-362.

Charles C, Gafni A, Whelan T (1997). Shared decision-making in the medical encounter: What does it mean? (Or it takes at least two to tango). Soc Sci Med 44.681-692.

Charman RA (1989). Pain theory and physiotherapy. Physiotherapy 75.247-254.

Chavannes AW, Gubbels J, Post D, Rutten G, Thomas S (1986). Acute low back pain: patients' perceptions of pain four weeks after initial diagnosis and treatment in general practice. J Royal Coll GP 36.271-273.

Cherkin DC, MacCornack FA (1989). Patient evaluations of low back care from family physicians and chiropractors. West J Med 150.351-355.

Cherkin D, Deyo RA, Berg AO (1991). Evaluation of a physician education intervention to improve primary care for low-back pain. 2: Impact on patients. Spine 16.1173-1178.

Cherkin DC, Deyo RA, Loeser JD, Bush T, Waddell G (1994a). An international comparison of back surgery rates. Spine 19.1201-1206.

Cherkin DC, Deyo RA, Wheeler K, Ciol MA (1994b). Physician variation in diagnostic testing for low back pain. What you see is what you get. Arthritis & Rheumatism 37.15-22.

Cherkin DC, Deyo RA, Street JH, Barlow W (1996a). Predicting poor outcomes for back pain seen in primary care using patients' own criteria. Spine 21.2900-2907.

Cherkin DC, Deyo RA, Street JH, Hunt M, Barlow W (1996b). Pitfalls of patient education. Limited success of a program for back pain in primary care. Spine 21.345-355.

Cherkin DC, Deyo RA, Battie M, Street J, Barlow W (1998). A comparison of physical therapy, chiropractic manipulation, and provision of an educational booklet for the treatment of patients with low back pain. NEJM 339.1021-1029.

Choudhury AR, Taylor JC (1980). Cauda equina syndrome in lumbar disc disease. Acta Orthop Scand 51.493-499.

Cibulka MT, Delitto A, Koldehoff RM (1988). Changes in innominate tilt after manipulation of the sacroiliac joint in patients with low back pain. Phys Ther 68.9.1359-1363.

Cibulka MT, Koldehoff R (1999). Clinical usefulness of a cluster of sacroiliac tests in patients with and without low back pain. JOSPT 29.83-92.

Ciullo JV, Jackson DW (1985). Pars interarticularis stress reaction, spondylolysis, and spondylolisthesis in gymnasts. Clin Sports Med 4.95-109.

Clark S, Chritiansen A, Hellman DF, Hugunin JW, Hurst KM (1999). Effects of ipsilateral anterior thigh soft tissue stretching on passive unilateral straight-leg raise. JOSPT 29.4-9.

Cloward RB (1952). Anterior herniation of a ruptured lumbar intervertebral disc. A.M.A. Archives of Surgery 64.457-463.

Cloward RB (1959). Cervical discography. A contribution to the aetiology and mechanism of neck, shoulder and arm pain. Ann Surg 150.1052-1064.

Cohen JE, Goel V, Frank JW, Bombardier C, Pelosos P, Guilleman F (1994). Group education interventions for people with low back pain. An overview of the literature. Spine 19.1214-1222.

Colhoun E, McCall IW, Williams L, Cassar Pullicino VN (1988). Provocation discography as a guide to planning operations on the spine. JBJS 70B.267-271.

Collier BD, Johnson RP, Carrera GF et al. (1985). Painful spondylolysis or spondylolisthesis studied by radiography and single-photon emission computed tomography. Radiology 154.207-211.

Comstock CP, Carragee EJ, O'Sullivan GS (1994). Spondylolisthesis in the young athlete. Physician SportsMed 22.39-46.

Congeni J, McCulloch J, Swanson K (1997). Lumbar spondylolysis. A study of natural progression in athletes. Am J Sports Med 25.248-253.

Cooper RG, Freemont AJ, Hoyland JA *et al.* (1995). Herniated intervertebral disc-associated periradicular fibrosis and vascular abnormalities occur without inflammatory cell infiltration. Spine 20.591-598.

Coppes MH, Marani E, Thomeer RTWM, Groen GJ (1997). Innervation of "painful" lumbar discs. Spine 22.2342-2350.

Corrigan B, Maitland GD (1983). *Practical Orthopaedic Medicine.* Butterworth-Heinemann, Oxford.

Coste J, Delecoeuillerie G, Cohen de Lara A, Le Parc JM, Paolaggi JB (1994). Clinical course and prognostic factors in acute low back pain: an inception cohort study in primary care practice. BMJ 308.577-580.

Cousins M (1994). Acute and postoperative pain. In: Eds Wall PD, Melzack R. *Textbook of Pain* (3rd ed). Churchill Livingstone, Edinburgh.

Crock HV (1970). A reappraisal of intervertebral disc lesions. Med J Aus, May 983-989.

Crock HV (1986). Internal disc disruption. A challenge to disc prolapse fifty years on. Spine 11.650-653.

Croft P, Papageorgiou A, Ferry S, Thomas E, Jayson MIV, Silman AJ (1996). Psychologic distress and low back pain. Evidence from a prospective study in the general population. Spine 20.2731-2737.

Croft P, Papageorgiou A, McNally R (1997). *Low Back Pain – Health Care Needs Assessment* Radcliffe Medical Press, Oxford.

Croft PR, Macfarlane GJ, Papageoorgiou AC, Thomas E, Silman AJ (1998). Outcome of low back pain in general practice: a prospective study. BMJ 316.1356-1359.

Croft P, Papageorgiou A, Thomas E, Macfarlane GJ, Silman AJ (1999). Short-term physical risk factors for new episodes of low back pain. Prospective evidence from the south Manchester back pain study. Spine 24.1556-1561.

Crook J, Weir R, Tunks E (1989). An epidemiological follow-up survey of persistent pain sufferers in a group family practice and speciality pain clinic. Pain 36.49-61.

CSAG (1994). *Clinical Standards Advisory Group: Back Pain.* HMSO, London.

Cutler RB, Fishbain DA, Rosomoff HL, Abdel-Moty E, Khalil TM, Rosomoff RS (1994). Does nonsurgical pain centre treatment of chronic pain return patients to work? A review and meta-analysis of the literature. Spine 19.643-652.

Cyriax J (1982). *Textbook of Orthopaedic Medicine* (8th ed). Bailliere Tindall, London.

Cyron BM, Hutton WC, Troup JDG (1976). Spondylolytic fractures. JBJS 58B.462-466.

Cyron BM, Hutton WC (1978). The fatigue strength of the lumbar neural arch in spondylolysis. JBJS 60B.234-238.

Dalton M, Coutts A (1994). The effect of age on cervical posture in a normal population. In: Boyling JD, Palastanga N (Eds). *Grieve's Modern Manual Therapy* (2nd ed). Churchill Livingstone, Edinburgh.

Damkot DK, Pope MH, Lord J, Frymoyer JW (1984). The relationship between work history, work environment and low back pain in men. Spine 9.395-399.

Danielsen JM, Johnsen R, Kibsgaard SK, Hellevik E (2000). Early aggressive exercise for postoperative rehabilitation after discectomy. Spine 25.1015-1020.

Danielson BI, Frennered AK, Irstam LKH (1991). Radiologic progression of isthmic lumbar spondylolisthesis in young patients. Spine 16.422-425.

Davies JR, Gibson T, Tester L (1979). The value of exercise in the treatment of low back pain. Rheumatol Rehab 18.243-247.

Davis P, Lentle BC (1978). Evidence for sacroiliac disease as a common cause of low backache in women. Lancet ii.496-497.

de Bie RA, Verhagen AP, Lenssen AF *et al.* (1998). Efficacy of 904nm laser therapy in the management of musculoskeletal disorders: a systematic review. Phys Ther Rev 3.59-72.

Delaney PM, Hubka MJ (1999). The diagnostic utility of McKenzie clinical assessment for lower back pain. J Manipulative & Physiological Therapeutics 22.628-630.

Delauche-Cavallier MC, Budet C, Laredo JD *et al.* (1992). Lumbar disc herniation. Computed tomography scan changes after conservative treatment of nerve root compression. Spine17. 927-933.

Delitto A, Cibulka MT, Erhard RE, Bowling RW, Tenhula JA (1993). Evidence for use of an extension-mobilisation category in acute low back syndrome: a prescriptive validation pilot study. Physical Therapy 73.216-228.

Delitto A, Erhard RE, Bowling RW (1995). A treatment-based classification approach to low back syndrome: Identifying and staging patients for conservative treatment. Physical Therapy 75.470-489.

Derby R, Howard MW, Grant JM, Lettice JJ, van Peteghem PK, Ryan DP (1999). The ability of pressure-controlled discography to predict surgical and nonsurgical outcomes. Spine 24.364-372.

Dettori JR, Bullock SH, Sutlive TG, Franklin RJ, Patience T (1995). The effects of spinal flexion and extension exercises and their associated postures in patients with caute low back pain. Spine 20.2303-2312.

Deutman R, Diercks RL, de Jong TEAM, van Woerden HH (1995). Isthmic lumbar spondylolisthesis with sciatica: the role of the disc. Eur Spine J 4.136-138.

Deville WLJM, ven der Windt DAWM, Dzaferagic A, Bezemer PD, Bouter LM (2000). The test of Lasegue. Systematic review of the accuracy in diagnosing herniated discs. Spine 25.1140-1147.

DeWald RL, Bridwell KH, Prodromas C, Rodts MF (1985). Reconstructive spinal surgery as palliation for metastatic malignancies of the spine. Spine 10.21-26.

Deyo RA (1982). Compliance with therapeutic regimens in arthritis: Issues, current status, and a future agenda. Seminars in Arth & Rheum 12.233-244.

Deyo RA (1983). Conservative treatment for low back pain. Distinguishing useful from useless therapy. JAMA 250.1057-1062.

Deyo RA, Diehl AK (1986). Patient satisfaction with medical care for low-back pain. Spine 11.28-30.

Deyo RA, Tsui-Wu YJ (1987). Descriptive epidemiology of low-back pain and its related medical care in the United States. Spine 12.264-268.

Deyo RA, Diehl AK (1988a). Psychosocial predictors of disability in patients with low back pain. J Rheum 15.1557-1564.

Deyo RA, Diehl AK (1988b). Cancer as a cause of back pain: frequency, clinical presentation, and diagnostic strategies. J Gen Int Med 3.230-238.

Deyo RA, Loeser JD, Bigos SJ (1990). Herniated lumbar intervertebral disc. Ann Int Med 112.598-603.

Deyo RA, Rainville J, Kent DL (1992). What can the history and physical examination tell us about low back pain? JAMA 268.760-765.

Deyo RA (1993). Practice variations, treatment fads, rising disability. Spine 18.2153-2162.

Deyo RA (1996). Drug therapy for back pain. Which drugs help which patients? Spine 21.2840-2850.

Dieck GS, Kelsey Jl, Goel VK, Panjabi MM, Walter SD, Laprade MH (1985). An epidemiologic study of the relationship between postural asymmetry in the teen years and subsequent back and neck pain. Spine 10.872-877.

Dieppe P (1995). Management of hip osteoarthritis. BMJ 311.853-853.

Di Fabio RP (1992). Efficacy of manual therapy. Physical Therapy 72.853-864.

Di Fabio RP (1995). Efficacy of comprehensive rehabilitation programs and back school for patients with low back pain: a meta-analysis. Physical Therapy 75.865-878.

Digby JM, Kersley JB (1979). Pyogenic non-tuberculous spinal infection. An analysis of thirty cases. JBJS 61B.47-55.

DIHTA (1999). *Danish Institute for Health Technology Assessment: Low-Back Pain. Frequency, Management and Prevention from an HTA perspective*. Danish Health Technology Assessment. 1(1).

Dillane JB, Fry J, Kalton G (1966). Acute back syndrome – A study from general practice. BMJ 2.82-84.

Dixon M, Sweeney K (2000). *The Human Effect in Medicine. Theory, Research and Practice*. Radcliffe Medical Press, Oxford.

Dockrell S (1988). An investigation of the use of verbal and non-verbal communication skills by final-year physiotherapy students. Physiotherapy 74.52-55.

Dodd T (1997). *The Prevalence of Back Pain in Great Britain in 1996*. The Stationery Office, London.

Doita M, Kanatani T, Harada T, Mizuno K (1996). Immunohistologic study of the ruptured intervertebral disc of the lumbar spine. Spine 21.235-241.

Dolan P, Adams MA, Hutton WC (1988). Commonly adopted postures and their effect on the lumbar spine. Spine 13.197-201.

Dolan P (1998). Associations between mechanical loading, spinal function and low back pain. In: *Proceedings Third Interdisciplinary World Congress on Low Back & Pelvic Pain*, November, Vienna. Eds Vleeming A, Mooney V, Tilscher H, Dorman T, Snijders C.

Dolan P, Greenfield K, Nelson RJ, Nelson IW (2000). Can exercise therapy improve the outcome of microdiscectomy? Spine 25.1523-1532.

Donahue MS, Riddle DL, Sullivan MS (1996). Intertester reliability of a modified version of McKenzie's lateral shift assessments obtained on patients with low back pain. Physical Therapy 76.706-726.

Donatelli R, Owens-Burkhart H (1981). Effects of immobilization on the extensibility of periarticular connective tissue. JOSPT 3.67-72.

Donelson R, Silva G, Murphy K (1990). Centralization phenomenon. Its usefulness in evaluating and treating referred pain. Spine 15.211-213.

Donelson R, Grant W, Kamps C, Medcalf R (1991). Pain response to sagital end-range spinal motion. A prospective, randomised, multicentered trial Spine 16. S206-S212.

Donelson R, Aprill C, Medcalf R, Grant W (1997). A prospective study of centralization of lumbar and referred pain. A predictor of symptomatic discs and annular competence. Spine 22.1115-1122.

Don Tigny RL (1990). Anterior dysfunction of the sacroiliac joint as a major factor in the etiology of idiopathic low back pain syndrome. Physical Therapy 70.250-265.

Don Tigny RL (1997). Mechanics and treatment of the sacroiliac joint. In: Eds Vleeming A, Mooney V, Dorman T, Snijders C, Stoeckart R. *Movement, Stability & Low Back Pain. The Essential Role of the Pelvis.* Churchill Livingstone, New York.

Dougados M, van der Linden S, Juhlin R *et al.* (1991). The European spondylarthropathy study group preliminary criteria for the classification of spondylarthropathy. Arth & Rheum 34.1218-1227.

Dreyer SJ, Dreyfuss PH (1996). Low back pain and the zygapophyseal (facet) joints. Arch Phys Med Rehabil 77.290-300.

Dreyfuss P, Dreyer S, Griffin J, Hoffman J, Walsh N (1994). Positive sacroiliac screening tests in asymptomatic adults. Spine 19.10.1138-1143.

Dreyfuss P, Michaelsen M, Pauza K, McLarty J, Bogduk N (1996). The value of medical history and physical examination in diagnosing sacroiliac joint pain. Spine 21.22.2594-2602.

Dubner R (1991). Neuronal plasticity and pain following peripheral tissue inflammation or nerve injury. In *Proceedings of the Sixth World Congress on Pain*, Eds Bond MR, Charlton JE, Woolf CJ. Elsevier Publishers BV.

Duggleby T, Kumar S (1997). Epidemiology of juvenile low back pain: a review. Dis & Rehab 19.505-512.

Dumas GA, Reid JG, Wolfe LA, Griffin MP, McGrath MJ (1995). Exercise, posture, and back pain during pregnancy. Part 1. Exercise and posture. Clin Biomech 10.98-103.

Dupuis PR, Yong-Hing K, Cassidy JD, Kirkaldy-Willis WH (1985). Radiologic diagnosis of degenerative lumbar spinal instability. Spine 10.262-276.

Dvorak J, Gauchat MH, Valach L (1988). The outcome of surgery for lumbar disc herniation. 1. A 4-17 years' follow-up with emphasis on somatic aspects. Spine 13.1418-1422.

Dzioba RB, Doxey NC (1984). A prospective investigation into the orthopaedic and psychologic predictors of outcome of first lumbar surgery following industrial injury. Spine 9.614-623.

Edmondston SJ, Song S, Bricknell RV *et al.* (2000). MRI evaluation of lumbar spine flexion and extension in asymptomatic individuals. Manual Therapy 5.158-164.

Egan D, Cole J, Twomey L (1996). The standing forward flexion test: An inaccurate determinant of sacroiliac joint dysfunction. Physio 82.4.236-242.

Eisenstein SM, Ashton IK, Roberts S *et al.* (1994). Innervation of the spondylolysis "ligament". Spine 19.912-916.

Eklund JAE, Corlett EN (1987). Evaluation of spinal loads and chair design in seated work tasks. Clin Biomech 2.27-33.

Ellenberg MR, Ross ML, Honet JC, Schwartz M, Chodoroff G, Enochs S (1993). Prospective evaluation of the course of disc herniations in patients with proven radiculopathy. Arch Phys Med Rehabil 74.3-8.

Elnaggar IM, Nordin M, Sheikhzadeh A, Parnianpour M, Kahanovitz N (1991). Effects of spinal flexion and extension exercises on low-back pain and spinal mobility in chronic mechanical low-back pain patients. Spine 16.967-972.

Ensink FBM, Saur PMM, Frese K, Seeger D, Hildebrandt J (1996). Lumbar range of motion: influence of time of day and individual factors on measurements. Spine 21.1339-1343.

Enwemeka CS (1989). Inflammation, cellularity, and fibrillogenesis in regenerating tendon: implications for tendon rehabilitation. Physical Therapy 69.816-825.

Erhard RE, Delitto A, Cibulka MT (1994). Relative effectiveness of an extension program and a combined program of manipulation and flexion and extension exercises in patients with acute low back syndrome. Physical Therapy 74.1093-1100.

Evans G, Richards SH (1996). *Low Back Pain: An Evaluation of Therapeutic Interventions*. University of Bristol.

Evans P (1980). The healing process at cellular level: a review. Physiotherapy 66.256-259.

Evans RB (1989). Clinical application of controlled stress to the healing extensor tendon: a review of 112 cases. Physical Therapy 69.1041-1049.

Ezzo J, Berman B, Hadhazy VA, Jadad AR, Lao L, Singh BB (2000). Is acupuncture effective for the treatment of chronic pain? A systematic review. Pain 86.217-225.

Faas A (1996). Exercises: which ones are worth trying, for which patients, and when? Spine 21.2874-2879.

Fahey V, Opeskin K, Silberstein M, Anderson R, Briggs C (1998). The pathogenesis of Schmorl's nodes in relation to acute trauma. An autopsy study. Spine 23.2272-2275.

Fairbank JCT, Couper J, Davies JB, O'Brien JP (1980). The Oswestry low back pain disability questionnaire. Physiotherapy 66.271-273.

Fairbank JCT, Park WM, McCall IW, O'Brien JP (1981). Apophyseal injection of local anesthetic as a diagnostic aid in primary low-back pain syndromes. Spine 6.598-605.

Fairbank JCT, Pynsent PB (1992). Syndromes of back pain and their classification. In: Ed. Jayson MIV. *The Lumbar Spine and Back Pain* (4th ed). Churchill Livingstone, Edinburgh.

Falconer MA, Glasgow GL, Cole DS (1947). Sensory disturbances occurring in sciatica due to intervertebral disc protrusions: some observations on the fifth lumbar and first sacral dermatomes. J Neurol Neurosurg & Psychiat 10.72-84.

Falconer MA, McGeorge M, Begg AC (1948). Observations on the cause and mechanism of symptom-production in sciatica and low-back pain. J Neurol Neurosurg & Psychiat 11.13-26.

Fanciullacci F, Sandri S, Politi P, Zanollo A (1989). Clinical, urodynamic and neurophysiological findings in patients with neuropathic bladder due to lumbar intervertebral disc protrusion. Paraplegia 27.354-358.

Fardon DF, Milette PC, Faciszewski T et al. (2001). Nomenclature and classification of lumbar disc pathology. Recommendations of the combined task forces of the North American Spine Society, Americal Society of Spine Radiology, and Americal Society of Neuroradiology. Spine 26.E93-E113.

Fast A, Shapiro D, Ducomunn EJ et al. (1987). Low-back pain in pregnancy. Spine 12.368-371.

Fast A, Weiss L, Ducommun EJ, Medina E, Butler JG (1990). Low-back pain in pregnancy. Abdominal muscles, sit-up performance, and back pain. Spine 15.28-30.

Feinstein B, Langton JNK, Jameson RM, Schiller F (1954). Experiments on pain referred from deep somatic tissues. JBJS 36A.981-997.

Felson DT (1988). Epidemiology of hip and knee osteoarthritis. Epidemiologic Reviews 10.1-28.

Fennell AJ, Jones AP, Hukins DWL (1996). Migration of the nucleus pulposus within the intervertebral disc during flexion and extension of the spine. Spine 21.2753-2757.

Ferguson SA, Marras WS (1997). A literature review of low back disorder surveillance measures and risk factors. Clin Biomech 12.211-226.

Ferguson SA, Marras WS, Gupta P (2000). Longitudinal quantitative measures of the natural course of low back pain recovery. Spine 25.1950-1956.

Fernand R, Fox DE (1985). Evaluation of lumbar lordosis. Spine 10.799-803.

Fernstrom U (1960). A discographical study of ruptured lumbar intervertebral discs. Acta Chir Scand S258.1-73.

Findlay GFG (1992). Tumours of the lumbar spine. In: Ed. Jayson MIV. *The Lumbar Spine and Back Pain* (4th ed). Churchill Livingstone, Edinburgh.

Fitzpatrick RM, Bury M, Frank AO, Donnelly T (1987). Problems in the assessment of outcome in a back pain clinic. International Disability Studies 9.161-165.

Floman Y (2000). Progression of lumbosacral isthmic spondylolisthesis in adults. Spine 25.342-347.

Flor H, Fydrich T, Turk DC (1992). Efficacy of multidisciplinary pain treatment centres: a meta-analytic review. Pain 49.221-230.

Fordyce WE, Atkinson RE, Battie M et al. (1995). *Back Pain in the Workplace. Management of Disability in Nonspecific Conditions*. IASP Press, Seattle.

Fortin JD, Dwyer AP, West S, Pier J (1994). Sacroiliac joint: Pain referral maps upon applying a new injection/arthrography technique. Part 1: Asymptomatic volunteers. Spine 19.13.1475-1482.

Foster D, John D, Elliott B, Ackland T, Fitch K (1989). Back injuries to fast bowlers in cricket: a prospective study. Br J Sports Med 23.150-154.

Foster NE, Thompson KA, Baxter GD, Allen JM (1999). Management of non-specific low back pain by physiotherapists in Britain and Ireland. A descriptive questionnaire of current clinical practice. Spine 24.1332-1342.

Fowler B, Oyekoya O (1995). The therapeutic efficacy of McKenzie concept in the management of low back pain. *Proceedings 12th International Congress of World Confederation for Physical Therapy*. June 25-30, 1995, Washington DC, USA. Abstract 1093.

Frank C, Woo SLY, Amiel D, Harwood F, Gomez M, Akeson W (1983). Medial collateral ligament healing. A multidisciplinary assessment in rabbits. Am J Sports Med 11.379-389.

Frank JW, Kerr MS, Brooker AS *et al.* (1996). Disability resulting from occupational low back pain. Part 1: What do we know about primary prevention? A review of the scientific evidence on prevention before disability begins. Spine 21.2908-2917.

Fraser R (2001). Point of view. Spine 26.2652.

Freburger JK, Riddle DL (1999). Measurement of sacroiliac joint dysfunction: a multicenter intertester reliability study. Physical Therapy 79.1134-1141.

Freburger JK, Riddle DL (2001). Using published evidence to guide the examination of the sacroiliac joint region. Physical Therapy 81.1135-1143.

Fredrickson BE, Baker D, McHolick WJ, Yuan HA, Lubicky JP (1984). The natural history of spondylolysis and spondylolisthesis. JBJS 66A.699-707.

Freemont AJ, Peacock TE, Goupille P, Hoyland JA, O'Brien J, Jayson MIV (1997). Nerve in growth into diseased intervertebral disc in chronic back pain. Lancet 350.178-181.

Frennered AK, Danielson BI, Nachemson AL, Nordwall AB (1991). Midterm follow-up of young patients fused *in situ* for spondylolisthesis. Spine 16.409-416.

Friberg O (1983). Clinical symptoms and biomechanics of lumbar spine and hip joint in leg length inequality. Spine 8.643-650.

Friberg O (1987). Lumbar instability: a dynamic approach by traction-compression radiography. Spine 12.119-129.

Fries JW, Abodeely DA, Vijungco JG, Yeager VL, Gaffey WR (1982). Computed tomography of herniated and extruded nucleus pulposus. J Computer Assisted Tomography 6.874-887.

Fritz JM, Erhard RE, Vignovic M (1997). A nonsurgical treatment approach for patients with lumbar spinal stenosis. Physical Therapy 77.962-973.

Fritz JM, Delitto A, Welch WC, Erhard RE (1998). Lumbar spinal stenosis: A review of current concepts in evaluation, management, and outcome measurements. Arch Phys Med Rehabil 79.700-708.

Fritz JM, George S (2000). The use of a classification approach to identify subgroups of patients with acute low back pain. Spine 25.106-114.

Fritz JM, Delitto A, Vignovic M, Busse RG (2000a). Interrater reliability of judgements of the centralization phenomenon and status change during movement testing in patients with low back pain. Arch Phys Med Rehabil 81.57-61.

Fritz JM, Wainner RS, Hicks GE (2000b). The use of nonorganic signs and symptoms as a screening tool for return-to-work in patients with acute low back pain. Spine 25.1925-1931.

Fritz JM, George SZ, Delitto A (2001). The role of fear-avoidance beliefs in acute low back pain: relationships with current and future disability and work status. Pain 94.7-15.

Frost H, Klaber Moffett JA, Moser JS, Fairbank JCT (1995). Randomised controlled trial for evaluation of fitness programme for patients with chronic low back pain. BMJ 310.151-154.

Frost H, Lamb SE, Klaber Moffett JA, Fairbank JCT, Moser (1998). A fitness programme for patients with chronic low back pain: 2-year follow-up of a randomised controlled trial. Pain 75.273-279.

Frymoyer JW, Pope MH, Clements JH *et al.* (1983). Risk factors in low-back pain. JBJS 65A.213-218.

Frymoyer JW, Newberg A, Pope MH, Wilder DG, Clements J, MacPherson B (1984). Spine radiographs in patients with low-back pain. JBJS 66A.1048-1055.

Fuchioka M, Nakai O, Yamaura I, Ohkawa J (1993). Perforating patterns of nucleus pulposus in the lumbar disc herniation. McKenzie Institute (UK) Newsletter 1.3.3-10.

Funk D, Swank AM, Adams KJ, Treolo D (2001). Efficacy of moist heat pack application over static stretching on hamstring flexibility. J Strength & Conditioning Res 15.123-126.

Gaines WG, Hegmann KT (1999). Effectiveness of Waddell's nonorganic signs in predicting a delayed return to regular work in patients experiencing acute occupational low back pain. Spine 24.396-401.

Gallagher J, di Vadi PLP, Wedley JR *et al.* (1994). Radiofrequency facet joint denervation in the treatment of low back pain: a prospective controlled double-blind study to assess its efficacy. The Pain Clinic 7.193-198.

Gam AN, Johannsen F (1995). Ultrasound therapy in musculoskeletal disorders: a meta-analysis. Pain 63.85-91.

Gamsa A (1990). Is emotional disturbance a precipitator or a consequence of chronic pain? Pain 42.183-195.

Garfin SR, Rydevik B, Lind B, Massie J (1995). Spinal nerve root compression. Spine 20.1810-1820.

Gatchel RJ, Polatin PB, Mayer TG (1995). The dominant role of psychosocial risk factors in the development of chronic low back pain disability. Spine 20.2702-2709.

Gauvin MG, Riddle DL, Rothstein JM (1990). Reliability of clinical measurements of forward bending using the modified finger-to-floor method. Physical Therapy 70.443-447.

Gebhardt WA (1994). Effectiveness of training to prevent job-related back pain: a meta-analysis. Br J Clin Psychology 33.571-574.

Gelberman RH, Amiel D, Gonsalves M, Woo S, Akeson WH (1981). The influence of protected passive mobilisation on the healing of flexor tendons: A biochemical and micoangiographic study. Br Soc for Surg Hand 13.120-128.

Gelberman GH, Woo SLY, Lothringer K, Akeson WH, Amiel D (1982). Effects of early intermittent passive mobilisation on healing canine flexor tendons. J Hand Surg 4.170-175.

Gertzbein SD, Holtby R, Tile M, Kapasouri A, Chan KW, Cruikshank B (1984). Determination of a locus of instantaneous centers of rotation of the lumbar disc by Moire fringes. Spine 9.409-413.

Gertzbein SD, Seligman J, Holtby R *et al.* (1985). Centrode patterns and segmental instability in degenerative disc disease. Spine 10.257-261.

Getty J (1990). Laminectomies. In: *The Lumbar Spine*. Eds Weinstein JN, Wiesel SW. WB Saunders Company, Philidelphia.

Gibson JNA, Grant IC, Waddell G (1999). The Cochrane review of surgery for lumbar disc prolapse and degenerative lumbar spondylosis. Spine 24.1820-1832.

Gifford L (1998a). The 'central' mechanisms. In: Ed. Gifford L. *Topical Issues in Pain*. NOI Press, Falmouth.

Gifford L (1998b). Pain, the tissues and the nervous system: A conceptual model. Physiotherapy 84.27-36.

Gill K, Krag MH, Johnson GB, Haugh LD, Pope MH (1988). Repeatability of four clinical methods for assessment of lumbar spinal motion. Spine 13.50-53.

Gillan MGC, Ross JC, McLean IP, Porter RW (1998). The natural history of trunk list, its associated disability and the influence of McKenzie management. Eur Spine J 7.480-483.

Gleave JRW, Macfarlane R (1990). Prognosis for recovery of bladder function following lumbar central disc prolapse. Br J Neurosurg 4.205-210.

Goertz MN (1990). Prognostic indicators for acute low-back pain. Spine15.1307-1310.

Goldby L (1995). A randomised controlled trial comparing the McKenzie method of mechanical diagnosis and therapy with a non-prescriptive exercise regime in the conservative treatment of chronic low back pain. *Proceedings 4th McKenzie Institute International Conference*, Cambridge, England, 16-17 September 1995.

Gonnella C, Paris SV, Kutner M (1982). Reliability in evaluating passive intervertebral motion. Physical Therapy 62.436-444.

Goodacre JA, Mander M, Dick WC (1991). Patients with ankylosing spondylitis show individual patterns of variation in disease activity. Br J Rheum 30.336-338.

Gordan SJ, Yang KH, Mayer PJ, Mace AH, Kish VL, Radin EL (1991). Mechanism of disc rupture. A preliminary report. Spine 16.450-456.

Gran JT (1985). An epidemiological survey of the signs and symptoms of ankylosing spondylitis. Clin Rheum 4.161-169.

Gran JT, Husby G, Hordvik M (1985). Prevalence of ankylosing spondylitis in males and females in a young middle-aged population of Tromso, northern Norway. Ann Rheum Dis 44.359-367.

Gray JAM (1997). *Evidence-based Healthcare. How to Make Health Policy and Management Decisions*. Churchill Livingstone, New York.

Greene G (2001). 'Red Flags': essential factors in recognising serious spinal pathology. Manual Therapy 6.253-255.

Greenfield S, Anderson H, Winickoff RN, Morgan A, Komaroff AL (1975). Nurse-protocol management of low back pain. Outcomes, patient satisfaction, and efficiency of primary care. West J Med 123.350-359.

Grobler LJ, Novotny JE, Wilder DG, Frymoyer JW, Pope MH (1994). L4-5 isthmic spondylolisthesis. A biomechanical analysis comparing stability in L4-5 and L5-S1 isthmic spondylolisthesis. Spine 19.222-227.

Gronblad M, Virri J, Tolonen J *et al.* (1994). A controlled immunohistochemical study of inflammatory cells in disc herniation tissue. Spine 19.2744-2751.

Grubb SA, Lipscomb HJ, Guilford WB (1987). The relative value of lumbar roentgenograms, metrizamide myelography, and discography in the assessment of patients with chronic low-back syndrome. Spine 12.282-286.

Grundy PF, Roberts CJ (1984). Does unequal leg length cause back pain? A case-control study. Lancet ii.256-258.

Hackett GI, Bundred P, Hutton JL, O'Brien J, Stanley IM (1993). Management of joint and soft tissue injuries in 3 general practices: value of on-site physiotherapy. Br J General Practice 43.61-64.

Hadler NM (1997). Back pain in the workplace. Spine 22.935-940.

Hagen KB, Thune O (1998). Work incapacity from low back pain in the general population. Spine 23.2091-2095.

Hagen KB, Hilde G, Jamtvedt G, Winnem MF (2000). The Cochrane review of bed rest for acute low back pain and sciatica. Spine 25.2932-2939.

Haigh R, Clarke AK (1999). Effectiveness of rehabilitation for spinal pain. Clin Rehab 13.S1.63-81.

Haldeman S, Rubinstein SM (1992). Cauda equina syndrome in patients undergoing manipulation of the lumbar spine. Spine 17.1469-1473.

Hall H, McIntosh G, Wilson L, Melles T (1998). Spontaneous onset of back pain. Clin J Pain 14.129-133.

Hall JA, Dornan MC (1988). What patients like about their medical care and how often are they asked: A meta-analysis of the satisfaction literature. Soc Sci Med 27.935-939.

Hall S, Bartleson JD, Onofrio BM et al. (1985). Lumbar spinal stenosis. Clinical features, diagnostic procedures, and results of surgical treatment in 68 patients. Ann Int Med 103.271-275.

Hamanishi C, Kawabata T, Yosii T, Tanaka S (1994). Schmorl's nodes on magnetic resonance imaging. Their incidence and clinical relevance. Spine 19.450-453.

Hampton D, Laros G, McCarron R, Franks D (1989). Healing potential of the anulus fibrosus. Spine 14.398-401.

Hanai F, Matsui N, Hongo N (1996). Changes in response of wide dynamic range neurons in the spinal dorsal horn after dorsal root or dorsal root ganglion compression. Spine 21.1408-1415.

Hansson T, Bigos S, Beecher P, Wortley M (1985). The lumbar lordosis in acute and chronic low-back pain. Spine 10.154-155.

Harada Y, Nakahara S (1989). A pathologic study of lumbar disc herniation in the elderly. Spine 14.1020-1024.

Harada M, Abumi K, Ito M, Kaneda K (2000). Cineradiographic motion analysis of normal lumbar spine during forward and backward flexion. Spine 25.1932-1937.

Hardcastle P, Annear P, Foster DH et al. (1992). Spinal abnormalities in young fast bowlers. JBJS 74B.421-425.

Hardcastle PH (1993). Repair of spondylolysis in young fast bowlers. JBJS 75B.398-402.

Hardy MA (1989). The biology of scar formation. Physical Therapy 69.1014-1024.

Hardy GLH, Napier JK (1991). Inter and intratherapist reliability of passive accessory movement technique. NZ J Physio December 22-24.

Harms M (1990). Effect of wheelchair design on posture and comfort of users. Physiotherapy 76.266-271.

Harms-Ringdahl K (1986). On assessment of shoulder exercise and load-elicited pain in the cervical spine. Scand J Rehab Med S14.1-40.

Harreby M, Hesselsoe G, Kjer J, Neergaard K (1997). Low back pain and physical exercise in leisure time in 38-year-old men and women: a 25-year prospective cohort study of 640 school children. Eur Spine J 6.181-186.

Harris IE, Weinstein SL (1987). Long-term follow-up of patients with grade-III and IV spondylolisthesis. JBJS 69A.960-969.

Harrison DD, Harrison SO, Croft AC, Harrison DE, Troyanovich SJ (1999). Sitting biomechanics part 1: review of the literature. J Manip Physiological Therapeutics 22.594-609.

Harrison DD, Harrison SO, Croft AC, Harrison DE, Troyanovich SJ (2000). Sitting biomechanics part 2: Optimal car driver's seat and optimal driver's spinal model. J Manip Physiological Therapeutics 23.37-47.

Hart LG, Deyo RA, Cherkin DC (1995). Physician office visits for low back pain. Spine 20.11-19.

Hartvigsen J, Bakketeig LS, Leboeuf-Yde C, Engberg ME, Lauritzen T (2001). The association between physical workload and low back pain clouded by the "healthy worker" effect. Spine 26.1788-1793.

Harvey CJ, Richenberg JL, Saifuddin A, Wolman RL (1998). Pictorial review: The radiological investigation of lumbar spondylolysis. Clin Rad 53.723-728.

Hasenbring M, Marienfeld G, Kuhlendahl D, Soyka D (1994). Risk factors of chronicity in lumbar disc patients. A prospective investigation of biologic, psychologic, and social predictors of therapy outcome. Spine 19.2759-2765.

Haswell K, Gilmour J (1997). Basic interviewing skills: how they are used by manipulative physiotherapists. NZ J Physiotherapy August 11-14.

Hayes MA, Howard TC, Gruel CR, Kopta JA (1989). Roentenographic evaluation of lumbar spine flexion-extension in asymptomatic individuals. Spine 14.327-331.

Hazard RG, Reid S, Haugh LD, McFarlane G (2000). A controlled trial of an educational pamphlet to prevent disability after occupational low back injury. Spine 25.1419-1423.

Hedman TP, Fernie GR (1997). Mechanical response of the lumbar spine to seated postural loads. Spine 22.734-743.

Heggeness M, Esses SI (1991). Degenerative spinal stenosis. Current Orthopaedics 5.119-124.

Heiberg E, Aarseth SP (1997). Epidemiology of pelvic pain and low back pain in pregnant women. In: Eds Vleeming A, Mooney V, Dorman T, Snijders C, Stoeckart R. *Movement, Stability & Low Back Pain. The Essential Role of the Pelvis*. Churchill Livingstone, New York.

Helbig T, Lee CK (1988). The lumbar facet syndrome. Spine 13.61-64.

Helewa A, Goldsmith CH, Lee P, Smythe HA, Forwell L (1999). Does strengthening the abdominal muscles prevent low back pain – A randomised controlled trial. J Rheumatol 26.1808-1815.

Heliovaara M, Impivaara O, Sievers K, Melkas T, Knekt P, Korpi J, Aromaa A (1987). Lumbar disc syndrome in Finland. J Epidem & Comm Health 41.251-258.

Heliovaara M, Sievers K, Impivaara O *et al.* (1989). Descriptive epidemiology and public health aspects of low back pain. Annals of Medicine 21.327-333.

Hellsing AL, Linton SJ, Kalvemark M (1994). A prospective study of patients with acute back and neck pain in Sweden. Physical Therapy 74.116-128.

Henricson AS, Fredriksson K, Persson I, Pereira R, Rostedt Y, Westlin NE (1984). The effect of heat and stretching on the range of hip motion. JOSPT 6.110-115.

Henry JL (1989). Concepts of pain sensation and its modulation. J Rheumatology Supp 19.16.104-112.

Hensinger RN (1989). Current concepts review. Spondylolysis and spondylolisthesis in children and adults. JBJS 71A.1098-1107.

Henson J, McCall IW, O'Brien JP (1987). Disc damage above a spondylolisthesis. Br J Radiology 60.69-72.

Herkowitz HN (1995). Spine update. Degenerative lumbar spondylolisthesis. Spine 20.1084-1090.

Heszen-Klemens I, Lapinska E (1984). Doctor-patient interaction, patients' health behavior and effects of treatment. Soc Sci Med 19.9-18.

Hickey DS, Hukins DWL (1980). Relation between the structure of the annulus fibrosus and the function and failure of the intervertebral disc. Spine 5.106-116.

Hilde G, Bo K (1998). Effect of exercise in the treatment of chronic low back pain: a systematic review, emphasising type and dose of exercise. Phys Ther Rev 3.107-117.

Hill P (1998). Fear-avoidance theories. In: Ed. Gifford L. *Topical Issues in Pain.* NOI Press, Falmouth.

Hillman M, Wright A, Rajaratnam G, Tennant A, Chamberlain MA (1996). Prevalence of low back pain in the community: implications for service provision in Bradford, UK. J Epidem Comm Health 50.347-352.

Hilton RC, Ball J, Bemm RT (1976). Vertebral end-plate lesions (Schmorl's nodes) in the dorsolumbar spine. Ann Rheum Dis 35.127-132.

Hirsch C, Schajowicz F (1953). Studies on structural changes in lumbar anulus fibrosus. Acta Orth Scand 22.184-231.

Hoffman RM, Wheeler KJ, Deyo RA (1993). Surgery for herniated lumbar discs: a literature synthesis. J Gen Intern Med 8.487-496.

Hollenberg GM, Beattie PF, Meyers SP, Weinberg EP, Adams MJ (2002). Stress reactions of the lumbar pars interarticularis. The development of a new MRI classification system. Spine 27.181-186.

Holmes MAM, Rudland JR (1991). Clinical trials of ultrasound treatment in soft tissue injury: A review and critique. Physio Theory & Practice 7.163-175.

Hopayian K, Mugford M (1999). Conflicting conclusions from two systematic reviews of epidural steroid injections for sciatica: which evidence should general practitioners heed? Br J Gen Pract 49.57-61.

Hoogendoorn WE, van Poppel MNM, Bongers PM, Koes BW, Bouter LM (1999). Physical load during work and leisure time as risk factors for back pain. Scand J Work Environ Health 25.387-403.

Hoogendoorn WE, Bongers PM, de Vet *et al.* (2000a). Flexion and rotation of the trunk and lifting at work are risk factors for low back pain. Results of a prospective cohort study. Spine 25.3087-3092.

Hoogendoorn WE, van Poppel MNM, Bongers PM, Koes BW, Bouter LM (2000b). Systematic review of psychosocial factors at work and private life as risk factors for back pain. Spine 25.2114-2125.

Horton WC, Daftari TK (1992). Which disc as visualised by MRI is actually a source of pain? A correlation between MRI and discography. Spine 17.S164-S171.

Howe JF, Loeser JD, Calvin WH (1977). Mechanosensitivity of dorsal root ganglia and chronically injured axons: a physiological basis for the radicular pain of nerve root compression. Pain 3.25-41.

Hsu KY, Zucherman JF, Derby R, White AH, Goldthwaite N, Wynne G (1988). Painful lumbar end-plate disruptions: a significant discographic finding. Spine 13.76-78.

Hubley CL, Kozey JW, Stanish WD (1984). The effects of static stretching exercises and stationary cycling on range of motion at the hip joint. JOSPT 6.104-109.

Hunter G (1994). Specific soft tissue mobilisation in the treatment of soft tissue lesions. Physiotherapy 80.15-21.

Huskisson EC (1974). Measurement of pain. Lancet 2.1127-1131.

Indahl A, Velund L, Reikeraas O (1995). Good prognosis for low back pain when left untampered. Spine 20.473-477.

Indahl A, Haldorsen EH, Holm S, Reikeras O, Ursin H (1998). Five-year follow-up study of a controlled clinical trial using light mobilisation and an informative approach to low back pain. Spine 23.2625-2630.

Inman VT, Saunders JBCM (1947). Anatomicophysiological aspects of injuries to the intervertebral disc. JBJS 29.461-475.

Ito T, Takano Y, Yuasa N (2001). Types of lumbar herniated disc and clinical course. Spine 26.648-651.

Iversen MD, Katz JN (2001). Examination findings and self-reported walking capacity in patients with lumbar spinal stenosis. Physical Therapy 81.1296-1306.

Jackson DW, Wiltse LL, Crincione RJ (1976). Spondylolysis in the female gymnast. Clin Orth & Rel Res 117.68-73.

Jackson DW (1979). Low back pain in young athletes: evaluation of stress reaction and discogenic problems. Am J Sports Med 7.364-366.

Jackson RP, Glah JJ (1987). Foraminal and extraforaminal lumbar disc herniation: diagnosis and treatment. Spine 12.577-585.

Jackson RP, Jacobs RR, Montesano PX (1988). Facet joint injection in low-back pain. A prospective statistical study. Spine 13.966-971.

Jackson RP, McManus AC (1994). Radiographic analysis of sagital plane alignment and balance in standing volunteers and patients with low back pain matched for age, sex, and size. A prospective controlled clinical study. Spine 19.1611-1618.

Jadad AR, McQuay HJ (1993). The measurement of pain. In *Outcome Measures in Orthopaedics*. Eds Pynsent PB, Fairbank JCT, Carr A. Butterworth Heinemann, Oxford.

Jaffray D, O'Brien JP (1986). Isolated intervertebral disc resorption. A source of mechanical and inflammatory back pain? Spine 11.397-401.

Jason H (1997). Manual skills and good judgement are vital but insufficient: clinicians must also be effective educators. J Manual & Manip Therapy 5.178.

Jellema P, van Tulder MW, van Poppel MNM, Nachemson AL, Bouter LM (2001). Lumbar supports for prevention and treatment of low back pain. A systematic review within the framework of the Cochrane Back Review Group. Spine 26.377-386.

Jenis LG, An HS (2000). Spine Update. Lumbar foraminal stenosis. Spine 25.389-394.

Jensen MC, Brant-Zawadzki MN, Obuchowski N, Modic MT, Malkasian D, Ross JS (1994). Magnetic resonance imaging of the lumbar spine in people without back pain. NEJM 331.69-73.

Jensen MP, Turner JA, Romano JM, Karoly P (1991). Coping with chronic pain: a critical review of the literature. Pain 47.249-283.

Jette AM, Smith K, Haley SM, Davis KD (1994). Physical therapy episodes of care for patients with low back pain. Physical Therapy 74.101-115.

Jette MA, Delitto A (1997). Physical therapy treatment choices for musculoskeletal impairments. Physical Therapy 77.145-154.

Jinkins JR, Whittemore AR, Bradley WG (1989). The anatomic basis of vertebrogenic pain and the autonomic syndrome associated with lumbar disc extrusion. AJR 152.1277-1289.

Johnson MI (1997). The physiology of the sensory dimensions of clinical pain. Physiotherapy 83.526-536.

Johnson RJ (1993). Low-back pain in sports. Managing spondylolysis in young patients. Physician & Sportsmed 21.53-59.

Johnsson KE, Uden A, Rosen I (1991). The effect of decompression on the natural course of spinal stenosis. A comparison of surgically treated and untreated patients. Spine 16.615-619.

Johnsson KE, Rosen I, Uden A (1992). The natural course of lumbar spinal stenosis. Clin Orth & Rel Res 279.82-86.

Johnsson KE (1995). Lumbar spinal stenosis. Acta Orthop Scand 66.403-405.

Jones M, Butler D (1991). Clinical reasoning. In: Butler DS, *Mobilisation of the Nervous System*. Churchill Livingstone, Melbourne.

Jones M, Christensen N, Carr J (1994). Clinical reasoning in orthopaedic manual therapy. In: Ed. Grant R. *Physical Therapy of the Cervical and Thoracic Spine (2nd)*. Churchill Livingstone, New York.

Jones MA (1992). Clinical reasoning in manual therapy. Physical Therapy 72.875-884.

Jonsson B, Stromqvist B (1993). Symptoms and signs in degeneration of the lumbar spine. JBJS 75B.381-385.

Jonsson B, Stromqvist B (1996). Neurologic signs in lumbar disc herniation. Preoperative affliction and postoperative recovery in 150 cases. Acta Orthop Scand 67.466-469.

Jonsson B, Stromqvist B (1996b). Clinical appearance of contained and noncontained lumbar dsic herniations. J Spinal Disorders 9.32-38.

Jonsson B, Annertz M, Sjoberg C, Stromqvist B (1997a). A prospective and consecutive study of surgically treated lumbar spinal stenosis. Part i: Clinical features related to radiographic findings. Spine 22.2932-2937.

Jonsson B, Annertz M, Sjoberg C, Stromqvist B (1997b). A prospective and consecutive study of surgically treated lumbar spinal stenosis. Part ii: Five-year follow-up by an independent observer. Spine 22.2938-2944.

Jonsson B, Johnsson R, Stromqvist B (1998). Contained and noncontained lumbar disc herniation in the same patient. Two case reports. Spine 23.277-280.

Jorring K (1980). Osteoarthritis of the hip. Acta Orthop Scand 51.523-530.

Jull G, Bogduk N, Marsland A (1988). The accuracy of manual diagnosis for zygapophysial joint pain syndromes. Med J Aus 148.233-236.

Kaapa E, Han X, Holm S, Peltonen J, Takala T, Vanharanta H (1995). Collagen synthesis and types I, III, IV, and VI collagens in an animal model of disc degeneration. Spine 20.59-67.

Kadish LJ, Simmons EH (1984). Anomalies of the lumbosacral nerve roots. An anatomical investigation and myelographic study. JBJS 66B.411-416.

Kaneda K, Satoh S, Nohara Y, Oguma T (1985). Distraction rod instrumentation with posterolateral fusion in isthmic spondylolisthesis. Spine 10. 383-389.

Karas BE, Conrad KM (1996). Back injury prevention interventions in the workplace. An integrative review. AAOHN 44.189-196.

Karas R, McIntosh G, Hall H, Wilson L, Melles T (1997). The relationship between nonorganic signs and centralization of symptoms in the prediction of return to work for patients with low back pain. Physical Therapy 77.354-360.

Karppinen J, Malmivaara A, Kurunlahti M *et al.* (2001a). Periradicular infiltration for sciatica. A randomized controlled trial. Spine 26.1059-1067.

Karppinen J, Ohinmaa A, Malmivaara A *et al.* (2001b). Cost effectiveness of periradicular infiltration for sciatica. Subgroup analysis of a randomized controlled trial. Spine 26.2587-2595.

Katz JN, Lipson SJ, Larson MG, McInnes JM, Fossel AH, Liang MH (1991). The outcome of decompressive laminectomy for degenerative lumbar stenosis. JBJS 73A.809-816.

Katz JN, Dalgas M, Stucki G *et al.* (1995). Degenerative lumbar spinal stenosis. Diagnostic value of the history and physical examination. Arthritis & Rheumatism 38.1236-1241.

Katz JN, Lipson SJ, Chang LC, Levine SA, Fossel AH, Liang MH (1996). Seven to 10-year outcome of decompressive surgery for degenerative lumbar spinal stenosis. Spine 21.92-98.

Kay MA, Helewa A (1994). The effects of Maitland and McKenzie techniques in the musculoskeletal management of low back pain: a pilot study. Physical Therapy 74.5S.S59 (abstract).

Keegan JJ (1953). Alterations of the lumbar curve related to posture and seating. JBJS 35A.589-603.

Keim HA, Reina EG (1975). Osteoid-osteoma as a cause of scoliosis. JBJS 57A.159-163.

Kellgren JH (1939). On the distribution of pain arising from deep segmental somatic structures with charts of segmental pain areas. Clin Sci 4.35-46.

Kellgren JH (1977). The anatomical source of back pain. Rheum & Rehab 16.3-12.

Kelsey JL (1975). An epidemiological study of acute herniated lumbar intervertebral discs. Rheumatology & Rehabilitation 14.144-159.

Kelsey JL, Githens PB, White AA *et al.* (1984a). An epidemiological study of lifting and twisting on the job and risk for acute prolapsed lumbar intervertebral disc. J Orthop Res 2.61-66.

Kelsey JL, Githens PB, O'Connor T (1984b). Acute prolapsed lumbar intervertebral disc. An epidemiological study with special reference to driving automobiles and cigarette smoking. Spine 9.608-613.

Kendall N, Watson P (2000). Identifying psychosocial yellow flags and modifying management. In: Ed. Gifford L. *Topical Issues in Pain 2. Biopsychosocial Assessment and Management.* Physiotherapy Pain Association, CNS Press, UK.

Kendall PH, Jenkins JM (1968). Exercises for backache: A double-blind controlled trial. Physiotherapy 54.154-157.

Kent DL, Haynor DR, Larson EB, Deyo RA (1992). Diagnosis of lumbar spinal stenosis in adults: a metaanalysis of the accuracy of CT, MR, and myelography. AJR 158.1135-1144.

Key JA, Ford LT (1948). Experimental intervertebral disc lesions. JBJS 30A.621-630.

Khuffash B, Porter RW (1989). Cross leg pain and trunk list. Spine 14.602-603.

Kilby J, Stigant M, Roberts A (1990). The reliability of back pain assessment by physiotherapists, using a 'McKenzie algorithm'. Physiotherapy 76.579-583.

Kilpikoski S, Airaksinen O, Kankaanpaa M, Leminen P, Videman T, Alen M (2002). Inter-tester reliability of low back pain assessment using the McKenzie method. Spine 27.E207-E214.

Kjellby-Wendt G, Styf J (1998). Early active training after lumbar discectomy. A prospective, randomised, and controlled study. Spine 23.2345-2351.

Klaber Moffett JA, Richardson PH (1995). The influence of psychological variables on the development and perception of musculoskeletal pain. Physio Theory & Pract 11.3-11.

Klaber Moffett J, Richardson G, Sheldon TA, Maynard A (1995). *Back Pain: Its Management and Cost to Society.* NHS Centre for Reviews and Dissemination, University of York.

Klapow JC, Slater MA, Patterson TL, Doctor JN, Atkinson JH, Garfin SR (1993). An empirical evaluation of multidimensional clinical outcome in chronic low back pain patients. Pain 55.107-118.

Klenerman L, Slade PD, Stanley IM *et al.* (1995). The predication of chronicity in patients with an acute attack of low back pain in a general practice setting. Spine 20.478-484.

Knutsson B, Lindh K, Telhag H (1966). Sitting – an electromyographic and mechanical study. Acta Orthop Scand 37.415-428.

Koes BW, Bouter LM, Beckerman H, van der Heijden GJMG, Knipschild PG (1991). Physiotherapy exercises and back pain: a blinded review. BMJ 302.1572-1576.

Koes BW, van Tulder MW, van der Windt DAWM, Bouter LM (1994). The efficacy of back schools: a review of randomized clinical trials. J Clin Epidem 47.851-862.

Koes BW, Scholten RJPM, Mens JMA, Bouter LM (1995). Efficacy of epidural steroid injections for low back pain and sciatica: a systematic review of randomised clinical trials. Pain 63.279-288.

Koes BW, van den Hoogen (1994). Efficacy of bed rest and orthosis of low-back pain. A review of randomised clinical trials. Eur J Phys Med Rehabil 4.86-93.

Koes BW, Assendelft WJJ, van der Heijden GJMG, Bouter LM (1996). Spinal manipulation for low back pain. An updated systematic review of randomized clinical trials. Spine 21.2860-2873.

Koes BW, Scholten RJPM, Mens JMA, Bouter LM (1997). Efficacay of NSAIDs for low back pain: a systematic review of randomised clinical trials. Ann Rheum Dis 56.214-223.

Kokmeyer DJ, van der Wurff P, Aufdemkampe G, Fickenscher TCM (2002). The reliability of multitest regimens with sacroiliac pain provocation tests. J Manip Physiol Ther 25.42-48.

Komori H, Shinomiya K, Nakai O, Yamaura I, Takeda S, Furuya K (1996). The natural history of herniated nucleus pulposus with radiculopathy. Spine 21.225-229.

Kopec JA, Esdaile JM, Abrahamowicz M *et al.* (1995). The Quebec back pain disability scale. Measurement properties. Spine 20.341-352.

Kopp JR, Alexander AH, Turocy RH, Levrini MG, Lichtman DM (1986). The use of lumbar extension in the evaluation and treatment of patients with acute herniated nucleus pulposus. A preliminary report. Clin Orthop & Rel Res 202:211-218.

Kortelainen P, Puranen J, Koivisto E, Lahde S (1985). Symptoms and signs of sciatica and their relation to the localization of the lumbar disc herniation. Spine 10.88-92.

Kostuik JP, Harrington I, Alexander D, Rand W, Evans D (1986). Cauda equina syndrome and lumbar disc herniation. JBJS 68A.386-391.

Krag MH, Seroussi RE, Wilder DG, Pope MH (1987). Internal displacement distribution from in vitro loading of human thoracic and lumbar spinal motion segments: Experimental results and theoretical predictions. Spine 12.1001-1007.

Krag MH, Cohen MC, Haugh LD, Pope MH (1990). Body height change during upright and recumbent posture. Spine 15.202-207.

Kramer J (1990). *Intervertebral Disk Diseases. Causes, Diagnosis, Treatment and Prophylaxis.* (2nd ed.). Thieme Medical Publishers, New York.

Kramer J (1995). Presidential address: Natural course and prognosis of intervertebral disc diseases. ISSLS, Seattle, Washington, June 1994. Spine 20.635-639.

Krause N, Ragland DR, Greiner BA, Fisher JM, Holman BL, Selvin S (1997). Physical workload and ergonomic factors associated with prevalence of back and neck pain in urban transit operators. Spine 22.211-2127.

Krause N, Ragland DR, Fisher JM, Syme SL (1998). Psychosocial job factors, physical workload, and incidence of work-related spinal injury: a 5-year prospective study of urban transit operators. Spine 23.2507-2516.

Kristiansson P, Svardsudd K (1996). Discriminatory power of tests applied in back pain during pregnancy. Spine 21.2337-2344.

Kristiansson P, Svardsudd K, von Schoultz B (1996a). Back pain during pregnancy. A prospective study. Spine 21.702-709.

Kristiansson P, Svardsudd K, von Schoultz B (1996b). Serum relaxin, symphyseal pain, and back pain during pregnancy. Am J Obstet Gynecol 175.1342-1347.

Kristiansson P (1997). S-Relaxin and pelvic pain in pregnant women. In: Eds Vleeming A, Mooney V, Dorman T, Snijders C, Stoeckart R. *Movement, Stability & Low Back Pain. The Essential Role of the Pelvis.* Churchill Livingstone, New York.

Kristiansson P, Nilsson-Wikmar L, von Schoultz B, Svardsudd K, Wramsby H (1998). Back pain in IVF-induced and spontaneous pregnancies. In: Eds Vleeming A, Mooney V, Tilscher H, Dorman T, Snijders C. *3rd Interdisciplinary World Congress on Low Back and pelvic pain.* November 19-21, 1998, Vienna, Austria.

Krogsgaard MR, Wagn P, Bengtsson J (1998). Epidemiology of acute vertebral osteomyelitis in Denmark. Acta Orthop Scand 69.513-517.

Kunogi JI, Hasue M (1991). Diagnosis and operative treatment of intraforaminal and extraforaminal nerve root compression. Spine 16.1312-1320.

Kuslich SD, Ulstrom CL, Michael CJ (1991). The tissue origin of low back pain and sciatica: A report of pain response to tissue stimulation during operations on the lumbar spine using local anaesthesia. Orth Clin Nth Am 22.181-187.

Lahad A, Malter AD, Berg AO, Deyo RA (1994). The effectiveness of four interventions for the prevention of low back pain. JAMA 272.1286-1291.

Lane JM, Riley EH, Wirganowicz PZ (1996). Osteoporosis: diagnosis and treatment. JBJS 78A.618-632.

Lanier DC, Stockton P (1988). Clinical predictors of outcomes of acute episodes of low back pain. J Family Pract 27.483-489.

Lansbury G (2000). Chronic pain management: a qualitative study of elderly people's preferred coping strategies and barriers to management. Disability & Rehab 22.2-14.

LaRocca H (1992). Taxonomy of chronic pain syndromes. Spine 17.S344-S355.

Laslett M, Michaelsen DJ (1991). A survey of patients suffering mechanical low back pain syndrome or sciatica treated with the "McKenzie method". NZ J Physiotherapy 24-32.

Laslett M, Schreck R, Williams M, Foley K, Fellows D (1992). The relationship between lumbar list and the topographical position of herniated nucleus pulposus (abstract). *International Federation of Orthopaedic Manipulative Therapists (IFOMT)*, June 1-5, Vail, Colorado. McKenzie Institute (UK) Newsletter 1.2.32.

Laslett M, Williams M (1994). The reliability of selected pain provocation tests for sacroiliac joint pathology. Spine 19.11.1243-1249.

Laslett M (1997). Pain provocation sacroiliac joint tests: reliability and prevalence. In *Movement, Stability & Low Back Pain. The essential role of the pelvis*. Eds Vleeming A, Mooney V, Dorman T, Snijders C, Stoeckart R, Churchill Livingstone, New York.

Latza U, Kohlmann T, Deck R, Raspe H (2000). Influence of occupational factors on the relation between socio-economic status and self-reported back pain in a population-based sample of German adults with back pain. Spine 25.1390-1397.

Lawrence RC, Helmick CG, Arnett FC, Deyo RA *et al.* (1998). Estimates of the prevalence of arthritis and selected musculoskeletal disorders in the United States. Arthr & Rheum 41.778-799.

Leboeuf-Yde C, Klougart N, Lauritzen T (1996). How common is low back pain in the Nordic population? Data from a recent study on a middle-aged general Danish population and four surveys previously conducted in the Nordic countries. Spine 21.1518-1526.

Leboeuf-Yde C, Kyvik KO (1998). At what age does low back pain become a common problem? A study of 29,424 individuals aged 12-41 years. Spine 23.228-234.

Leclaire R, Blier F, Fortin L, Proulx (1997). A cross-sectional study comparing the Oswestry and Roland-Morris functional disability scales in two populations of patients with low back pain of different levels of severity. Spine 22.68-71.

Leclaire R, Fortin L, Lambert R, Bergeron YM, Rossignol M (2001). Radiofrequency facet joint denervation in the treatment of low back pain. A placebo-controlled clinical trial to assess efficacy. Spine 26.1411-1417.

Lee D (1997). Treatment of pelvic instability. In: Eds Vleeming A, Mooney V, Dorman T, Snijders C, Stoeckart R. *Movement, Stability & Low Back Pain. The Essential Role of the Pelvis.* Churchill Livingstone, New York.

Lee R, Evans J (1994). Towards a better understanding of spinal posteroanterior mobilisation. Physiotherapy 80.68-73.

Lehmann TR, Brand RA (1983). Instability of the lower lumbar spine. Orthop Trans 7.97.

Lehmann TR, Russell DW, Spratt KF (1983). The impact of patients with nonorganic physical findings on a controlled trial of transcutaneous electrical nerve stimulation and electroacupuncture. Spine 8.625-634.

Lentell G, Hetherington T, Eagan J, Morgan M (1992). The use of thermal agents to influence the effectiveness of a low-load prolonged stretch. JOSPT 16.200-207.

Lethem J, Slade PD, Troup JDG, Bentley G (1983). Outline of a fear-avoidance model of exaggerated pain perception – 1. Behavioural Research Therapy 21.401-408.

Levangie PK (1999a). Four clinical tests of sacroiliac joint dysfunction: the association of test results with innominate torsion among patients with and without low back pain. Physical Therapy 79.1043-1057.

Levangie PK (1999b). The association between static pelvic asymmetry and low back pain. Spine 24.1234-1242.

Levine J, Taiwo Y (1994). Inflammatory pain. In: Eds Wall PD, Melzack R. *Textbook of Pain* (3rd ed.), 45-56. Churchill Livingstone, Edinburgh.

Light KE, Nuzik S, Personius W, Barstrom A (1984). Low-load prolonged stretch vs. high-load brief stretch in treating knee contractures. Physical Therapy 64.330-333.

Lilius G, Laasonen EM, Myllynen P, Harilainen A, Gronlund G (1989). Lumbar facet joint syndrome. A randomised clinical trial. JBJS 71B.681-684.

Lindgren KA, Sihvonen T, Leino E, Pitkanen M, Mannien H (1993). Exercise therapy effects on functional radiographic findings and segmental electromyographic activity in lumbar spine instability. Arch Phys Med Rehabil 74.933-939.

Lindsay DM, Meeuwisse WH, Mooney ME, Summersides J (1995). Interrater reliability of manual therapy assessment techniques. Physio Canada 47.173-180.

Linssen ACG, Spinhoven P (1992). Multimodal treatment programmes for chronic pain: a quantitative analysis of existing research data. J Pysch Res 36.275-286.

Linton SJ, Kamwendo K (1987). Low back schools. A critical review. Physical Therapy 67.1375-1383.

Linton SJ (1996). Early interventions for the secondary prevention of chronic musculoskeletal pain. In: Ed. Campbell JN. *Pain 1996 – An Updated Review.* IASP, Seattle.

Linton SJ, Hellsing AL, Hallden K (1998). A population-based study of spinal pain among 35-45-year-old individuals. Spine 23.1457-1463.

Linton SJ (1998). The socioeconomic impact of chronic back pain: Is anyone benefitting? Pain 75.163-168.

Linton SJ (2000a). A review of psychological risk factors in back and neck pain. Spine 25.1148-1156.

Linton SJ (2000b). Psychological risk factors for neck and back pain. In: Eds Nachemson AL, Jonsson E. *Neck and Back Pain. The Scientific Evidence of Causes, Diagnosis, and Treatment*. Lippincott Williams & Wilkins, Philadelphia.

Linton SJ, van Tulder MW (2000). Preventive interventions for back and neck pain. In: Eds Nachemson AL, Jonsson E. *Neck and Back Pain. The Scientific Evidence of Causes, Diagnosis, and Treatment*. Lippincott Williams & Wilkins, Philadelphia.

Linton SJ, Ryberg M (2001). A cognitive-behavioral group intervention as prevention for persistent neck and back pain in a non-patient population: a randomised controlled trial. Pain 90.83-90.

Linton SJ, van Tulder MW (2001). Preventive interventions for back and neck pain. What is the evidence? Spine 26.778-787.

Little H (1988). The natural history of ankylosing spondylitis. J Rheum 15.1179-1180.

Little P, Roberts L, Blowers H *et al.* (2001). Should we give detailed advice and information booklets to patients with back pain? A randomized controlled factorial trial of a self-management booklet and doctor advice to take exercise for back pain. Spine 26.2065-2072.

Locker D, Dunt D (1978). Theoretical and methodological issues in sociological studies of consumer satisfaction with medical care. Soc Sci Med 12.283-292.

Long AL (1995). The centralization phenomenon. Its usefulness as a predictor of outcome in conservative treatment of chronic low back pain (a pilot study). Spine 20.2513-2521.

Lonstein JE (1992). Spinal deformities. In: Ed. Jayson MIV. *The Lumbar Spine and Back Pain* (4th ed.). Churchill Livingstone, Edinburgh.

Lonstein JE (1999). Spondylolisthesis in children. Cause, natural history, and management. Spine 24.2640-2648.

Lord MJ, Small JM, Dinsay JM, Watkins RG (1997). Lumbar lordosis. Effects of sitting and standing. Spine 22.2571-2574.

Lorig K, Lubeck D, Kraines RG, Seleznick M, Holman HR (1985). Outcomes of self-help education for patients with arthritis. Arth & Rheum 28.680-685.

Lorig KR, Mazonson PD, Holman HR (1993). Evidence suggesting that health education for self-management in patients with chronic arthritis has sustained health benefits while reducing health care costs. Arth & Rheum 36.439-446.

Lorig K (1995). Patient education: Treatment or nice extra. Br J Rheum 34.703-704.

Lorio MP, Bernstein AJ, Simmons EH (1995). Sciatic spinal deformity – lumbosacral list: an "unusual" presentation with review of the literature. J Spinal Disorders 8.201-205.

Lorish CD, Boutagh ML (1997). Patient education in rheumatology. Current Opinion in Rheum 9.106-111.

Loupasis GA, Stamos K, Katonis PG, Sapkas G, Korres DS, Hartofilakidis G (1999). Seven- to 20-year outcome of lumbar discectomy. Spine 24.2313-2317.

Lovell FW, Rothstein JM, Personius WJ (1989). Reliability of clinical measurements of lumbar lordosis taken with a flexible rule. Physical Therapy 69.96-105.

Lowe J, Schachner E, Hirschberg E, Shapiro Y, Libson E (1984). Significance of bone scintigraphy in symptomatic spondylolysis. Spine 9.653-655.

Lowe RW, Hayes TD, Kaye J, Bagg RJ, Luekens CA (1976). Standing roentgenograms in spondylolisthesis. Clin Orth & Rel Res 117.80-84.

Lu YM, Hutton WC, Gharpuray VM (1996). Do bending, twisting, and diurnal fluid changes in the disc affect the propensity to prolapse? A viscoelastic finite element model. Spine 21.2570-2579.

Maclennan AH, Nicholson R, Green RC, Bath M (1986). Serum relaxin and pelvic pain of pregnancy. Lancet 243-245.

Macnab I, McCulloch J (1990). *Backache* (2nd ed.). Williams & Wilkins, Baltimore.

Maezawa S, Muro T (1992). Pain provocation at lumbar discography as analyzed by computed tomography/discography. Spine 17.1309-1315.

Magni G, Caldieron C, Rigatti-Luchini S, Merskey H (1990). Chronic musculoskeletal pain and depressive symptoms in the general population. An analysis of the 1st National Health and Nutritional Examination Survey data. Pain 43.299-307.

Magnusson ML, Bishop JB, Hasselquist L, Spratt KF, Szpalski M, Pope MH (1998a). Range of motion and motion patterns in patients with low back pain before and after rehabilitation. Spine 23.2631-2639.

Magnusson SP, Aagard P, Simonsen E, Bojsen-Moller F (1998b). A biomechanical evaluation of cyclic and static stretch in human skeletal muscle. Int J Sports Med 19.310-316.

Magora A (1972). Investigation of the relation between low back pain and occupation. Industrial Medicine 41.5-9.

Magora A (1973). Investigation of the relation between low back pain and occupation. Physical requirements: bending, rotation, reaching and sudden maximal effort. Scandinavian J Rehab Med 5.186-190.

Magora A (1975). Investigation of the relation between low back pain and occupation. Scand J Rehab Med 7.146-151.

Magora A, Schwartz A (1976). Relation between the low back pain syndrome and x-ray findings. 1. Degenerative osteoarthritis. Scand J Rehab Med 8.115-125.

Maher C, Latimer J (1992). Pain or resistance – the manual therapists' dilemma. Aus J Physio 38.257-260.

Maher C, Adams R (1994). Reliability of pain and stiffness assessments in clinical manual lumbar spine examination. Physical Therapy 74.801-811.

Maher C, Adams R (1995). Is the clinical concept of spinal stiffness multidimensional? Physical Therapy 75.854-864.

Maher C, Latimer J, Refshauge K (1999). Prescription of activity for low back pain: What works? Aus J Physio 45.121-132.

Maher CG (2000). A systematic review of workplace interventions to prevent low back pain. Aus J Physio 46.259-269.

Main CJ, Waddell G (1998). Spine Update. Behavioural responses to examination. A reappraisal of the interpretation of "nonorganic signs". Spine 23.2367-2371.

Maitland GD (1986). *Vertebral Manipulation* (5th ed.). Butterworths, London, p 21.

Maitland GD (1991). *Peripheral Manipulation* (3rd ed.). Butterworth Heinemann, Oxford, pp221-224.

Maigne JY, Rime B, Deligne B (1992). Computed tomographic follow-up study of forty-eight cases of nonoperatively treated lumbar intervertebral disc herniation. Spine17.1071-1074.

Maigne J-Y, Aivalikilis A, Pfefer F (1996). Results of sacroiliac joint double block and value of sacroiliac pain provocation tests in 54 patients with low back pain. Spine 21.16.1889-1892.

Maistrelli GL, Vaughan PA, Evans DC, Barrington TW (1987). Lumbar disc herniations in the elderly. Spine 12.63-66.

Majeske C, Buchanan C (1984). Quantitative description of two sitting postures, with and without a lumbar support pillow. Physical Therapy 64.1531-1533.

Malmivaara A, Hakkinen U, Aro T *et al.* (1995). The treatment of acute low back pain – bed rest, exercises, or ordinary activity? NEJM 332.351-355.

Mandal AC (1984). The correct height of school furniture. Physiotherapy 70.48-53.

Maniadakis N, Gray A (2000). The economic burden of back pain in the UK. Pain 84.95-103.

Mann M, Glasheen-Wray M, Nyberg R (1984). Therapist agreement for palpation and observation of iliac crest heights. Physical Therapy 64.334-338.

Manniche C, Skall HF, Braendhot L *et al.* (1993a). Clinical trial of postoperative dynamic back exercises after first lumbar discectomy. Spine 18.92-97.

Manniche C, Asmussen K, Lauritsen B *et al.* (1993b). Intensive dynamic back exercises with or without hyperextension in chronic back pain after surgery for lumbar disc protrusion. A clinical trial. Spine 18.560-567.

Mannion AF, Dolan P, Adams MA (1996). Psychological questionnaires: Do "abnormal" scores precede or follow first-time low back pain? Spine 21.2603-2611.

Mantle MJ, Greenwood RM, Currey HLF (1977). Backache in pregnancy. Rheum & Rehab 16.95-101.

Mantle MJ, Holmes J, Currey HLF (1981). Bachache in pregnancy 2: Prophylactic influence of back care classes. Rheum & Rehab 20.227-232.

Marhold C, Linton SJ, Melin L (2001). A cognitive-behavioral return-to-work program: effects on pain patients with a history of long-term versus short-term sick leave. Pain 91.155-163.

Marks R (1989). Distribution of pain provoked from lumbar facet joints and related structures during diagnostic spinal infiltration. Pain 39.37-40.

Marras WS, Lavender SA, Leurgens SE *et al.* (1993). The role of dynamic three-dimensional trunk motion in occupationally-related low back disorders. Spine 18.617-628.

Massett D, Malchaire J (1994). Low back pain. Epidemiologic aspects and work-related factors in the steel industry. Spine 19.143-146.

Matsubara Y, Kato F, Mimatsu K, Kajino G, Nakamura S, Nitta H (1995). Serial changes on MRI in lumbar disc herniations treated conservatively. Neuroradiology 37.378-383.

Matsui H, Ohmori K, Kanamori M, Ishihara H, Tsuji H (1998). Significance of sciatic scoliotic list in operated patients with lumbar disc herniation. Spine 23.338-342.

Matyas TA, Bach TM (1985). The reliability of selected techniques in clinical arthrometrics. Aus J Physio 31.175-199.

Mau W, Zeidler H, Mau R, Majewski A, Freyschmidt J, Deicher H (1987). Outcome of possible ankylosing spondylitis in a 10 years' follow-up study. Clin Rheum 6.S2.60-66.

Mau W, Zeidler H, Mau R et al. (1988). Clinical features and prognosis of patients with possible ankylosing spondylitis. Results of a 10-year follow up. J Rheumatol 15.1109-1114.

May S (1998). A qualitative study into patients' satisfaction with physiotherapy care for low back pain, and patients' opinions about self-management for back pain. MSc, Sheffield University.

May S (2001). Patient satisfaction with management of back pain. Part 2: An explorative, qualitative study into patients' satisfaction with physiotherapy. Physiotherapy 87.10-20.

Mazzuca SA, Brandt KD, Katz BP, Chambers M, Byrd D, Hanna M (1997). Effects of self-care education on the health status of inner-city patients with osteoarthritis of the knee. Arth & Rheum 40.1466-1474.

McCall IW, Park WM, O'Brien JP, Seal V (1985). Acute traumatic intraosseous disc herniation. Spine 10.134-137.

McCarron RF, Wimpee MW, Hudkins PG, Laros GS (1987). The inflammatory effect of nucleus pulposus. A possible element in the pathogenesis of low-back pain. Spine 12.760-764.

McCarthy C, Cushnaghan J, Dieppe P (1994). Osteoarthritis. In *Textbook of Pain* (3rd ed.). Eds Wall PD, Melzack R. Churchill Livingstone, Edinburgh.

McCombe PF, Fairbank JCT, Cockersole BC, Pynsent PB (1989). Reproducibility of physical signs in low-back pain. Spine 14.9.908-918.

McCulloch JA, Waddell G (1980). Variation of the lumbosacral myotomes with bony segmental anomalies. JBJS 62B.475-480.

McFadden JW (1988). The stress lumbar discogram. Spine 13.931-933.

McGill SM, Brown S (1992). Creep response of the lumbar spine to prolonged full flexion. Clin Biomech 7.43-46.

McGorry RW, Webster BS, Snook SH, Hsiang SM (2000). The relation between pain intensity, disability, and the episodic nature of chronic and recurrent low back pain. Spine 25.834-841.

McGregor AH, McCarthy ID, Hughes SPF (1995). Motion characteristics of normal subjects and people with low back pain. Physiotherapy 81.632-637.

McGuirk B, King W, Govind J, Lowry J, Bogduk N (2001). Safety, efficacy, and cost effectiveness of evidence-based guidelines for the mangement of acute low back pain in primary care. Spine 26.2615-2622.

McKenzie AM, Taylor NF (1997). Can physiotherapists locate lumbar spinal levels by palpation? Physiotherapy 83.235-239.

McKenzie RA (1972). Manual correction of sciatic scoliosis. NZ Med J 76.194-199.

McKenzie RA (1979). Prophylaxis in recurrent low back pain. NZ Med J 89.22-23.

McKenzie RA (1981). *The Lumbar Spine. Mechanical Diagnosis and Therapy*. Spinal Publications, New Zealand.

McKenzie R (1989). A perspective on manipulative therapy. Physiotherapy 75.440-444.

McKenzie R (1997). *Treat Your Own Back* (5th ed.). Spinal Publications New Zealand Ltd.

McKenzie R, May S (2000). *The Human Extremities Mechanical Diagnosis and Therapy*. Spinal Publications New Zealand Ltd.

McKinnon ME, Vickers MR, Ruddock VM, Townsend J, Meade TW (1997). Community studies of the health service implications of low back pain. Spine 22.2161-2166.

McLean IP, Gillan MGC, Ross JC, Aspden RM, Porter RW (1996). A comparison of methods for measuring trunk list. A simple plumbline is the best. Spine 21.1667-1670.

McNair PJ, Dombroski EW, Hewson DJ, Stanley SN (2000). Stretching at the ankle joint: viscoelastic responses to holds and continuous passive motion. Med Sci Sports Exerc 33.354-358.

McNally DS, Adams MA (1992). Internal intervertebral disc mechanics as revealed by stress profilometry. Spine 17.66-73.

McNally DS, Adams MA, Goodship AE (1993). Can intervertebral disc prolapse be predicted by disc mechanics? Spine 18.1525-1530.

McNally DS, Shackleford IM, Goodship AE, Mulholland RC (1996). *In vivo* stress measurement can predict pain on discography. Spine 21.2580-2587.

Meijne W, van Neerbos K, Aufdemkampe G, van der Wurff P (1999). Intraexaminer and interexaminer reliability of the Gillet test. J Manip Physiol Thera 22. 4-9.

Melton LJ (1997). Epidemiology of spinal osteoporosis. Spine 22.2S-11S.

Melzack R, Wall P (1988). *The Challenge of Pain* (2nd ed.) Penguin Books.

Mens JMA, Vleeming A, Stoeckart R, Stam HJ, Snijders CJ (1996). Understanding peripartum pain. Implications of a patient survey. Spine 21.1363-1370.

Mens JMA, Snijders CJ, Stam HJ (2000). Diagonal trunk muscle exercises in peripartum pelvic pain: a randomized clinical trial. Physical Therapy 80.1164-1173.

Merrilees MJ, Flint MH (1980). Ultrastructural study of tension and pressure zones in a rabbit flexor tendon. Am J Anat 157.87-106.

Merskey H (1975). Pain terms: a list with definitions and notes on usage. Pain 6.249-252.

Meyer RA, Campbell JN, Raja SN (1994). Peripheral neural mechanisms of nociception. In: *Textbook of Pain* (3rd ed.). Eds Wall PD, Melzack R. Churchill Livingstone, Edinburgh.

Michel A, Kohlmann T, Raspe H (1997). The association between clinical findings on physical examination and self-reported severity in back pain. Results of a population-based study. Spine 22.296-304.

Micheli L, Wood R (1995). Back pain in young athletes: significant differences from adults in causes and patterns. Arch Pediatr Adol Med 149.15-18.

Micheli LJ, Yancey RA (1996). Overuse injuries of the spine. In: Eds Harries M, Williams C, Stanish WD, Micheli LJ. *Oxford Textbook of Sports Medicine*. OUP, Oxford.

Miedema HS, Chorus AMJ, Wevers CWJ, van der Linden S (1998). Chronicity of back problems during working life. Spine 23.2021-2029.

Mielenz TJ, Carey TS, Dyrek DA, Harris BA, Garrett JM, Darter JD (1997). Physical therapy utilization by patients with acute low back pain. Physical Therapy 77.1040-1051.

Milette PC, Fontaine S, Lepanto L, Breton G (1995). Radiating pain to the lower extremities caused by lumbar disc rupture without spinal nerve root involvement. Am Soc Neurorad 16.1605-1613.

Milette PC (1997). The proper terminology for reporting lumbar intervertebral disk disorders. Am J Neurorad 18.1859-1866.

Milette PC, Fontaine S, Lepanto L, Cardinal E, Breton G (1999). Differentiating lumbar disc protrusions, disc bulges, and discs with normal contour but abnormal signal intensity. MRI with discographic correlations. Spine 24.44-53.

Milne S, Welch V, Brosseau L *et al.* (2001). Transcutaneous electrical nerve stimulation (TENS) for chronic low back pain (Cochrane Review). In: The Cochrane Library, Issue 2, 2001. Oxford: Update Software.

Minor SD (1996). Use of back belts in occupational settings. Physical Therapy 76.403-408.

Mior SA, McGregor M, Schut B (1990). The role of experience in clinical accuracy. J Manip Physio Thera 13.68-71.

Mitchell SL, Creed G, Thow M *et al.* (1999). *Physiotherapy Guidelines for the Management of Osteoporosis.* CSP, London.

Moller H, Sundin A, Hedlund R (2000). Symptoms, signs, and functional disability in adult spondylolisthesis. Spine 25.683-689.

Moller H, Hedlund R (2000). Surgery versus conservative management in adult isthmic spondylolisthesis. A prospective randomised study: part 1. Spine 25.1711-1715.

Moneta GB, Videman T, Kaivanto K, Aprill C *et al.* (1994). Reported pain during lumbar discography as a function of anular ruptures and disc degeneration. Spine 19.1968-1974.

Mooney V, Robertson J (1976). The facet syndrome. Clin Orth & Rel Res 115.149-156.

Moore JE, von Korff M, Cherkin D, Saunders K, Lorig K (2000). A randomized trial of a cognitive-behavioral program for enhancing back pain self care in a primary care setting. Pain 88.145-153.

Moore K, Dumas GA, Reid JG (1990). Postural changes associated with pregnancy and their relationship with low-back pain. Clin Biomechanics 5.169-174.

Moore RJ, Vernon-Roberts B, Fraser RD, Osti OL, Schembri (1996). The origin and fate of herniated lumbar intervertebral disc tissue. Spine 21.2149-2155.

Mootz RD, Keating JC, Kontz HP, Milus TB, Jacobs GE (1989). Intra and interobserver reliability of passive motion mobilisation of the lumbar spine. J Manip Physio Thera 12.440-445.

Moran R, O'Connell D, Walsh MG (1988). The diagnostic value of facet joint injections. Spine 13.1407-1410.

Morita T, Ikata T, Katoh S, Miyake R (1995). Lumbar spondylolysis in children and adolescents. JBJS 77B.620-625.

Moriwaki K, Yuge O (1999). Topographical features of cutaneous tactile hypoesthetic and hyperesthetic abnormalities in chronic pain. Pain 81.1-6.

Morley S, Eccleston C, Williams A (1999). Systematic review and meta-analysis of randomized controlled trials of cognitive behaviour therapy and behaviour therapy for chronic pain in adults, excluding headache. Pain 80.1-13.

Mullen PD, Laville EA, Biddle AK, Lorig K (1987). Efficacy of psychoeducational interventions on pain, depression, and disability in people with arthritis: a meta analysis. J Rheumatol S15.14.33-39.

Muller CF, Monrad T, Biering-Sorensen F, Darre E, Deis A, Kryger P (1999). The influence of previous low back trouble, general health, and working conditions on future sick-listing because of low back trouble. Spine 24.1562-1570.

Mulvein K, Jull G (1995). Kinematic analysis of the lumbar lateral flexion and lumbar lateral shift movement techniques. J Manual & Manip Therapy 3.104-109.

Mundt DJ, Kelsey JL, Golden AL *et al.* (1993)An epidemiological study of non-occupational lifting as a risk factor for herniated lumbar intervertebral disc. Spine 18.595-602.

Murphey F (1968). Sources and patterns of pain in disc disease. Clin Neurosurg 15.343-351.

Murphy PL, Volinn E (1999). Is occupational low back pain on the rise? Spine 24.691-697.

Murphy-Cullen CL, Larsen LC (1984). Interaction between the socio-demographic variables of physicians and their patients: its impact upon patient satisfaction. Soc Sci Med 19.163-166.

Nachemson A, Morris JM (1964). *In vivo* measurements of intradiscal pressure. JBJS 46A.1077-1092.

Nachemson A, Elfstrom G (1970). Intravital dynamic pressures in lumbar discs. Scand J Rehab Med S1.1-40.

Nachemson A (1992). Lumbar mechanics as revealed by lumbar intradiscal pressure measurements. In: Ed. Jayson MIV. *The Lumbar Spine and Back Pain* (4ᵗʰ ed.). Churchill Livingstone, Edinburgh.

Nachemson A (1999a). Back pain: Delimiting the problem in the next millennium. Int J Law Psychiatry 22.473-490.

Nachemson A (1999b). Failed Back Surgery Syndrome is syndrome of failed back surgeons. Pain Clinic 11.271-284.

Nachemson A, Vingard E (2000). Influences of individual factors and smoking on neck and low back pian. In: Eds Nachemson AL, Jonsson E. *Neck and Back Pain. The Scientific Evidence of Causes, Diagnosis, and Treatment*. Lippincott Williams & Wilkins, Philadelphia.

Nachemson A, Waddell G, Norlund AI (2000). Epidemiology of neck and back pain. In: Eds Nachemson AL, Jonsson E. *Neck and Back Pain. The Scientific Evidence of Causes, Diagnosis, and Treatment*. Lippincott Williams & Wilkins, Philadelphia.

Natarajan R, Andersson G (1994). A model to study the disc degeneration process. Spine 19.259-265.

Nelemans PJ, de Bie RA, de Vet HCW, Sturmans F (2001). Injection therapy for subacute and chronic benign low back pain. Spine 26.501-515.

Nelson MA, Allen P, Clamp SE, de Dombal FT (1979). Reliability and reproducibility of clinical findings in low-back pain. Spine 4.97-101.

Nelson MA (1992). Surgery – an overview. In: Ed. Jayson MIV. *The Lumbar Spine and Back Pain* (4th ed.). Churchill Livingstone, Edinburgh.

Newton M, Waddell G (1991). Reliability and validity of clinical measurements of the lumbar spine in patients with chronic low back pain. Physiotherapy 77.796-800.

Nicholas MK (1996). Theory and practice of cognitive-behavioural programs. IN Pain 1996 – An Updated Review. ED Campbell JN. IASP, Seattle.

Nichols PJR (1960). Short-leg syndrome. BMJ i.1863-1865.

Niggemeyer O, Strauss JM, Schulitz KP (1997). Comparison of surgical procedures for degenerative lumbar spinal stenosis: a meta-analysis of the literaure from 1975 to 1995. Eur Spine J 6.423-429.

Ninomiya M, Muro T (1992). Pathoanatomy of lumbar disc herniation as demonstrated by CT/Discography. Spine 17.1316-1322.

Nitta H, Tajima T, Sugiyama H, Moriyama A (1993). Study on dermatomes by means of selective lumbar spinal nerve block. Spine 18.1782-1786.

Nordin M, Campello M (1999). Physical therapy. Exercise and the modalities: when, what and why? Neuro Clin Nth Am 17.75-89.

Noren L, Ostgaard S, Nielsen TF, Ostgaard HC (1997). Reduction of sick leave for lumbar back and posterior pelvic pain in pregnancy. Spine 22.2157-2160.

Norland AI, Waddell G (2000). Cost of back pain in some OECD countries. In: Eds Nachemson AL, Jonsson E. *Neck and Back Pain. The Scientific Evidence of Causes, Diagnosis, and Treatment*. Lippincott Williams & Wilkins, Philadelphia.

Nwuga G, Nwuga V (1985). Relative therapeutic efficacy of the Williams and McKenzie protocols in back pain management. Physiotherapy Practice 4.99-105.

Nykvist F, Hurme M, Alaranta H, Kaitsaari M (1995). Severe Sciatica – A Thirteen Year Follow up of 342 Patients. (Abstract). ISSLS Conference, Helsinki, 18-22 June 1995.

O'Brien Cousins S (1998). *Exercise, Aging & Health. Overcoming Barriers to an Active Old Age*. Brunner/Mazel, Philadelphia.

O'Connell JEA (1943). Sciatica and the mechanism of the production of the clinical syndrome in protrusions of the lumbar intervertebral discs. Br J Surg 30.315-327.

O'Connell JEA (1951). Protrusions of the lumbar intervertebral discs. JBJS 33B.8-30.

O'Connell JEA (1955). Involvement of the spinal cord by intervertebral disc protrusions. Br J Surg 43.225-247.

Oda H, Taguchi T, Fuchigami Y (1999). Mini-symposium: Lumbar spinal canal stenosis. (2) Conservative treatment. Current Orthop 13.178-183.

O'Haire C, Gibbons P (2000). Inter-examiner and intra-examiner agreement for assessing sacroiliac anatomical landmarks using palpation and observation: pilot study. Manual Therapy 5.13-20.

O'Hara LJ, Marshall RW (1997). Far lateral lumbar disc herniation. JBJS 79B. 943-947.

Ohmori K, Ishida Y, Takatsu T, Inoue H, Suzuki K (1995). Vertebral slip in lumbar spondylolysis and spondylolisthesis. Long-tepm follow-up of 22 adult patients. JBJS 77B.771-773.

Ohnmeiss DD, Vanharanta H, Ekholm J (1997). Degree of disc disruption and lower extremity pain. Spine 22.1600-1605.

O'Leary A (1985). Self-efficacy and health. Behav Res Ther 23.437-451.

Oliver J, Middleditch A (1991). *Functional Anatomy of the Spine*. Butterworth-Heinemann, Oxford.

Olmarker K, Rydevik BL (1991). Pathophysiology of sciatica. Orth Clin Nth Am 22.223-234.

Olmarker K, Rydevik BL, Nordburg N (1993). Autologus nuclear pulposus induces neurophysiological and histologic changes in porcine cauda equina nerve roots. Spine 18.1425-1432.

Onel D, Sari H, Donmez C (1993). Lumbar spinal stenosis: Clinical/radiologic therapeutic evaluation in 145 patients. Conservative treatment or surgical intervention? Spine 18.291-298.

Ong LML, de Haes CJM, Hoos AM, Lammes FB (1995). Doctor-patient communication: A review of the literature. Soc Sci Med 40.903-918.

Osterbauer PJ, De Boer KF, Widmaier R, Petermann E, Fuhr AW (1993). Treatment and biomechanical assessment of patients with chronic sacroiliac syndrome. J Manip Physio Thera 16.82-90.

Osterman K, Schlenzka D, Poussa M, Seitsalo S, Virta L (1993). Isthmic spondylolisthesis in symptomatic and asymptomatic subjects, epidemiology, and natural history with special reference to disk abnormality and mode of treatment. Clin Orth & Rel Res 297.65-70.

Ostgaard HC, Andersson GBJ, Karlsson K (1991). Prevalence of back pain during pregnancy. Spine 16.549-552.

Ostgaard HC, Andersson GBJ (1991). Previous back pain and risk of developing back pain in a future pregnancy. Spine 16.432-436.

Ostgaard HC, Andersson GBJ, Schultz AB, Miller JAA (1993). Influence of some biomechanical factors on low-back pain in pregnancy. Spine 18.61-65.

Ostgaard HC, Zetherstrom G, Roos-Hansson E, Svanberg B (1994a). Reduction of back and posterior pelvic pain in pregnancy. Spine 19.894-900.

Ostgaard HC, Zetherstrom G, Roos-Hansson E (1994b). The posterior pelvic pain provocation test in pregnant women. Eur Spine J 3.258-260.

Ostgaard HC, Roos-Hansson E, Zetherstrom G (1996). Regression of back and posterior pelvic pain after pregnancy. Spine 21.2777-2780.

Ostgaard HC, Zetherstrom G, Roos-Hansson E (1997). Back pain in relation to pregnancy. A 6-year follow-up. Spine 22.2945-2950.

Ostgaard HC (1997). Lumbar back and posterior pelvic pain in pregnancy. In: Eds: Vleeming A, Mooney V, Dorman T, Snijders C, Stoeckart R. *Movement, Stability & Low Back Pain. The Essential Role of the Pelvis*. Churchill Livingstone, New York.

Osti OL, Vernon-Roberts B, Moore RJ, Fraser RD (1992). Annular tears and disc degeneration in the lumbar spine. JBJS 74B.678-682.

O'Sullivan PB, Twomey LT, Allison GT (1997). Evaluation of specific stabilizing exercise in the treatment of chronic low back pain with radiologic diagnosis of spondylolysis or spondylolisthesis. Spine 22.2959-2967.

Overman SS, Larson JW, Dickstein DA, Rockey PH (1988). Physical therapy care for low back pain. Physical Therapy 68.199-207.

Painting S, Chester T (1996). The effect of positions and movements on low back pain. McKenzie Institute (UK) Newsletter 4.8-11.

Papageorgiou AC, Rigby AS (1991). Low back pain. Br. J Rheum. 30.208-210.

Papageorgiou AC, Croft PR, Ferry S, Jayson MIV, Silman AJ (1995). Estimating the prevalence of low back pain in the general population. Spine 20.1889-1894.

Papageorgiou AC, Croft PR, Thomas E, Ferry S, Jayson MIV, Silman AJ (1996). Influence of previous pain experience on the episode incidence of low back pain: results from the south Manchester back pain study. Pain 66.181-185.

Papanicolaou N, Wilkinson RH, Emans JB, Treves S, Micheli LJ (1985). Bone scintigraphy and radiography in young athletes with low back pain. AJR 145.1039-1044.

Paquet N, Malouin F, Richards CL (1994). Hip-spine movement interaction and muscle activation patterns during sagital trunk movements in low back pain patients. Spine 19.596-603.

Park WM, McCall IW, O'Brien JP, Webb JK (1979). Fissuring of the posterior annulus fibrosus in the lumbar spine. Br J Rad 52.382-387.

Parke WW, Watanabe R (1990). Adhesions of the ventral lumbar dura. An adjunct source of discogenic pain? Spine 15.300-303.

Patrick BS (1975). Extreme lateral ruptures of lumbar intervertebral discs. Surg Neurol 3.301-304.

Payne WK, Oglivie JW (1996). Back pain in children and adolescents. Ped Clinics Nth Am 43.899-917.

Pearcy M, Portek I, Shepherd J (1985). The effect of low-back pain on lumbar spinal movements measured by three-dimensional x-ray analysis. Spine 10.150-153.

Pearcy MJ, Bogduk N (1988). Instantaneous axes of rotation of the lumbar intervertebral joints. Spine 13.1033-1041.

Pedersen PA (1981). Prognostic indicators in low back pain. J Roy Coll Gen Pract 31.209-216.

Pellecchia GL (1994). Lumbar traction: a review of the literature. JOSPT 20.262-267.

Penning L, Blickman JR (1980). Instability in lumbar spondylolisthesis: a radiologic study of several concepts. AJR 134.293-301.

Penning L, Wilmink JT (1987). Posture-dependent bilateral compression of L4 or L5 nerve roots in facet hypertrophy. A dynamic CT-myelographic study. Spine12.488-500.

Penning L (1992). Functional pathology of lumbar spinal stenosis. Clinical Biomechanics 7.3-17.

Pheasant S (1998). *Bodyspace. Anthropometry, Ergonomics and the Design of Work* (2nd ed.). Taylor & Francis, London.

Philadelphia Panel (2001a). Philadelphia Panel evidence-based clinical practice guidelines on selected rehabilitation interventions for low back pain. Physical Therapy 81.1641-1674.

Philadelphia Panel (2001b). Philadelphia Panel evidence-based clinical practice guidelines on selected rehabilitation interventions: overview and methodology. Physical Therapy 81.1629-1640.

Philips HC (1987). Avoidance behaviour and its role in sustaining chronic pain. Behav Res Ther 25.273-279.

Philips HC, Grant L (1991). The evolution of chronic back pain problems: A longitudinal study. Behav Res Ther 29.435-441.

Philips HC, Grant L, Berkowitz J (1991). The prevention of chronic pain and disability: a preliminary investigation. Behav Res Ther 29.443-450.

Pitkanen M, Manninen HI, Lindgren KA, Turunen M, Airaksinen O (1997). Limited usefulness of traction-compression films in the radiographic diagnosis of lumbar spinal instability. Comparison with flexion-extension films. Spine 22.193-197.

Polatin PB, Cox B, Gatchel RJ, Mayer TG (1997). A prospective study of Waddell signs in patients with chronic low back pain. When they may not be predictive. Spine 22.1618-1621.

Ponte DJ, Jensen GJ, Kent BE (1984). A preliminary report on the use of the McKenzie protocol versus Williams protocol in the treatment of low back pain. JOSPT 6.130-139.

Pope MH, Bevins T, Wilder DG, Frymoyer JW (1985). The relationship between anthrometric, postural, muscular, and mobility characteristics of males ages 18-55. Spine 10.644-648.

Pope MH, DeVocht JW, McIntyre DR, Marker TK (2000). The thoracolumbar spine. In: Eds: Mayer TG, Gatchel RJ, Polatin PB. *Occupational Musculoskeletal Disorders. Function, Outcomes & Evidence*. Lippincott Williams & Wilkins, Philadelphia.

Pople IK, Griffith HB (1994). Prediction of an extruded fragment in lumbar disc patients from clinical presentations. Spine 19.156-158.

Porter RW, Hibbert CS (1984). Symptoms associated with lysis of the pars interarticularis. Spine 9.755-758.

Porter RW, Hibbert C, Evans C (1984). The natural history of root entrapment syndrome. Spine 9.418-421.

Porter RW, Miller CG (1986). Back pain and trunk list. Spine 11.596-599.

Porter RW (1989). Mechanical disorders of the lumbar spine. Annals of Medicine 21.361-366.

Porter RW (1993). *Management of Back Pain* (2nd ed.). Churchill Livingstone, Edinburgh.

Postacchini F (1996). Spine Update. Results of surgery compared with conservative management for lumbar disc herniations. Spine 21.1383-1387.

Postacchini F, Cinotti G, Gumina S (1998). Microsurgical excision of lateral lumbar disc herniation through an interlaminar approach. JBJS 80B. 201-207.

Potter NA, Rothstein JM (1985). Intertester reliability for selected clinical tests of the sacroiliac joint. Physical Therapy 65.11.1671-1675.

Potter RG, Jones JM (1992). The evolution of chronic pain among patients with musculoskeletal problems: a pilot study in primary care. Br J Gen Pract 42.462-464.

Potter RG, Jones JM, Boardman AP (2000). A prospective study of primary care patients with musculoskeletal pain: the identification of predictive factors for chronicity. Br J Gen Pract 50.225-227.

Poyanli A, Poyanli O, Akan K, Sencer S (2001). Pneumococcal vertebral oteomyelitis. Spine 26.2397-2399.

Prendeville K, Dockrell S (1998). A pilot survey to investigate the incidence of low back pain in school children. Physio Ireland 19.3-7.

Punnett L, Fine LJ, Keyserling WM, Herrin GD, Chaffin DB (1991). Back disorders and nonneutral trunk postures of automobile assembly workers. Scand J Work Environ Health 17.337-346.

Pynt J, Higgs J, Mackey M (2001). Seeking the optimal posture of the seated lumbar spine. Physio Theory & Practice 17.5-21.

Quinnell RC, Stockdale HR (1983). Observations of pressures within normal discs in the lumbar spine. Spine 8.166-169.

Rainville J, Sobel JB, Hartigan C (1994). Comparison of total lumbosacral flexion and true lumbar flexion measured by a dual inclinometer technique. Spine 19.2698-2701.

Rankine JJ, Fortune DG, Hutchinson CE, Hughes DG, Main CJ (1998). Pain drawings in the assessment of nerve root compression: A comparative study with lumbar spine magnetic resonance imaging. Spine 23.1668-1676.

Rankine JJ, Gill KP, Hutchinson CE, Ross ERS, Williamson JB (1999). The clinical significance of the high-intensity zone on lumbar spine magnetic resonance imaging. Spine. 24.1913-1920.

Rantanen P, Airaksinen O (1989). Poor agreement between so-called sacroiliac joint tests in ankylosing spondylitis patients. J Manual Med 4.62-64.

Raspe HH (1993). Back pain. In: Eds Silman AJ, Hochberg MC. *Epidemiology of the Rheumatic Diseases*. Oxford University Press, Oxford.

Rath W, Rath JD (1996). Outcome assessment in clinical practice. McKenzie Institute (USA) Journal 4.9-16.

Raymond J, Dumas JM (1984). Intraarticular facet block: diagnostic test or therapeutic procedure? Radiology 151.333-336.

Razmjou H, Kramer JF, Yamada R (2000a). Intertester reliability of the McKenzie evaluation in assessing patients with mechanical low-back pain. JOSPT 30.368-389.

Razmjou H, Kramer JF, Yamada R, Spratt KF (2000b). Author response. JOSPT 30.386-389.

Rebbeck T (1997). The efficacy of the McKenzie regimen – a meta-analysis of clinical trials. Conference Proceedings: 10th Biennial Conference of Manipulative Physiotherapists Association of Australia, Nov 26-29, Melbourne, Australia, 156-161.

Rekola KE, Keinanen-Kiukaanniemi S, Takala J (1993). Use of primary health services in sparsely populated country districts by patients with musculoskeletal symptoms: consultations with a physician. J Epidem Comm Health 47.153-157.

Resnick D, Niwayama G (1978). Intravertebral disk herniations: cartilaginous (Schmorl's) nodes. Radiology 126. 57-65.

Revel ME, Listrat VM, Chevalier XJ et al. (1992). Facet joint block for low back pain: identifying predictors of a good response. Arch Phys Med Rehabil 73.824-828.

Revel M, Poiraudeau S, Auleley GR *et al.* (1998). Capacity of the clinical picture to characterize low back pain relieved by facet joint injection. Proposed criteria to identify patients with painful facet joints. Spine 23.1972-1977.

Reynolds PMG (1975). Measurement of spinal mobility: a comparison of three methods. Rheum & Rehab 14.180-185.

Richardson C, Jull G, Hodges P, Hides J (1999). *Therapeutic Exercise for Spinal Segmental Stabilization in Low Back Pain. Scientific Basis and Clinical Approach.* Churchill Livingstone, Edinburgh.

Ricketson R, Simmons JW, Hauser BO (1996). The prolapsed intervertebral disc. The high-intensity zone with discography correlation. Spine 21.2758-2762.

Riddle DL, Rothstein JM (1993). Intertester reliability of McKenzie's classification of the syndrome types present in patients with low back pain. Spine 18.1333-1344.

Riddle DL (1998). Classification and low back pain: A review of the literature and critical analysis of selected systems. Physical Therapy 78.708-737.

Rigby AS (1991). Review of UK data on the rheumatic diseases – 5. Ankylosing spondylitis. Br J Rheum 30.50-53.

Roach KE, Brown M, Ricker E, Altenburger P, Tompkins J (1995). The use of patient symptoms to screen for serious back problems. JOSPT 21.2-6.

Roberts A (1991). The Nottingham acute back pain study. Thesis. Nottingham, England.

Robertson VJ, Baker KG (2001). A review of therapeutic ultrasound: effectiveness studies. Physical Therapy 81.1339-1350.

Robinson M (1994). The McKenzie method of spinal pain management. In: Boyling JD, Palastanga N. *Grieve's Modern Manual Therapy* (2nd ed.), 753-769. Churchill Livingstone, Edinburgh.

Rodichok LD, Ruckdeschel JC, Harper GR *et al.* (1986). Early detection and treatment of spinal epidural metastases: the role of myelography. Ann Neurol 20.696-702.

Roland M, Morris R (1983). A study of the natural history of back pain. Part 1: Development of a reliable and sensitive measure of disability in low-back pain. Spine 8.141-144.

Roland M, Dixon M (1989). Randomized controlled trial of an educational booklet for patients presenting with back pain in general practice. J Royal College GP 39.244-246.

Roland M, van Tulder (1998). Should radiologists change the way they report plain radiography of the spine? Lancet 352.229-230.

Rollnick S, Mason P, Butler C (1999). *Health Behavior Change. A Guide for Practitioners.* Churchill Livingstone, Edinburgh.

Rose MJ, Reilly JP, Pennie B, Bowen-Jones K, Stanley IM, Slade PD (1997). Chronic low back pain rehabilitation programs. Spine 22.2246-2253.

Rosenberg NJ, Bargar WL, Friedman B (1981). The incidence of spondylolysis and spondylolisthesis in non-ambulatory patients. Spine 6.35-38.

Rothwell RS, Davis P, Lentle BC (1981). Radionuclide bone scanning in females with chronic low back pain. Ann Rheum Dis 40.79-82.

Ruff RL, Lanska DJ (1989). Epidural metastases in prospectively evaluated veterans with cancer and back pain. Cancer 63.2234-2241.

Russell AS, Maksymowych W, LeClercq S (1981). Clinical examination of the sacroiliac joints: a prospective study. Arth & Rheum 24.1575-1577.

Rydevik B, Brown MD, Lundborg G (1984). Pathoanatomy and pathophysiology of nerve root compression. Spine 9.7-15.

Rydevik BL, Myers RR, Powell HC (1989). Pressure increase in the dorsal root ganglion following mechanical compression. Spine 14.574-576.

Saal JA, Saal JS (1989). Nonoperative treatment of herniated lumbar intervertebral disc with radiculopathy. An outcome study. Spine 14.431-437.

Saal JA, Saal JS, Herzog RJ (1990). The natural history of lumbar intervertebral disc extrusions treated nonoperatively. Spine 15.683-686.

Saal JS (1995). The role of inflammation in lumbar pain. Spine 20.1821-1827.

Saal JS (1996). Natural history and nonoperative treatment of lumbar disc herniation. Spine 21.2S-9S.

Sachs BL, Vanharanta H, Spivey MA *et al.* (1987). Dallas discogram description. A new classification of CT/discography in low back disorders. Spine 12.287-294.

Safran MR, Seaber AV, Garrett WE (1989). Warm-up and muscular injury prevention. An update. Sports Med 8.239-249.

Saifuddin A, White J, Tucker S, Taylor BA (1998). Orientation of lumbar pars defects. Implications for radiological detection and surgical management. JBJS 80B.208-211.

Sala DS (1997). Notes from a fringe watcher. Physio Theory & Practice 13.113-115.

Sanderson PL, Fraser RD (1996). The influence of pregnancy on the development of degenerative spondylolisthesis. JBJS 78B.951-954.

Sanderson PL, Getty CJM (1996). Long-term results of partial undercutting facetectomy for lumbar lateral recess stenosis. Spine 21.1352-1356.

Santos-Eggimann B, Wietlisbach V, Rickenbach M, Paccaud F, Gutzwiller F (2000). One-year prevalence of low back pain in two Swiss regions. Spine 25.2473-2479.

Sato H, Kikuchi S (1993). The natural history of radiographic instability of the lumbar spine. Spine 18.2075-2079.

Sato K, Kikuchi S, Yonezawa T (1999). *In vivo* intradiscal pressure measurement in healthy individuals and in patients with ongoing back problems. Spine 24.2468-2474.

Scalzitti DA (1997). Screening for psychological factors in patients with low back problems: Waddell's nonorganic signs. Physical Therapy 77.306-312.

Scavone JG, Latshaw RF, Weidner WA (1981a). Anteroposterior and lateral radiographs: an adequate lumbar spine examination. AJR 136.715-717.

Scavone JG, Latshaw RF, Rohrer GV (1981b). Use of lumbar spine films. JAMA 246.1105-1108.

Schaberg J, Gainor BJ (1985). A profile of metastatic carcinoma of the spine. Spine 10.19-20.

Schade V, Semmer N, Main CJ, Hora J, Boos N (1999). The impact of clinical, morphological, psychosocial and work-related factors on the outcome of lumbar discectomy. Pain 80.239-249.

Schaller JG (1979). The seronegative spondyloarthropathies of childhood. Clin Orth & Rel Res 143.76-83.

Scheer SJ, Radack KL, O'Brien DR (1996). Randomized controlled trials in industrial low back pain relating to return to work. Part 2. Discogenic low back pain. Arch Phys Med Rehabil 77.1189-1197.

Schellhas KP, Pollei SR, Gundry CR, Heithoff KB (1996). Lumbar disc high-intensity zone. Correlation of MRI and discography. Spine 21.79-86

Schenk R (2000). A randomised clinical trial comparing therapeutic interventions for low back pain (abstract). Proceedings McKenzie North American Conference, Orlando, Florida, June 2-4, 90.

Schers H, Braspenning J, Drijver R, Wensing M, Grol R (2000). Low back pain in general practice: reported management and reasons for not adhering to the guidelines in the Netherlands. Br J Gen Pract 50.640-644.

Schnebel BE, Simmons JW, Chowning J, Davidson R (1988). A digitizing technique for the study of movement of intradiscal dye in response to flexion and extension of the lumbar spine. Spine 13.309-312.

Schnebel BE, Watkins RG, Dillin W (1989). The role of spinal flexion and extension in changing nerve root compression in disc herniations. Spine 14.835-837.

Schneiderman GA, McLain RF, Hambly MF, Nielsen SL (1995). The pars defect as a source of pain. A histologic study. Spine 20.1761-1764.

Schwarzer AC, Wang S, Laurent R, McNaught P, Brooks PM (1992). The role of the zygapophyseal joint in chronic low back pain. Aust NZ J Med 22.185.

Schwarzer AC, Aprill CN, Derby R, Fortin J, Kine G, Bogduk N (1994a). The false-positive rate of uncontrolled diagnostic blocks of the lumbar zygapophyseal joints. Pain 58.195-200.

Schwarzer AC, Aprill CN, Derby R, Fortin J, Kine G, Bogduk N (1994b). Clinical features of patients with pain stemming from the lumbar zygapophyseal joints. Is the lumbar facet syndrome a clinical entity? Spine 19.1132-1137.

Schwarzer AC, Derby R, Aprill CN, Fortin J, Kine G, Bogduk N (1994c). Pain from the lumbar zygapophyseal joints: a test of two models. J Spinal Dis 7.331-336.

Schwarzer AC, Aprill CN, Derby R, Fortin J, Kine G, Bogduk N (1994d). The relative contributions of the disc and zygapophyseal joint in chronic low back pain. Spine 19.801-806.

Schwarzer AC, Aprill CN, Bogduk N (1995a). The sacroiliac joint in chronic low back pain. Spine 20.1.31-37.

Schwarzer AC, Wang S, Bogduk N, McNaught P, Laurent R (1995b). Prevalence and clinical features of lumbar zygapophyseal joint pain: a study in an Australian population with chronic low back pain. Ann Rheum Dis 54.100-106.

Schwarzer AC, Wang S, O'Driscoll D, Harrington T, Bogduk N, Laurent R (1995c). The ability of computed tomography to identify a painful zygapophyseal joint in patients with chronic low back pain. Spine 20.907-912.

Schwarzer AC, Aprill CN, Derby R, Fortin J, Kine G, Bogduk N (1995d). The prevalence and clinical features of internal disc disruption in patients with chronic low back pain. Spine 20.1878-1883.

Scrimshaw SV, Maher CG (2001). Randomized controlled trial of neural mobilization after spinal surgery. Spine 26.2647-2652.

Seitsalo S (1990). Operative and conservative treatment of moderate spondylolisthesis in young patients. JBJS 72B.908-913.

Seitsalo S, Osterman K, Hyvarinen H, Schlenzka D, Poussa M (1990). Severe spondylolisthesis in children and adolescents. JBJS 72B.259-265.

Seitsalo S, Osterman K, Hyvarinen H, Tallroth K, Schlenzka D, Poussa M (1991). Progression of spondylolisthesis in children and adolescents. A long-term follow-up of 272 patients. Spine 16.417-421.

Selim AJ, Ren XS, Fincke G, Deyo RA *et al.* (1998). The importance of radiating leg pain in assessing health outcomes among patients with low back pain. Spine 23.470-474.

Shaffer WO, Spratt KF, Weinstein J, Lehmann TR, Goel V (1990). The consistency and accuracy of roentgenograms for measuring sagital translation in the lumbar vertebral motion segment. An experimental model. Spine 15.741750.

Shah JS, Hampson WGJ, Jayson MIV (1978). The distribution of surface strain in the cadaveric lumbar spine. JBJS 60B.246-251.

Shapiro S (2000). Medical realities of cauda equina syndrome secondary to lumbar disc herniation. Spine 25.348-352.

Shekelle PG, Adams AH, Chassin MR, Hurwitz EL, Brook RH (1992). Spinal manipulation for low-back pain. Ann Int Med 117.590-598.

Shekelle PG, Markovitch M, Louie R (1995). Comparing the costs between provider types of episodes of back pain care. Spine 20.221-227.

Shekelle P (1997). The epidemiology of low back pain. In: *Low Back Pain*, Eds Giles LGF, Singer KP, Butterworth Heineman, Oxford.

Shepperd J (1995). In vitro study of segmental motion in the lumbar spine. JBJS 77B.Supp2.161.

Shepperd JAN, Rand C, Knight G, Wetheral G (1990). Patterns of internal disc dynamic, cadaver motion studies. Orthop Trans 14.321.

Shipley JA, Beukes CA (1998). The nature of the spondylolytic defect. Demonstration of a communicating synovial pseudoarthrosis in the pars interarticularis. JBJS 80B.662-664.

Shirazi-Adl A (1989). Strain in fibres of a lumbar disc. Analysis of the role of lifting in producing disc prolapse. Spine 14.96-103.

Shirazi-Adl A (1994). Biomechanics of the lumbar spine in sagital/ lateral movements. Spine 19.2407-2414.

Shrier I, Gossal K (2000). Myths and truths of stretching. Physician & Sportsmed 28.57-63.

Siddall PJ, Cousins MJ (1997). Spine Update. Spinal pain mechanisms. Spine 22.98-104.

Sihvonen T, Lindgren KA, Airaksinen O, Mannien H (1997). Movement disturbance of the lumbar spine and abnormal back muscle electromyographic findings in recurrent low back pain. Spine 22.289-295.

Sikorski JM (1985). A rationalized approach to physiotherapy for low-back pain. Spine 10.571-579.

Silvers HR, Lewis PJ, Clabeaux DE, Asch HL (1994). Lumbar disc excisions in patients under the age of 21 years. Spine 19.2387-2392.

Sim J, Waterfield J (1997). Validity, reliability and responsiveness in the assessment of pain. Physio Theory & Practice 13.23-37.

Simmonds MJ, Kumar S, Lechelt E (1995). Use of a spinal model to quantify the forces and motion that occur during therapists' tests of spinal motion. Physical Therapy 75.212-222.

Simmons JW, Emery SF, McMillin JN, Landa D, Kimmich SJ (1991). Awake discography. A comparison study with magnetic resonance imaging. Spine 16.S6.S216-S221.

Simotas AC, Dorey FJ, Hansraj KK, Cammisa F (2000). Nonoperative treatment for lumbar spinal stenosis. Clinical and outcome results and a 3-year survivorship analaysis. Spine 25.197-204.

Simotas AC (2001). Nonoperative treatment for lumbar spinal stenosis. Clin Orth & Rel Res 384.153-161.

Simpson SR (1989). Evaluation of a flexible ruler technique for measuring lumbar lordosis in the clinical assessment of low back pain. J Soc Occup Med 39.25-29.

Simunic DI, Broom ND, Robertson PA (2001). Biomechanical factors influencing nuclear disruption of the intervertebral disc. Spine 26.1223-1230.

Sinaki M, Mikkelsen BA (1984). Postmenopausal spinal osteoporosis: flexion versus extension exercises. Arch Phys Med Rehabil 65.593-596.

Sinaki M, Lutness MP, Ilstrup DM, Chu CP, Gramse RR (1989). Lumbar spondylolisthesis: retrospective comparison and three-year follow-up of two conservative treatment programmes. Arch Phys Med Rehabil 70.594598.

Sitzia J, Wood N (1997). Patient satisfaction: A review of issues and concepts. Soc Sci Med 45.1829-1843.

Skelton AM, Murphy EA, Murphy RJL, O'Dowd TC (1996). Patients' views of low back pain and its management in general practice. Br J General Practice 46.153-156.

Skovron ML, Szpalski M, Nordin M, Melot C, Cukier D (1994). Sociocultural factors and back pain: a population-based study in Belgian adults. Spine 19.129-137.

Skytte L (2001). The prognostic value of the centralization phenomenon on a patient population with subacute radiating symptoms. 7th McKenzie Institute International Conference, August 17-19, 2001, Ottawa, 228-232.

Slipman CW, Sterenfeld EB, Chou LH, Herzog R, Vresilovic E (1998). The predictive value of provocative sacroiliac joint stress maneuvers in the diagnosis of sacroiliac joint syndrome. Arch Phys Med Rehabil 79.288-292.

Slipman CW, Jackson HB, Lipetz JS, Chan KT, Lenrow D, Vresilovic EJ (2000). Sacroiliac joint pain referral zones. Arch Phys Med Rehabil 81.334-338.

Sluijs EM, Kok GJ, van der Zee J (1993). Correlates of exercise compliance in physical therapy. Physical Therapy 73.771-786.

Smedley J, Egger P, Cooper C, Coggon D (1997). Prospective cohort study of predictors of incident low back pain in nurses. BMJ 314.1225-1228.

Smedley J, Inskip H, Cooper C, Coggon D (1998). Natural history of low back pain. A longitudinal study in nurses. Spine 23.2422-2426.

Smith BMT, Hurwitz EL, Solsberg D *et al.* (1998). Interobserver reliability of detecting lumbar intervertebral disc high-intensity zone on magnetic resonance imaging and association of high-intensity zone with pain and annular disruption. Spine 23.2074-2080.

Smith CA (1994). The warm-up procedure: To stretch or not to stretch. A brief review. JOSPT 19.12-17.

Smith JA, Hu SS (1999). Management of spondylolysis and spondylolisthesis in the pediatric and adolescent population. Orth Clin Nth Am 30.487-499.

Smith JW, Walmsley R (1951). Experimental incision of the intervertebral disc. JBJS 33B.612-625.

Smith R (2000). Metabolic disorders of the spine. In: Eds Bartley R, Coffey P. *Management of Low Back Pain in Primary Care.* Butterworth Heinemann, Oxford.

Smyth MJ, Wright V (1958). Sciatica and the intervertebral disc. An experimental study. JBJS 40A.1401-1418.

Snook SH, Webster BS, McGorry RW, Fogleman MT, McCann KB (1998). The reduction of chronic non-specific low back pain through the control of early morning lumbar flexion. A randomised controlled trial. Spine 23.2601-2607.

Snook SH (2000). The reduction of chronic non-specific low back pain through the control of early morning lumbar flexion. Follow-up. Report McKenzie North American Conference, Orlando, Florida, USA.

Soler T, Calderon C (2000). The prevalence of spondylolysis in the Spanish elite athlete. Am J Sports Med 28.57-62.

Soukka A, Alaranta H, Tallroth KAJ, Heliovaara M (1991). Leg-length inequality in people of working age. The association between mild inequality and low-back pain is questionable. Spine 16.429-431.

Spencer DL (1990). Mechanisms of nerve root compression due to a herniated disc. In: Eds: Weinstein JN, Wiesel SW. *The Lumbar Spine.* WB Saunders Co, Philaidelphia pp141-145.

Spiliopoulou I, Korovessis P, Konstantinou D, Dimitracopoulos G (1994). IgG and IgM concentration in the prolapsed human intervertebral disc and sciatica etiology. Spine 19.1320-1323.

Spitzer WO, LeBlanc FE, Dupuis M *et al.* (1987). Scientific approach to the activity assessment and management of activity-related spinal disorders. Spine 12.7.S1-S55.

Spratt KF, Lehmann TR, Weinstein JN, Sayre HA (1990). A new approach to the low-back physical examination. Behavioural assessment of mechanical signs. Spine 15.96-102.

Spratt KF, Weinstein JN, Lehmann TR, Woody J, Sayre H (1993). Efficacy of flexion and extension treatments incorporating braces for low-back pain patients with retrodisplacement, spondylolisthesis, or normal sagital translation. Spine 18.1839-1849.

Spurling RG, Grantham EG (1940). Neurologic picture of herniations of the nucleus pulposus in the lower part of the lumbar region. Archives of Surgery 40.375-388.

Stankovic R, Johnell O (1990). Conservative treatment of acute low-back pain. A prospective randomised trial: McKenzie method of treatment versus patient education in "mini back school". Spine 15.120-123.

Stankovic R, Johnell O (1995). Conservative treatment of acute low-back pain. A 5-year follow-up study of two methods of treatment. Spine 20.469-472.

Stankovic R, Johnell O, Maly P, Willner S (1999). Use of lumbar extension, slump test, physical and neurological examination in the evaluation of patients with suspected herniated nucleus pulposus. A prospective clinical study. Manual Therapy 4.25-32.

Steiner ME, Micheli LJ (1985). Treatment of symptomatic spondylolysis and spondylolisthesis with the modified Boston brace. Spine 10.937-943.

Stewart MA (1984). What is a successful doctor-patient interview? A study of interactions and outcomes. Soc Sci Med 19.167-175.

Stinson JT (1993). Spondylolysis and spondylolisthesis in the athlete. Clin Sports Med 12.517-528.

Stokes IAF, Frymoyer JW (1987). Segmental motion and instability. Spine 12.688-691.

Strender LE, Sjoblom A, Sundell K, Ludwig R, Taube A (1997). Interexaminer reliability in physical examinations of patients with low back pain. Spine 22.814-820.

Streiner DL, Norman GR (1996). *PDQ Epidemiology* (2nd ed.). Mosby, St Louis.

Sturesson B (1997). Movement of the sacroiliac joint: a fresh look. In: Eds Vleeming A, Mooney V, Dorman T, Snijders C, Stoeckart R. *Movement, Stability & Low Back Pain. The Essential Role of the Pelvis.* Churchill Livingstone, New York.

Sturesson B, Uden G, Uden A (1997). Pain pattern in pregnancy and "catching" of the leg in pregnant women with posterior pelvic pain. Spine 22.1880-1884.

Sturesson B, Uden A, Vleeming A (2000a). A radiostereometric analysis of movements of the sacroiliac joints during the standing hip flexion test. Spine 25.364-368.

Sturesson B, Uden A, Vleeming A (2000b). A radiostereometric analysis of movements of the sacroiliac joints in the reciprocal straddle position. Spine 25.214-217.

Sufka A, Hauger B, Trenary M *et al.* (1998). Centralisation of low back pain and perceived functional outcome. JOSPT 27.205-212.

Suk KS, Lee HM, Moon SH, Kim NH (2001). Lumbosacral scoliotic list by lumbar disc herniation. Spine 26.667-671.

Sullivan MS, Dickinson CE, Troup JDG (1994). The influence of age and gender on lumbar spine sagital plane range of motion. A study of 1126 healthy subjects. Spine 19.682-686.

Sundararajan V, Konrad TR, Garrett J, Carey T (1998). Patterns and determinants of multiple provider use in patients with acute low back pain. J Gen Intern Med 13.528-533.

Szpalski M, Nordin M, Skovron ML, Melot C, Cukier D (1995). Health care utilisation for low back pain in Belgium. Spine 20.431-442.

Taimela S, Kujala UM, Salminen JJ, Viljanen T (1997). The prevalence of low back pain among children and adolescents. A nationwide, cohort-based questionnaire survey in Finland. Spine 22.1132-1136.

Taimela S, Diederich C, Hubsch M, Heinricy M (2000). The role of physical exercise and inactivity in pain recurrence and absenteeism from work after active outpatient rehabilitation for recurrent or chronic low back pain. A follow up study. Spine 25.1809-1816.

Takahashi K, Kagechika K, Takino T, Matsui T, Miyazaki T, Shima I (1995a). Changes in epidural pressure during walking in patients with lumbar spinal stenosis. Spine 20.2746-2749.

Takahashi K, Miyazaki T, Takino T, Matsui T, Tomita K (1995b). Epidural pressure measurements. Relationship between epidural pressure and posture in patients with lumbar spinal stenosis. Spine 20.650-653.

Takahashi H, Suguro T, Okazima Y, Motegi M, Okada Y, Kakiuchi T (1996). Inflammatory cytokines in the herniated disc of the lumbar spine. Spine 21.218-224.

Takahashi K, Shima I, Porter RW (1999). Nerve root pressure in lumbar disc herniation. Spine 24.2003-2006.

Takala EP, Viikari-Juntura E (2000). Do functional tests predict low back pain? Spine 25.2126-2132.

Tay ECK, Chacha PB (1979). Midline prolapse of a lumbar intervertebral disc with compression of the cauda equina. JBJS 61B.43-46.

Taylor JR, Twomey LT (1994). The effects of ageing on the intervertebral discs. In: Boyling JD, Palastanga N. Eds. *Grieve's Modern Manual Therapy* (2nd ed.). Churchill Livingstone, Edinburgh.

Taylor VM, Deyo RA, Cherkin DC, Kreuter W (1994). Low back pain hospitalization. Spine 19.1207-1213.

Taylor BF, Waring CA, Brashear TA (1995). The effects of therapeutic application of heat or cold followed by static stretch on hamstring muscle length. JOSPT 21.283-286.

Tenhula JA, Rose SJ, Delitto A (1990). Association between direction of lateral lumbar shift, movement tests, and side of symptoms in patients with low back pain syndrome. Physical Therapy 70.480-486.

Teplick JG, Haskin ME (1985). Spontaneous regression of herniated nucleus pulposus. AJR 145.371-375.

Terry W, Higgs J (1993). Educational programmes to develop clinical reasoning skills. Aus J Physio 39.47-51.

Thelander U, Fagerlund M, Friberg S, Larsson S (1994). Describing the size of lumbar disc herniations using computed tomography. A comparison of different size index calculations and their relation to sciatica. Spine 19.1979-1984.

Thomas E, Silman AJ, Papageorgiou AC, Macfarlane GJ, Croft PR (1998). Association between measures of spinal mobility and low back pain. An analysis of new attenders in primary care. Spine 23.343-347.

Thomas E, Silman AJ, Croft PR, Papageorgiou AC, Jayson MIV, Macfarlane GJ (1999). Predicting who develops chronic low back pain in primary care: A prospective study. BMJ 318.1662-1667.

Thomas KB (1987). General practice consultations: is there any point in being positive? BMJ 294.1200-1202.

Threlkeld AJ, Currier DP (1988). Osteoarthritis. Effects on synovial joint tissues. Physical Therapy 68.364-370.

Thorbjornsson CB, Alfredsson L, Fredriksson K et al. (2000). Physical and psychosocial factors related to low back pain during a 24-year period. A nested case-control study. Spine 25.369-375.

Timm KE (1994). A randomised-control study of active and passive treatments for chronic low back pain following L5 laminectomy. JOSPT 20.276-286.

Torgerson WR, Dotter WE (1976). Comparative roentgenographic study of the asymptomatic and symptomatic lumbar spine. JBJS 58A.850-853.

Toroptsova NV, Benevolenskaya LI, Karyakin AN, Sergeev IL, Erdesz S (1995). "Cross-sectional" study of low back pain among workers at an industrial enterprise in Russia. Spine 20.328-332.

Trede FV (2000). Physiotherapists' approaches to low back pain education. Physiotherapy. 86.427-433.

Triano JJ, Luttges MW (1982). Nerve irritation: a possible model of sciatic neuritis. Spine 7.129-136.

Troup JDG, Foreman TK, Baxter CE, Brown D (1987). The perception of back pain and the role of psychosocial tests of lifting capacity. Spine 12.645-657.

Tuite GF, Stern JD, Doran SE *et al.* (1994). Outcome after laminectomy for lumbar spinal stenosis. Part 1: Clinical correlations. J Neurosurg 81.699-706.

Turner JA, Ersek M, Herron L, Deyo R (1992). Surgery for lumbar spinal stenosis. Attempted meta-analysis of the literature. Spine 17.1-8.

Turner JA, Herron L, Deyo R (1993). Meta-analysis of the results of lumbar spine fusion. Acta Othop Scand S251.64.120-122.

Turner JA (1996). Educational and behavioural interventions for back pain in primary care. Spine 21.2851-2859.

Twomey LT, Taylor JR (1982). Flexion creep deformation and hysteresis in the lumbar vertebral column. Spine 7.116-122.

Twomey LT, Taylor JR, Oliver MJ (1988). Sustained flexion loading, rapid extension loading of the lumbar spine, and the physical therapy of related injuries. Physio Practice 4.129-138.

Twomey LT, Taylor JR (1994a). Factors influencing ranges of movement in the spine. In: Eds Boyling JD, Palastanga N. *Grieve's Modern Manual Therapy* (2nd ed.). Churchill Livingstone, Edinburgh.

Twomey LT, Taylor JR (1994b). Lumbar posture, movement, and mechanics. In: Eds Twomey LT, Taylor JR. *Clinics in Physical Therapy. Physical Therapy of the Low Back* (2nd ed.). Churchill Livingstone, New York.

Uden A, Landin LA (1987). Pain drawing and myelography in sciatic pain. Clin Orth & Rel Res 216. 124-130.

Udermann B, Tillotson J, Donelson R, Mayer J, Graves J (2000). Can an educational booklet change behaviour and pain in chronic low back pain patients? Abstract. 27th ISSLS, Adelaide, April 2000.

Udermann B, Spratt K, Donelson R, Tillotson J, Mayer J, Graves J (2001). Can an educational booklet change behaviour and pain in chronic low back pain patients? Abstract. 28th ISSLS, Edinburgh, June 2001

Underwood MR, Dawes P (1995). Inflammatory back pain in primary care. Br J Rheum 34.1074-1077.

Underwood MR, Morgan J (1998). The use of a back class teaching extension exercises in the treatment of acute low back pain in primary care. Family Practice 15.9-15.

Vad VB, Bhat AL, Lutz GE, Cammisa F (2002). Transforaminal epidural steroid injections in lumbosacral radiculopathy. A prospective randomized study. Spine 27.11-16.

van Baar ME, Dekker J, Bosveld W (1998). A survey of physical therapy goals and interventions for patients with back and knee pain. Physical Therapy 78.33-42.

van Deursen LLJM, Patijn J, Ockhuysen AL, Vortman BJ (1990). The value of some clinical tests of the sacroiliac joint. J Man Med 5.96-99.

van den Hoogen HMM, Koes BW, van Eijk JTM, Bouter LM (1995). On the accuracy of history, physical examination, and erythrocyte sedimentation rate in diagnosing low back pain in general practice. A criteria-based review of the literature. Spine 20.318-327.

van den Hoogen HJM, Koes BW, Deville W, Van Eijk JTM, Bouter LM (1997). The prognosis of low back pain in general practice. Spine 22.1515-1521.

van den Hoogen HJM, Koes BW, van Eijk JTM, Bouter LM, Deville W (1998). On the course of low back pain in general practice: A one year follow up study. Ann Rheum Dis 57.13-19.

van der Giezen AM, Bouter LM, Nijhuis FJN (2000). Prediction of return-to-work of low back pain patients sicklisted for 3-4 months. Pain 87.285-294.

Van der Heijden GJMG, Beurskens AJHM, Koes BW, Assendelft WJ, de Vet HC, Bouter LM (1995a). The efficacy of traction for back and neck pain: a systematic blinded review of randomised clinical trial methods. Physical Therapy 75.93-104.

Van der Heijden GJMG, Beurskens AJHM, Dirx MJM, Bouter LM, Lindeman E (1995b). Efficacy of lumbar traction: A randomised controlled trial. Physiotherapy 81.29-35.

van der Linden SM, Khan MA (1984). The risk of ankylosing spondylitis in HLA-B27 positive individuals: a reappraisal. J Rheumatol 11.727-728.

Van der Linden S, Valkenburg HA, Cats A (1984). Evaluation of diagnostic criteria for ankylosing spondylitis. Arth & Rheum 27.361-368.

Van der Windt DAWM, van der Heijden GJMG, van den Berg, ter Riet G, de Winter AF, Bouter LM (1999). Ultrasound therapy for musculoskeletal disorders: a systematic review. Pain 81.257-271.

van der Wurff P, Hagmeijer RHM, Meyne W (2000a). Clinical tests of the sacroiliac joint. A systematic methodological review. Part 1: reliability. Manual Therapy 5.30-36.

van der Wurff P, Meyne W, Hagmeijer RHM (2000b). Clinical tests of the sacroiliac joint. A systematic methodological review. Part 2: validity. Manual Therapy 5.89-96.

Van Dillen LR, Sahrmann SA, Norton BJ et al. (1998). Reliability of physical examination items used for classification of patients with low back pain. Physical Therapy 78.979-988.

Vanharanta H, Videman T, Mooney V (1986). McKenzie exercises, back trac, and back school in lumbar syndrome. *International Society for the Study of the Lumbar Spine,* Dallas, Texas, USA.

Vanharanta H, Sachs Bl, Spivey MA et al. (1987). The relationship of pain provocation to lumbar disc deterioration as seen by CT/Discography. Spine 12.295-298.

Vanharanta H, Guyer RD, Ohnmeiss DD et al. (1988). Disc deterioration in low-back syndromes. A prospective, multi-centre CT/Discrography study. Spine 13.1349-1351.

Vanharanta H, Ohnmeiss D, Rashbaum R *et al.* (1988). Effect of repeated trunk extension and flexion movements as seen by CT/discography. Clin. Trans 12.650-651.

van Kleef M, Barendse GAM, Kessels A *et al.* (1999). Randomized trial of radiofrequency lumbar facet denervation for chronic low back pain. Spine 24.1937-1942.

van Poppel MNM, Koes BW, Smid T, Bouter LM (1997). A systematic review of controlled clinical trials on the prevention of back pain in industry. Occupational & Environmental Med 54.841-847.

van Poppel MNM, Koes BW, Deville W, Smid T, Bouter LM (1998). Risk factors for back pain incidence in industry: a prospective study. Pain 77.81-86.

van Tulder MW, Koes BW, Bouter LM (1995). A cost-of-illness study of back pain in the Netherlands. Pain 62.233-240.

van Tulder MW, Koes BW, Bouter LM, Metsemakers JFM (1997a). Management of chronic nonspecific low back pain in primary care: A descriptive study. Spine 22.76-82.

van Tulder MW, Koes BW, Bouter LM (1997b). Conservative treatment of acute and chronic non-specific low back pain. A systematic review of randomised controlled trials of the most common interventions. Spine 22.2128-2156.

van Tulder MW, Assendelft WJJ, Koes BW, Bouter LM (1997c). Spinal radiographic findings and non-specific back pain. A systematic review of observational studies. Spine 22.427-434.

van Tulder MW, Cherkin DC, Berman B, Lao L, Koes BW (1999a). The effectiveness of acupuncture in the management of acute and chronic low back pain. A systematic review within the framework of the Cochrane collaboration back review group. Spine 24.1113-1123.

van Tulder MW, Esmail R, Bombardier C, Koes BW (1999b). Back schools for non-specific low back pain (Cochrane Review). In: *The Cochrane Library,* Issue 3, 1999. Oxford: Update Software.

van Tulder MW, Malmivaara A, Esmail R, Koes BW (2000a). Exercise therapy for low back pain. A systematic review within the framework of the Cochrane collaboration back review group. Spine 25.2784-2796.

van Tulder MW, Scholten RJPM, Koes BW, Deyo RA (2000b). Nonsteroidal anti-inflammatory drugs for low back pain. A systematic review within the framework of the Cochrane Collaboration Back Review Group. Spine 25.2501-2513.

van Tulder MW, Ostelo R, Vlaeyan JWS, Linton SJ, Morley SJ, Assendelft WJJ (2000c). Behavioiral treatment for chronic low back pain. A systematic review within the framework of the Cochrane Back Review Group. Spine 25.2688-2699.

Van Wijmen PM (1994). The use of repeated movements in the McKenzie method of spinal examination. In *Grieve's Modern Manual Therapy* (2nd ed.). Eds Boyling JD, Palastanga N. Churchill Livingstone, Edinburgh.

Videman T, Nurminen T, Tola *et al.* (1984). Low-back pain in nurses and some loading factors of work. Spine 9.400-404.

Videman T (1987). Connective tissue and immobilisation. Clin Orth & Rel Res 221.26-32.

Videman T, Rauhala H, Lindstrom K *et al.* (1989). Patient-handling skill, back injuries, and back pain. Spine 14.148-156.

Vincent-Smith B, Gibbons P (1999). Inter-examiner and intra-examiner reliability of the standing flexion test. Manual Therapy 4.87-93.

Vingard E, Nachemson A (2000). Work-related influences on neck and back pain. In: Eds: Nachemson AL, Jonsson E. *Neck and Back Pain. The Scientific Evidence of Causes, Diagnosis, and Treatment.* Lippincott Williams & Wilkins, Philadelphia.

Vingard E, Alfredsson L, Hagberg M *et al.* (2000). To what extent do current and past physical and psychosocial occupational factors explain care-seeking for low back pain in a working population. Spine 25.493-500.

Virri J, Gronblad M, Seitsalo S, Habtemariam A, Kaapa E, Karaharju E (2001). Comparison of the prevalence of inflammatory cells in subtypes of disc herniations and associations with straight leg raising. Spine 26.2311-2315.

Virta L, Ronnemaa T (1993). The association of mild-moderate isthmic lumbar spondylolisthesis and low back pain in middle-aged patients is weak and it only occurs in women. Spine 18.1496-1503.

Vlaeyen JWS, Linton SJ (2000). Fear-avoidance and its consequences in chronic musculoskeletal pain: a state of the art. Pain 85.317-332.

von Korff M, Dworkin SF, Le Resche L (1990). Graded chronic pain status: an epidemiological evaluation. Pain 40.279-291.

von Korff M, Ormel J, Keefe FJ, Dworkin SF (1992). Grading the severity of chronic pain. Pain 50.133-149.

von Korff M, Deyo RA, Cherkin DC, Barlow W (1993). Back pain in primary care. Spine 18.855-862.

von Korff M, Barlow W, Cherkin D, Deyo RA (1994). Effects of practice style in managing back pain. Ann Intern Med 121.187-195.

von Korff M, Saunders K (1996). The course of back pain in primary care. Spine 21.2833-2839.

von Korff M, Moore JE, Lorig K *et al.* (1998). A randomised trial of a lay person-led self-management group intervention for back pain patients in primary care. Spine 23.2608-2615.

Vroomen PCAJ, de Krom MCTFM, Wilmink JT, Kester ADM, Knottnerus JA (1999). Lack of effectiveness of bed rest for sciatica. N Eng J Med 340.418-423.

Vroomen PCAJ, de Krom MCTFM, Knottnerus JA (2000). Consistency of history taking and physical examination in patients with suspected lumbar nerve root involvement. Spine 25.91-97.

Vucetic N, Maattanen H, Svensson O (1995). Pain and pathology in lumbar disc hernia. Clin Orth & Rel Res 320.65-72.

Waddell G, McCulloch JA, Kummel E, Venner RM (1980). Nonorganic physical signs in low-back pain. Spine 5.117-125.

Waddell G, Main CJ, Morris EW, *et al.* (1982). Normality and reliability in the clinical assessment of backache. BMJ 284.1519-1523.

Waddell G, Main CJ (1984). Assessment of severity in low-back disorders. Spine 9.204-208.

Waddell G, Main CJ, Morris EW, Di Paola M, Gray ICM (1984). Chronic low-back pain, psychologic distress, and illness behaviour. Spine 9.209-213.

Waddell G, Morris EW, Di Paola MP *et al.* (1986). A concept of illness tested as an improved basis for surgical decisions in low-back disorders. Spine 11.712-719.

Waddell G (1987). A new clinical model for the treatment of low back pain. Spine 12.632-644.

Waddell G, Somerville D, Henderson I, Newton M (1992). Objective clinical evaluation of physical impairment in chronic low back pain. Spine 17.617-628.

Waddell G, Newton M, Henderson I, Somerville D, Main C (1993). A fear avoidance beliefs questionnaire (FABQ) and the role of fear avoidance beliefs in chronic low back pain and disability. Pain 52.157-168.

Waddell G (1994). *Epidemiology Review. Annex to CSAG Report on Back Pain.* HMSO, London.

Waddell G, Feder G, Lewis M (1997). Systematic reviews of bed rest and advice to stay active for acute low back pain. Br J Gen Pract 47.647-652.

Waddell G (1998). *The Back Pain Revolution.* Churchill Livingstone, Edinburgh.

Waddell G, McIntosh A, Hutchinson A, Feder G, Lewis M (1999). *Low Back Pain Evidence Review.* Royal College of General Practitioners, London.

Waddell G, Gibson JNA, Grant I (2000). Surgical treatment of lumbar disc prolapse and degenerative lumbar disc disease. In: Eds Nachemson AL, Jonsson E. *Neck and Back Pain. The Scientific Evidence of Causes, Diagnosis, and Treatment.* Lippincott Williams & Wilkins, Philadelphia.

Wainwright A (2000). Spinal infection. In: Eds Bartley R, Coffey P. *Management of Low Back Pain in Primary Care.* Butterworth Heinemann, Oxford.

Waldvogel FA, Vasey H (1980). Osteomyelitis: the past decade. New Eng J Med 303.360-370.

Walker JM (1992). The sacroiliac joint: A critical review. Physical Therapy 72.903-916.

Wallin D, Ekblom B, Grahn R, Nordenborg T (1985). Improvement in muscle flexibility. A comparison betrween two techniques. Am J Sports Med 13.263-268.

Walsh D (1991). Nociceptive pathways – Relevance to the physiotherapist. Physiotherapy 77.317-321.

Walsh K, Cruddas M, Coggon D (1992). Low back pain in eight areas of Britain. J Epidem Comm Health 46.227-230.

Walsh TR, Weinstein JN, Spratt KF, Lehmann TR, Aprill C, Sayre H (1990). Lumbar discography in normal subjects. A controlled, prospective study. JBJS72A.1081-1088.

Waters TR, Baron SL, Piacitelli LA *et al.* (1999). Evaluation of the revised NIOSH lifting equation. A cross-sectional epidemiologic study. Spine 24.386-395.

Watson J (1982). Pain mechanisms – A review. 3. Endogenous pain control mechanisms. Australian J Physiotherapy 28.38-45.

Watson PJ, Main CJ, Waddell G, Gales TF, Purcell-Jones G (1998). Medically certified work loss, recurrence and costs of wage compensation for back pain: a follow-up study of the working population of Jersey. Br J Rheum 37.82-86.

Watson P (2000). Psychosocial predictors of outcome from low back pain. In: Ed. Gifford L. *Topical Issues in Pain 2. Biopsychosocial Assessment and Management.* Physiotherapy Pain Association, CNS Press, UK.

Watson P, Kendall N (2000). Assessing psychosocial yellow flags. In: Ed. Gifford L. *Topical Issues in Pain 2. Biopsychosocial Assessment and Management.* Physiotherapy Pain Association, CNS Press, UK.

Watts RW, Silagy CA (1995). A meta-analysis on the efficacy of epidural corticosteroids in the treatment of sciatica. Anaesth Intensive Care 23.564-569.

Waxman R, Tennant A, Helliwell P (2000). A prospective follow-up study of low back pain in the community. Spine 25.2085-2090.

Weber H (1983). Lumbar disc herniation. A controlled, prospective study with ten years of observation. Spine 8.131-140.

Weber H, Holme I, Amlie E (1993). The natural course of acute sciatica with nerve root symptoms in a double-blind placebo-controlled trial evaluating the effect of piroxicam. Spine 18.1433-1438.

Weber H (1994). Spine update. The natural history of disc herniation and the influence of intervention. Spine 19.2234-2238.

Webster BS, Snook SH (1990). The cost of compensable low back pain. J Occupational Med 32.13-15.

Webster BS, Snook SH (1994). The cost of 1989 workers' compensation low back pain claims. Spine 19.1111-1116.

Weiler PJ, King GJ, Gertzbein SD (1990). Analysis of sagital plane instability of the lumbar spine in vivo. Spine 15.1300-1306.

Weinreb JC, Wolbarsht LB, Cohen JM, Brown CEL, Maravilla KR (1989). Prevalence of lumbosacral intervertebral disc abnormalities on MR images in pregnant and asymptomatic nonpregnant women. Radiology 170.125-128.

Weinstein JN (1992). The role of neurogenic and non-neurogenic mediators as they relate to pain and the development of osteoarthritis. Spine 17.S356-S361.

Weiser S, Cedraschi C (1992). Psychosocial issues in the prevention of chronic low back pain – a literature review. Bailliere's Clinical Rheumatology 6.657-684.

Weitz EM (1981). The lateral bending sign. Spine 6.388-397.

Wensing M, Grol R, Smits A (1994). Quality judgements by patients on general practice care: a literature analysis. Soc Sci Med 38.45-53.

Werneke MW, Harris DE, Lichter RL (1993). Clinical effectiveness of behavioral signs for screening chronic low-back pain patients in a work-oriented physical rehabilitation program. Spine 18.2412-2418.

Werneke M, Hart DL, Cook D (1999). A descriptive study of the centralization phenomenon. Spine 24.676-683.

Werneke M, Hart DL (2000). Role of the centralization phenomenon as a prognostic factor for chronic pain or disability. JOSPT 30.1. Abstract. A33. PL96.

Werneke M, Hart DL (2001). Centralization phenomenon as a prognostic factor for chronic low back pain and disability. Spine 26.758-765.

Wessling KC, DeVane DA, Hylton CR (1987). Effects of static stretch versus static stretch and ultrasound combined on triceps surae muscle extensibility in healthy women. Physical Therapy 67.674-679.

Wetzel FT, LaRocca SH, Lowery GL, Aprill CN (1994). The treatment of lumbar spinal pain syndromes diagnosed by discography. Lumbar arthrodesis. Spine 19.792-800.

Wheeler AH, Hanley EN (1995). Spine Update. Nonoperative treatment for low back pain. Rest to restoration. Spine 20.375-378.

Wiberg G (1949). Back pain in relation to the nerve supply of the intervertebral disc. Acta Orth Scand 19.211-221.

Wiesel SW, Tsourmas N, Feffer HL, Citrin CM, Patronas N (1984). A study of computer-assisted tomography. 1. The incidence of positive CAT scans in an asymptomatic group of patients. Spine 9.549-551.

Wilder DG, Pope MH, Frymoyer JW (1988). The biomechanics of lumbar disc herniation and the effect of overload and instability. J Spinal Disorders 1.16-32.

Wiley JJ, Macnab I, Wortzman G (1968). Lumbar discography and its clinical applications. Can J Surg 11.280-289.

Wilke HJ, Neef P, Caimi M, Hoogland T, Claes LE (1999). New *in vivo* measurements of pressure in the intervertebral disc in daily life. Spine 24.755-762.

Wilkinson A (1992). Stretching the truth. A review of the literature on muscle stretching. Aus J Physio 38.283-287.

Willen J, Danielson B, Gaulitz A, Niklason T, Schonstrom N, Hansson T (1997). Dynamic effects on the lumbar spinal canal. Axially loaded CT-Myelography and MRI in patients with sciatica and/or neurogenic claudication. Spine 22.2968-2976.

Williams PL, Warwick R (Eds) (1980). *Gray's Anatomy* (36th ed.). Churchill Livingstone, Edinburgh.

Williams MM, Hawley JA, McKenzie RA, van Wijmen PM (1991). A comparison of the effects of two sitting postures on back and referred pain. Spine 16.1185-1191.

Williams S, Weinman J, Dale J, Newman S (1995). Patient expectations: What do primary care patients want from their GP and how far does meeting expectations affect patient satisfaction? Family Practice 12.193-201.

Williams DA, Feuerstein M, Durbin D, Pezzullo J (1998a). Health care and indemnity costs across the natural history of disability in occupational low back pain. Spine 23.2329-2336.

Williams RA, Pruitt SD, Doctor JN *et al.* (1998b). The contribution of job satisfaction to the transition from acute to chronic low back pain. Arch Phys Med Rehabil 79.366-374.

Williams S, Weinman J, Dale J, Newman S (1995). Patient expectations: What do primary care patients want from the GP and how far does meeting expectations affect patient satisfaction? Family Practice 12.193-201.

Wilson L, Hall H, McIntosh G, Melles T (1999). Intetester reliability of a low back pain classification system. Spine 24.248-254.

Wiltse LL, Widell EH, Jackson DW (1975). Fatigue fracture: the basic lesion in isthmic spondylolisthesis. JBJS 57A.17-22.

Winkel J, Mathiassen SE (1994). Assessment of physical work load in epidemiologic studies: concepts, issues and operational considerations. Ergonomics 37.979-988.

Witte MB, Barbul A (1997). General principles of wound healing. Surg Clinics Nth Am 77.509-528.

Wolff I, van Croonenborg JJ, Kemper HC, Kostense PJ, Twisk JW (1999). The effect of exercise training programs on bone mass: a meta-analysis of published controlled trials in pre- and postmenopausal women. Osteoporosis International 9.1-12.

Woody J, Lehmann T, Weinstein J, Hayes M, Spratt K (1983). Excessive translation on flexion-extension radiographs in asymptomatic populations. Orthop Trans 12.3.603.

Woolf CJ (1991). Generation of acute pain: central mechanisms. Br Med Bull 47.523-533.

Woolf CJ, Bennett GJ, Doherty M *et al.* (1998). Towards a mechanism-based classification of pain? Pain 77.227-229.

Wordsworth BP, Mowat AG (1986). A review of 100 patients with ankylosing spondylitis with particular reference to socio-economic effects. Br J Rheum 25.175-180.

Worth DR (1994). Movements of the head and neck. In: Eds Boyling JD, Palastanga N. *Grieve's Modern Manual Therapy* (2nd ed.). Churchill Livingstone, Edinburgh.

Wright D, Barrow S, Fisher AD, Horsley SD, Jayson MIV (1995). Influence of physical, psychological and behavioural factors on consultations for back pain. Br J Rheum 34.156-161.

Wroblewski BM (1978). Pain in osteoarthritis of the hip. The Practitioner 1315.140-141.

Yasuma T, Makino E, Saito S, Inui M (1986). Histological development of intervertebral disc herniation. JBJS 68A.1066-1072.

Yasuma T, Koh S, Okamura, Yamauchi Y (1990). Histological changes in aging lumbar intervertebral discs. JBJS 72A.220-229.

Yildizhan A, Pasaoglu A, Okten T, Ekinci N, Aycan K, Aral O (1991). Intradural disc herniations. Pathogenesis, clinical picture, diagnosis and treatment. Acta Neurochir 110.160-165.

Yorimitsu E, Chiba K, Toyama Y, Hirabayashi K (2001). Long-term outcomes of standard discectomy for lumbar disc herniations. A follow-up study of more than 10 years. Spine 26.652-657.

Yoshizawa H, O'Brien JP, Smith WT, Trumper M (1980). The neuropathology of intervertebral discs removed for low-back pain. Pathology 132.95-104.

Yoshizawa H, Kobayashi S, Morita T (1995). Chronic nerve root compression. Pathophysiologic mechanism of nerve root dysfunction. Spine 20.397-407.

Yoshizawa H (1999). Mini-symposium: Lumbar spinal canal stenosis. 1. Clinical and radiological assessment. Curr Orthop 13.173-177.

Young G, Jewell D (1999). Interventions for preventing and treating backache in pregnancy. (Cochrane Review). In: The Cochrane Library, Issue 3, 1999, Oxford: Update Software.

Young S (1995). Spinal stenosis. McKenzie Institute UK Newsletter 4.1.3-7.

Young S, Laslett M, Aprill C, Donelson R, Kelly C (1998). The sacroiliac joint a study comparing physical examination and contrast enhance pain provocation/ anesthetic block arthrography. In: Eds Vleeming A, Mooney V, Tilscher H, Dorman T, Snijders C. *3rd Interdisciplinary World Congress on Low Back and Pelvic Pain.* November 19-21, 1998, Vienna, Austria.

Young S, Aprill C (2000). Characteristics of a mechanical assessment for chronic facet joint pain. J Manual & Manipulative Therapy 8.78-84.

Yu S, Sether LA, Ho PSP, Wagner M, Haughton VM (1988a). Tears of the anulus fibrosus: Correlation between MR and pathologic findings in cadavers. AJNR 9.367-370.

Yu S, Haughton VM, Ho PSP, Sether LA *et al.* (1988b). Progressive and regressive changes in the nucleus pulposus. Radiology 169.93-97.

Yu S, Haughton VM, Sether LA *et al.* (1989). Criteria for classifying normal and degenerated lumbar intervertebral discs. Radiology 170.523-526.

Zanoli G, Stromqvist B, Jonsson B (2001). Visual analogue scales for interpretation of back and leg pain intensity in patients operated for degenerative lumbar spine disorders. Spine 26.2375-2380.

Zimmerman M (1992). Basic neurophysiological mechanisms of pain and pain therapy. In: Ed Jayson MIV. *The Lumbar Spine and Back Pain.* Churchill Livingstone, Edinburgh.

Zimmerman T (1998). The effectiveness of different intervention strategies in preventing back pain in members of the nursing population and the general population. Work 11.221-231.

Zusman M (1992). Central nervous system contribution to mechanically produced motor and sensory responses. Aus J Physio 38.245-255.

Zusman M (1994). The meaning of mechanically produced responses. Aus J Physio 40.35-39.

Zwerling C, Ryan J, Schootman M (1993). A case-control study of risk factors for industrial low back injury. Spine 18.1242-1247.

Zylbergold RS, Piper MC (1981). Lumbar disc disease: comparative analysis of physical therapy treatments. Arch Phys Med Rehabil 62.176-179.

Anterior compartment

The compartment of the intervertebral segment that is compressed with flexion forces.

Centralisation

The phenomenon by which distal limb pain emanating from although not necessarily felt in the spine is immediately or eventually abolished in response to the deliberate application of loading strategies. Such loading causes an abolition of peripheral pain that appears to progressively retreat in a proximal direction. As this occurs there may be a simultaneous development or increase in proximal pain. The phenomenon only occurs in the derangement syndrome.

Curve reversal/obstruction to curve reversal

In an asymptomatic state, individuals can move from an extreme position of flexion to an extreme position of extension without impediment; in derangement this can become difficult or impossible. Following a period of loading or repeated movements in one direction the opposite movement may become obstructed, and recovery is slow, gradual and/or painful. Thus, after spending a period of time in flexion, as in bending or sitting, or after repeated flexion, the patient is unable to regain the upright position immediately or without pain. They are forced to gradually and painfully resume the erect posture or movements into extension. In severe derangements patients may have difficulty straightening after one flexion movement.

Deformity

The patient experiences a sudden onset of pain and immediately or subsequently develops a loss of movement and a deformity so severe that they are unable to move out of the abnormal posture. The patient is fixed in kyphosis, lateral shift or lordosis and is unable to self-correct this very visible anatomical misalignment. If they are able to correct the deformity, they cannot maintain the correction. This phenomenon only occurs in derangement and must be immediately recognised as it determines treatment.

- *Kyphotic deformity* – the patient is fixed in flexion and is unable to extend.

- *Lateral shift* – the patient is fixed in (for instance) right lateral shift and is unable to bring his hips back to the mid-line or assume a position of left lateral shift. In the case of a 'hard' deformity, the patient will need clinician assistance to correct it, while in the case of a 'soft' deformity, the patient may be able to self-correct with repeated movements.
- *Lordotic deformity* – the patient is fixed in extension and is unable to flex.

Derangement syndrome

Rapid and lasting changes, sometimes over a few minutes or a few days, in pain intensity and location. Mechanical presentation can occur in this syndrome with the performance of movements or the adoption of sustained postures. Loading strategies produce a decrease, abolition or centralisation of symptoms. Opposite loading strategies may cause production, worsening or peripheralisation of symptoms if prolonged over a sufficient time. A distinguishing set of characteristics will be found during the history-taking and physical examination. The conceptual model involves internal articular displacement that causes a disturbance in the joint, which produces pain and impairment.

Deviation

There are two types of deviation: a) postural b) on movement.

a) Postural deviations – patients may prefer to hold themselves shifted to one side or in a degree of flexion because this brings temporary easing of their condition. However, they are capable of straightening, which distinguishes this group from those with a deformity. Both occur only in derangement.

b) Deviation on movement – for instance, as the patient flexes, they deviate away from the pure sagittal plane to left or right. This is indicative of either an adherent nerve root or a derangement.

Directional preference

The phenomenon of preference for postures or movement in one direction that is a characteristic of the derangement syndrome. It describes the situation when postures or movements in one direction decrease, abolish or centralise symptoms and often increase a limitation of movement. Postures or movements in the opposite direction often cause these symptoms and signs to worsen. This does not always occur, and may be a product of the length of exposure to provocative loading.

Distal symptoms

The symptoms located furthest down the leg; these may be radicular or somatic referred pain, or paraesthesia. During the evaluation of symptomatic responses to mechanical loading, the most distal symptoms are closely monitored. Movements that decrease or abolish these symptoms are prescribed, while movements that increase or produce them are avoided.

Dysfunction syndrome

Pain from the dysfunction syndrome is caused by mechanical deformation of structurally impaired soft tissues. This abnormal tissue may be the product of previous trauma or degenerative processes and the development of imperfect repair. Contraction, scarring, adherence, adaptive shortening or imperfect repair tissue become the source of symptoms and functional impairment. Pain is felt when the abnormal tissue is loaded. A distinguishing set of characteristics will be found during the history-taking and physical examination. In spinal dysfunction pain, is consistently produced at restricted end-range, and abates once the loading is released. Dysfunction may affect contractile, peri-articular or neural structures, with the latter two occurring in the spine.

Extension principle

This principle of treatment encompasses procedures, both patient- and therapist-generated, that produce extension of the lumbar spine. In a posterior derangement these will be used to abolish, decrease or centralise symptoms. In an extension dysfunction, the extension principle is used for remodelling.

Flexion principle

This principle of treatment encompasses procedures, both patient- and therapist-generated, that produce flexion of the lumbar spine. In an anterior derangement these will be used to abolish, decrease or centralise symptoms. In a flexion or ANR dysfunction, the flexion principle is used for remodelling.

Force alternatives

A change in the manner in which a force may be applied during the exploration of loading strategies to reduce derangements. For instance, alternative start positions (standing or lying), force directions (sagittal or lateral), dynamic (repeated movements) or static forces (sustained positions).

Force progressions

Within each principle of treatment direction (extension, flexion, lateral), there is a range of loading strategies available. These involve greater or more specific forces, but are still in the same plane of movement. For instance, sustained mid-range positions, end-range patient-generated movement, patient-generated force with clinician overpressure, clinician-generated force, or repeated movements over several days. Force progressions are used to determine the correct directional preference and when lesser forces are not able to maintain improvements.

Kappa

The Kappa coefficient is commonly used in studies to address the reliability of two testers to come to the same conclusion about a test. It takes account of the fact that there is a 50% probability of chance agreement even if random judgements are made. It reports a numerical value, with 1.00 being perfect agreement and 0.00 for agreement no better than chance. Negative values imply that agreement is worse than what would be expected by chance alone.

Guide to Kappa values

Kappa value	Strength of agreement
<0.20	Poor
0.21-0.40	Fair
0.41-0.60	Moderate
0.61-0.80	Good
0.81-1.00	Very good

Source: Altman 1991

Lateral compartment

The compartment of the intervertebral segment that is compressed with lateral forces. The lateral compartment becomes relevant if lateral forces influence the patient's symptoms.

Relevant lateral component

This refers to patients with derangement who have unilateral or asymmetrical symptoms that do not improve with sagittal plane forces. When the lateral component is relevant, asymmetrical forces are necessary to achieve centralisation or decrease of symptoms.

Lateral principle

This principle of treatment encompasses procedures, both patient- and therapist-generated, that produce an asymmetrical force on the lumbar spine. In postero-lateral or antero-lateral derangement these will be used to abolish, decrease or centralise symptoms.

Loading strategies

Describes the applied movements, positions or loads required to stress particular structures, and may be dynamic or static – dynamic would be a repeated movement; static, a sustained posture. The significant loading strategies, postures and repeated movements are those that alter symptoms.

Mechanical presentation

The outward manifestations of a musculoskeletal problem such as deformity, loss of movement range, velocity of movement or movement deviations. Very important in re-assessment of treatment efficacy.

Mechanical response

Change in mechanical presentation, for instance an increase or decrease in range of movement in response to a particular loading strategy.

Mechanical syndromes

Refers to the three mechanical syndromes as described by McKenzie – derangement, dysfunction and posture, which describe the majority of non-specific spinal problems.

Non-mechanical factors

Factors that are non-mechanical in nature that may influence a patient's experience of pain. For instance, in the acute phase of a problem, the pain-generating mechanism may be primarily inflammatory. In the chronic stage, various non-mechanical factors, such as central or peripheral sensitisation or psychosocial factors, may influence pain modulation.

Pain

Acute pain

Pain of recent onset of less than seven days. This includes some with pain of an inflammatory nature, but many will experience pain of a mechanical nature due to derangement.

Sub-acute pain

Pain that has lasted between seven days and seven weeks. In some this may represent an interface between inflammatory and mechanical pain, but again, mechanical factors are likely to predominate.

Chronic pain

Pain that has lasted for longer than seven weeks. In the majority this will be mechanical in nature, and non-mechanical in a minority.

Chronic pain states

Pain of long duration in which non-mechanical factors are important in pain maintenance. These factors may relate to peripheral or central sensitisation or psychosocial factors, such as fear–avoidance, etc. Symptoms are often widespread and aggravated by all activity, and patients display exaggerated pain behaviour and mistaken beliefs about movement and pain.

Chemical or inflammatory pain

Pain mediated by the inflammatory chemicals released following tissue damage, or due to systemic pathology, such as ankylosing spondylitis.

Mechanical pain

Pain that results from mechanical deformation of tissues. This occurs with abnormal stresses on normal tissues, as in the postural syndrome, and normal stresses on abnormal tissues, such as in derangement and dysfunction.

Constant pain

Constant pain describes symptoms that are present throughout the patient's waking day, without any respite, even though it may vary in intensity. This may be chemical or mechanical in origin, and may also exist in chronic pain states.

Intermittent pain

This describes pain that comes and goes during the course of the day. Commonly this relates to intermittent mechanical deformation that results in pain. Pain may be momentary or appear and linger for varying amounts of time, but does at some point during the day completely stop.

Site and spread of pain

The area in which pain is perceived in terms of the extent of referral into the limb. The most distal site of pain is important to monitor regarding centralisation and peripheralisation. This information provides important information during assessment and re-assessment of the symptomatic presentation.

Severity of pain

This provides important information during assessment and re-assessment of the symptomatic presentation. Either the patient is asked on a one-to-ten scale about the intensity of the pain on different occasions, or in retrospect is asked to compare present pain to when they first attended.

Peripheralisation

Peripheralisation describes the phenomenon when pain emanating from the spine, although not necessarily felt in it, *spreads* distally into, or further down, the limb. This is the reverse of centralisation. In response to repeated movements or a sustained posture, if pain is produced and remains in the limb, spreads distally or increases distally, that loading strategy should be avoided. The phenomenon only occurs in the derangement syndrome. The temporary production of distal pain with end-range movement, which does not worsen, is not peripheralisation, as this response may occur with an adherent nerve root.

Posterior compartment

Describes the compartment of the intervertebral segment that is compressed with extension forces.

Postural syndrome

Mechanical deformation of normal soft tissues arising from prolonged postural stresses, affecting any articular structures and resulting in pain. A distinguishing set of characteristics is found during the history-taking and physical examination. If prolonged sitting produces pain, it will be abolished by posture correction. Range will be full and pain-free, and repeated movements have no effect.

Red flags

This refers to features of the history-taking that may indicate serious spinal pathology, such as cancer, cauda equina syndrome or fracture. If possible 'red flag' pathology is suspected, further mechanical therapy is contraindicated and the patient should be referred to a specialist.

Reliability

This is the characteristic of a test or measuring tool to give the same answer in different situations. Inter-tester reliability examines the degree of agreement between different clinicians on the same occasion; intra-tester reliability examines the degree of reliability of a single tester on different occasions. Results are presented in several ways: as a percentage agreement, correlation coefficients, or Kappa values.

Sensitivity

This is a characteristic of a clinical test used to diagnose a problem. The sensitivity is the ability of the test to be positive in all who have the problem. When a test is 100% sensitive, it is able to detect all who have the condition of interest. The sensitivity is the true positive rate. When sensitivity is extremely high (>0.95 or 95%), a negative test response rules out that disease. Poor sensitivity indicates a test that fails to identify many of those with the disease of interest.

Specificity

This is a characteristic of a clinical test used to diagnose a problem. The specificity is the ability of a test not to be positive in those who do not have the problem; it is thus the true negative rate. When a test is 100% specific it is able to identify all those who do not have the condition of interest. When specificity is extremely high (>0.95 or 95%) a positive test result gives a definite positive diagnosis. Poor specificity indicates a test that fails to exclude many individuals without the disease of interest.

Stage of condition

All musculoskeletal conditions can be anywhere on the continuum from acute to sub-acute to chronic. These stages are often of more significance to management than a structural diagnosis.

Standardised terms

These are used to make consistent descriptions of symptomatic responses to different loading strategies to judge their value for self-treatment. The description of symptoms during and *after* loading is significant in determining the management strategy to be applied. These are the words used to describe symptom response during the physical examination.

During loading:

Increase	Symptoms already present are increased in intensity.
Decrease	Symptoms already present are decreased in intensity.
Produce	Movement or loading creates symptoms that were not present prior to the test.
Abolish	Movement or loading abolishes symptoms that were present prior to the test.

Better	Symptoms produced on movement, decrease on repetition.
Centralises	Movement or loading abolishes the most distal symptoms.
Peripheralises	Movement or loading produces more distal symptoms. No effectMovement or loading has no effect on symptoms during testing.
End-range pain	Pain that only appears at end-range of movement disappears once end-range is released, and in which the range does not rapidly change. In end-range pain due to derangement, increased force reduces symptoms, while with end-range pain due to dysfunction, increased force will increase symptoms.

Pain during movement

Pain produced during the range of movement, but then subsides or remains when the individual moves further into the range of movement. In the three mechanical syndromes in the spine, this only occurs in derangements.

After loading

WorseSymptoms produced or increased with movement or loading remain aggravated following the test.

Not worse	Symptoms produced or increased with movement or loading return to baseline following the test.
Better	Symptoms decreased or abolished with movement or loading remain improved after testing.
Not better	Symptoms decreased or abolished with movement or loading return to baseline after testing.
Centralised	Distal symptoms abolished by movement or loading remain abolished after testing.
Peripheralised	Distal symptoms produced during movement or loading remain after testing.
No effect	Movement or loading has no effect on symptoms during or after testing.

State of tissues

This describes the different conditions that tissues could be in. They may be normal or abnormal. Abnormal tissues may be injured, healing, scarred or contracted, with healing suspended, hypersensitive to normal loading due to changes in the nervous system, degenerated or painful due to derangements.

Status of condition

This describes the direction of the condition relative to recovery. It may either be improving, worsening or unchanging. Its status is significant in decisions concerning management.

Symptomatic presentation

This describes the details of the patient's complaints and can be assessed and re-assessed regarding site, intermittency/constancy, diurnal variation, severity, consequent analgesic/NSAID consumption and self-reported functional disability. This is very important in re-assessment of treatment efficacy.

Symptomatic response

The behaviour of pain in response to a particular loading strategy, for instance centralisation, peripheralisation, worse or better.

Traffic light guide

Identification of patient's responses to loading strategies, using standardised terminology, determines the appropriateness of a management direction. If the patient remains worse afterwards, this is a 'red light' to that procedure; if the patient remains better, this is a 'green light' for that exercise; if there is no change, an 'amber light', a force progression or force alternative *may* be required. An 'amber' response is also a 'green light' in the presence of a dysfunction.

Treatment principle

The treatment principle defines the force direction used in management; they are termed extension, flexion or lateral. Each principle of treatment contains patient- and clinician-generated force progressions. In a derangement, the treatment principle is determined by the direction that causes a decrease, abolition or centralisation of pain. In a dysfunction, the treatment principle is determined by the direction that reproduces the relevant symptom.

Validity

This is the ability of a test to diagnose or measure what it is intended to diagnose or measure. There are various dimensions of validity, but criterion validity is critical to the accuracy of a diagnosis. This is the ability of a test to determine the presence or absence of a particular pathology. The value of a test is judged by its ability to diagnose the pathology compared to a 'gold standard'. The validity of the 'gold standard' is meant to be about 100%. Validity is measured by sensitivity and specificity.

Yellow flags

Term used to describe psychosocial risk factors for developing or perpetuating long-term disability or sick leave as a consequence of musculoskeletal symptoms. They include factors such as the attitudes and beliefs of the patient about their problem, their behavioural responses to it, compensation issues, inappropriate health care advice, information or treatment, emotions such as depression, anxiety and fear of movement, and relations with family and work.

Index